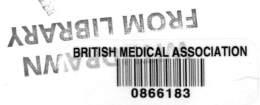

Handbook of Stroke

Second Edition

David O. Wiebers, M.D.
Professor of Neurology
Mayo Clinic College of Medicine
Consultant, Departments of Neurology and Health Sciences
   Research
Mayo Clinic and Mayo Foundation
Rochester, Minnesota

Valery L. Feigin, M.D., D.Sc.
Professor of Neurology
Associate Professor of Medicine
Clinical Trials Research Unit
School of Public Health
University of Auckland
Auckland, New Zealand

Robert D. Brown, Jr., M.D., M.P.H.
Professor of Neurology
Mayo Clinic College of Medicine
Consultant, Department of Neurology
Mayo Clinic and Mayo Foundation
Rochester, Minnesota

Foreword by

Jack P. Whisnant, M.D.
Emeritus Professor of Neurology
Mayo Clinic College of Medicine
Consultant Emeritus, Department of Health Sciences Research
Mayo Clinic and Mayo Foundation
Rochester, Minnesota

Lippincott Williams & Wilkins
a Wolters Kluwer business
Philadelphia · Baltimore · New York · London
Buenos Aires · Hong Kong · Sydney · Tokyo

Acquisitions Editor: Frances DeStefano
Developmental Editor: Louise Bierig
Managing Editor: Scott Scheidt
Project Manager: Alicia Jackson
Senior Manufacturing Manager: Benjamin Rivera
Cover Designer: Terry Mallon
Production Service: GGS Book Services
Printer: RR Donnelley—Crawfordsville

© 2006 by LIPPINCOTT WILLIAMS & WILKINS, a Wolters Kluwer business
530 Walnut Street
Philadelphia, PA 19106 USA
LWW.com

1st Edition, ©1997 Mayo Foundation, Rochester, Minnesota. Published by
Lippincott-Raven Publishers.

Library of Congress Cataloging-in-Publication Data

Wiebers, David O.
Handbook of stroke/David O. Wiebers, Valery L. Feigin, Robert D. Brown, Jr.;
foreword by Jack P. Whisnant.—2nd ed.
     p.; cm.
  Includes bibliographical references and index.
  ISBN 0-7817-8658-4
  1. Cerebrovascular disease—Handbooks, manuals, etc. I. Feigin, Valery L.
II. Brown, Robert D. (Robert Duane), 1961- III. Title.
  [DNLM: 1. Cerebrovascular Disorders—complications. 2. Cerebrovascular
Disorders—diagnosis. 3. Cerebrovascular Disorders—therapy. 4. Acute Disease—
therapy. WL 355 W642h 2006]
RC388.5.W463 2006
616.8'1—dc22
                                                              2005031125

   To purchase additional copies of this book, call our customer service department
at (800) 638-3030 or fax orders to (301) 223-2320. International customers should
call (301) 223-2300.

   Visit Lippincott Williams & Wilkins on the Internet at LWW.com. Lippincott
Williams & Wilkins customer service representatives are available from 8:30 am to
6 pm, EST.
                                          10 9 8 7 6 5 4 3 2 1

For our patients, our colleagues, and our families

Contents

VI.   Assessing and Discussing Prognosis and Natural History of Cerebrovascular Disorders

VII.   Management and Rehabilitation After Stroke

Appendixes

Foreword

During the first half of the 20th century, very little scientific attention was given to understanding the clinical characteristics of patients with different types of stroke, and no attention was directed at differentiating mechanisms. The nosologic term for stroke in mortality statistics in the early part of the 20th century was "apoplexy," from the Greek, "to strike down." The derivation of the generic clinical term "cerebrovascular accident" is obscure. This term helped to promote the idea that patients with stroke were victims and that somehow the disorder was providential and, therefore, not something that was subject to intervention by physicians or scientists. In teaching hospitals, patients with stroke were not considered appropriate for teaching of residents and students about disease processes. Patients with stroke either were not admitted to an acute care hospital or were admitted to a nonteaching service for maintenance care.

The last half of the 20th century began with a few clinicians calling attention to the importance of stroke as a clinical problem and providing leadership in efforts to understand the mechanisms of how some disorders lead to the occurrence of stroke. These early efforts led to increasing interest of clinicians and soon attracted clinical and laboratory research attention to this common clinical disorder.

Clinicians now recognize the importance of differentiating types of stroke and the pathophysiologic substrate when possible. Increasingly sophisticated imaging studies have greatly enhanced the ability of the neurologist or others to determine the type and characteristics of stroke. The goal of the clinician now is to assess the patient for management options, which could be medical, surgical, or other intervention.

Successful treatment until recently has centered around management of risk factors and comorbid conditions to prevent stroke. Attention now is focused on lysing thrombi in arteries that supply the circulation to the brain to prevent or lessen the damage from ischemia. The efforts to protect or preserve the integrity of the brain after ischemia have developed, but, thus far, they have not been successful. The need now is for clinicians to be aware of the need for urgent attention if treatments of stroke are to be effective.

Handbook of Stroke has been produced by experienced clinicians who have presented the topics in a unique fashion, following the thought processes that experienced neurovascular clinicians use. The emphasis on the importance of what can be learned from the history is almost unique in recent literature on stroke. The authors use clinical management algorithms that are helpful to clinicians of all types. They also have addressed when patients with stroke should be hospitalized and when they can be safely evaluated as outpatients. Telephone triage is considered part of the assessment.

Development of effective treatments for stroke aimed at preventing death and reducing impairment of function requires knowledgeable clinicians who put a high priority on attending to the care of patients with stroke immediately after the stroke is evident.

I know the authors well through personal interaction, and I am pleased that they have produced a volume that emphasizes the importance of clinical assessment of patients with stroke.

Jack P. Whisnant, M.D.

Preface

One of the most rewarding and fulfilling aspects of our work involves providing information to colleagues that can contribute to the care of their patients. It is a way for us to benefit many more patients than we could possibly see one on one in our offices. This potential for patient and physician benefit formed the impetus for our developing the first edition of the *Handbook of Stroke* and motivated us to produce a second edition.

It is particularly meaningful to us that the first edition was translated into several languages so that it could be shared with international colleagues. We have endeavored to make the second edition as user-friendly as possible for physicians and other health care professionals who see patients with cerebrovascular disorders. Specifically, the book has been oriented to provide clinical recommendations based on available evidence and clinical experience to address specific situations as the reader would encounter them.

We are again greatly indebted to numerous individuals who played major roles in developing and completing this book. From a professional standpoint, we recognize our numerous colleagues and trainees who provide us with a source for exchange of ideas, learning, and camaraderie. We express particular gratitude and indebtedness to Jack P. Whisnant, M.D., our beloved mentor and colleague, whose unselfish guidance and generosity over the years have been particular blessings. We wish it were possible for all physicians to work with someone like Jack during the course of their careers.

We also gratefully acknowledge the outstanding contributions of Roberta Schwartz for her editorial support at Mayo Clinic; Scott Scheidt, Fran DeStefano, and Anne Sydor for their editorial support at Lippincott Williams & Wilkins; Sandra Twaites for her secretarial support; Bob Benassi and John Hagen for their artistic expertise in illustrating the book; Glenn Forbes, M.D., and John Huston, M.D., for their radiologic expertise and assistance in providing radiographs; Brian Younge, M.D., for his support in providing neuro-ophthalmologic photographs; and Rita Jones, R.D., for her valuable assistance on dietary and nutritional issues.

We express deep thanks to our parents for teaching us the importance of caring for others, for developing our desire for knowledge, and for instilling within us the courage to dream and the will to succeed. We also thank our other cherished family members for their unfailing love and support. Finally, we thank our patients for their role in inspiring us to write this book, for teaching us so much over the years, and for allowing us to experience the profound satisfaction of assisting them.

D.O.W.
V.L.F.
R.D.B.

Handbook of Stroke

Second Edition

I

Clinical and Laboratory Assessment of Patients with Cerebrovascular Disease

NOTICE

The indications and dosages of all drugs in this book have been recommended in the medical literature and conform to the practices of the general medical community. The medications described do not necessarily have specific approval by the Food and Drug Administration for use in the diseases and dosages for which they are recommended. The package insert for each drug should be consulted for use and dosage as approved by the FDA. Because standards for usage change, it is advisable to keep abreast of revised recommendations, particularly those concerning new drugs.

Systematic Clinical Assessment

The clinician must call on comprehensive clinical assessment skills to provide the patient with an accurate and efficient diagnosis. Because many processes other than cerebrovascular disease may cause neurologic symptoms, differential diagnosis is important. A detailed clinical history and systematic neurologic, neurovascular, and general examinations are important aspects of the clinical assessment of patients with suspected cerebrovascular disease.

Although the clinical evaluation of patients with different forms of cerebrovascular disease varies somewhat (for example, with altered levels of consciousness or intellectual disturbances), most parts of the clinical assessment are uniform.

QUESTIONS TO ASK

It is important for the clinician to use a systematic approach to evaluate the patient with a potential cerebrovascular problem. In patients with transient neurologic dysfunction, it is useful to discuss in great detail from beginning to end at least one spell with the patient to clarify the diagnosis. For virtually all patients in whom cerebrovascular disorders are suspected, it is useful to direct the interview step by step to facilitate answering four fundamental questions:

1. Is the problem vascular?
2. Is the vascular problem one of hemorrhage or ischemia?
3. If the problem is hemorrhagic, what are the location and the cause?
4. If the problem is infarction, what is the arterial or venous distribution, and what is the underlying mechanism for the ischemia?

Is the Problem Vascular?

The answer to the first question is based primarily on the temporal profile of the patient's presenting symptoms. The classic vascular profile involves sudden onset with rapid progression to maximal deficit (instantaneously or in seconds). All the affected areas of the body are involved from the onset. The **rapid onset and evolution** usually apply to all types of cerebrovascular episodes, regardless of the total duration of symptoms. The prototype for brief ischemic spells is the **transient ischemic attack** (TIA), defined as a temporary episode of **focal** ischemic neurologic dysfunction that resolves completely within 24 hours. It is important to distinguish TIA from an episode of generalized cerebral ischemia (syncope) and from spells such as seizures or migraine, both of which may appear as episodes of transient focal neurologic dysfunction. The temporal profile of focal seizures generally involves progression and evolution within a few minutes (approximately 2 to 3 minutes), whereas the focal deficit that sometimes occurs with migraine usually builds or moves during 15 to 20 minutes (for example, increasing scintillating scotomata or marching numbness starting in one hand) before subsiding and is often associated with localized headache, normally occurring after the focal neurologic deficit. Migraine aura that occurs without subsequent headache is often referred to as a migraine equivalent.

Another distinguishing characteristic of vascular spells is that most tend to produce negative phenomena (for example, weakness, deadness, visual loss), but focal seizures tend to produce positive phenomena (for example, tonic-clonic movements, tingling, visual hallucinations, scintillating scotomata), and migraine may produce either phenomena (more commonly, positive).

There are rare exceptions to these guidelines. Some TIAs may present with rhythmic jerking of the arm or the leg, often occurring when the patient arises from a sitting or a lying position. A contralateral high-grade carotid stenosis or an occlusion is often detected (the so-called shaky-limb TIA). Likewise, seizures may present with speech arrest, or weakness may occur after a seizure (Todd's paralysis).

A focal neurologic deficit that lasts longer than 24 hours and is caused by brain ischemia is called a cerebral infarction (ischemic stroke). When such a deficit persists for longer than 24 hours but resolves within 3 weeks, the episode is considered a minor ischemic stroke but is sometimes called a **reversible ischemic neurologic deficit** (RIND).

An exception to the usual rapid evolution of ischemic cerebrovascular events occurs in patients who have increasing neurologic deficit for as long as 72 hours after the onset of symptoms. These patients are classified as having **progressing cerebral infarction**, a phenomenon that is more common in strokes involving the vertebrobasilar system. In this situation, the clinician should carefully consider the possibility of an underlying mass lesion (for example, subdural hematoma, neoplasm, abscess), a demyelinating disease, or a superimposed encephalopathy.

Is the Vascular Problem One of Hemorrhage or Ischemia?

Having determined that the problem is vascular, the clinician next must attempt to distinguish whether the main process is one of hemorrhage or ischemia. Overall, ischemic strokes comprise approximately 80% to 85% of all strokes; intracerebral hemorrhage and subarachnoid hemorrhage comprise approximately 10% and 5% of all strokes, respectively.

The onset of symptoms with headache or stiff neck favors a hemorrhagic process, as does early decreased level of consciousness in a patient with a presumed supratentorial lesion. Ischemia is more likely when the symptoms are consistent with neurologic dysfunction from a single arterial territory or when improvement occurs rapidly or early in the clinical course. Although the distinction between hemorrhage and ischemia is seldom difficult clinically, there are exceptions, and sometimes the two occur simultaneously (such as hemorrhagic infarction). Computed tomography has revolutionized the clinician's ability to distinguish between hemorrhage and infarction in emergency situations and thus has resolved virtually all cases in which uncertainty exists.

Ischemic lesions appear as normal areas or as areas of decreased attenuation within the first several hours after the onset of symptoms, whereas hemorrhagic lesions usually appear immediately as areas of increased attenuation. Rarely, magnetic resonance imaging may provide additional help with the distinction between hemorrhage and ischemia.

If the Problem Is Hemorrhagic, What Are the Location and the Cause?

If the problem is hemorrhagic, then the clinician must attempt to define the type, location, and cause of the hemorrhage to facilitate proper management (Table 1-1). It is important to determine location because this usually helps to define the cause of the hemorrhage. The five commonly defined locations, proceeding from external to internal, are (1) epidural and (2) subdural hematomas, both usually caused by head trauma; (3) subarachnoid hemorrhage, usually caused by aneurysm or arteriovenous malformation (AVM); and (4) intracerebral and (5) intraventricular hemorrhages, both often a result of hypertension, AVM, or aneurysm (Fig. 1-1).

If the Problem Is Infarction, What Is the Arterial or Venous Distribution, and What Is the Underlying Mechanism for the Ischemia?

If the problem is ischemic, the clinician first should attempt to define the location of the process within the patient's central nervous system. This involves localizing the neurologic dysfunction to one or more vascular territories and requires some knowledge of neuroanatomy, including the cerebral circulation. The **first step in localization** is to distinguish generalized ischemia (syncope, anoxic encephalopathy) from focal cerebral ischemia (TIA, reversible ischemic neurologic deficit, cerebral infarction, progressing cerebral infarction). Differentiation is particularly important because of the vastly different implications of

Table 1-1. Locations and associated causes of intracranial hemorrhage

Location	Cause
Epidural	Head trauma, tear in meningeal artery
Subdural	Head trauma, tear in bridging vein
Subarachnoid	Aneurysm or arteriovenous malformation
Intracerebral	Hypertension, arteriovenous malformation, aneurysm, amyloid angiopathy, primary and metastatic neoplasms, infections, hematologic disorders, use of anticoagulant or thrombolytic agents
Intraventricular	Hypertension, aneurysm, arteriovenous malformation, hematologic disorders, use of anticoagulant or thrombolytic agents (often an extension of deep intracerebral hemorrhage)

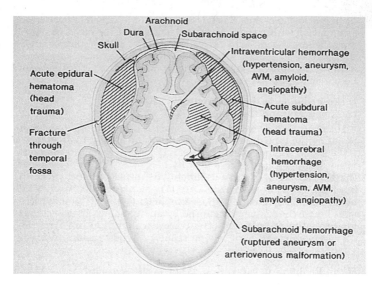

Figure 1-1.   Locations of intracranial hemorrhage. AVM = arteriovenous malformation.

the two ischemias in terms of cause, management, and prognosis. If the problem is focal (or multifocal), the **second step in localization** involves distinguishing anterior circulation (carotid system) from posterior circulation (vertebrobasilar system) processes. From there, the clinician can further subdivide the ischemic lesion into individual or multiple vascular territories by relating the clinical findings to the functional anatomy of the cerebral vessels (see Appendixes A-1 and A-2). If a patient has multiple vascular spells, then it is important to know whether all spells are similar (stereotyped) and to review at least one spell in great detail.

After localization of the process is clarified, one next should consider the underlying mechanism. Major categories of cerebral ischemic events relating to underlying pathophysiology, proceeding from proximal to distal in the arterial system, are (1) **cardiac disease**, (2) **large vessel disease** (craniocervical occlusive disease), (3) **small vessel disease**, and (4) **hematologic disease** (see Table 8-1). Another common but somewhat less clinically useful way to categorize ischemic stroke subtypes is to use the categories of **thrombotic infarction**, in which a locally decreased blood supply is caused by a blockage formed in situ in an artery; **embolic infarction**, referring to a blockage caused by a piece of material that has broken free from a more proximal site; and **lacunar infarction**, which is frequently but not always caused by thrombosis of one of the small penetrating branch arteries.

Historical Evaluation of Key Signs and Symptoms

A detailed history is the most important part of the evaluation of a patient with cerebrovascular disease. Initial attention should be directed toward identifying and characterizing (1) the patient's **chief complaints** or **main symptoms**; (2) the **time of onset** and possible **precipitating events**; (3) the features of the **circumstance of onset**, including the patient's activities, the **temporal profile** of the **onset of symptoms**, and the rapidity with which maximal deficit developed (a typical vascular profile involves sudden onset with rapid progression to maximal deficit with all of affected areas of the body involved from the onset); (4) the presence of focal or generalized **neurologic deficit** at the onset or alterations of **level of consciousness** at onset; (5) the presence of **headache**, **vomiting**, or **seizure activity** (focal or generalized); and (6) the **chronologic course of neurologic symptoms** after onset.

Frequently, the patient may not remember the precise details of the early temporal course and other important historical details. In this case, family members are often the best source of the information. The patient should be asked what is specifically meant by certain words that are used to describe symptoms (for example, "dizziness," "headache," and "poor vision") because these terms have a wide range of different meanings with different implications for diagnosis and management.

This chapter describes several symptoms that are particularly pertinent to patients with cerebrovascular disorders and addresses their application to the diagnosis of these conditions.

HEADACHE

Sudden severe headache that is described by the patient as "like being hit over the head by a hammer" (or some similar description) is suggestive of **subarachnoid hemorrhage**. This headache is usually associated with neck stiffness (meningismus) and may be localized to the posterior neck. However, as many as 30% of all subarachnoid hemorrhages present atypically, and a minor subarachnoid hemorrhage, especially in elderly individuals, may not present with severe headache, stiff neck, or catastrophic onset. In these cases, any element of abruptness in a new character of headache should always raise the possibility of subarachnoid or other intracranial hemorrhage.

Localized or pulsating headache associated with slowly progressive focal neurologic deficit may occur with growing intracranial **arteriovenous malformations** (which may produce pulsatile tinnitus with or without cranial bruit) **or aneurysms**. Aneurysms of the internal carotid artery (intracavernous part or near the petrous apex) may produce facial or retro-orbital pain. Aneurysms of the middle cerebral artery (lateral fissure) are sometimes associated with retro-orbital pain, aneurysms of the posterior cerebral artery are associated with retro-orbital or occipital pain, and aneurysms of the basilar artery may cause hemifacial pain.

The headache of **intracerebral hemorrhage** is usually sudden in onset and often associated with a progressive focal neurologic deficit, vomiting, and altered consciousness.

Patients with **cerebral infarction** uncommonly (20%) have headache at the onset of the episode (more commonly with embolic ischemic lesions). Occasionally, a patient with a large cerebral infarction may experience headache (caused by cerebral edema) beginning as long as a few days after the onset of stroke. However, this type of headache is usually temporary; more severe or persistent headache warrants further investigation for other underlying causes, such as tumor, abscess, vasculitis, or hemorrhagic infarct. Although few headache syndromes in the setting of cerebral infarction provide aid in localization, a focal supraorbital headache associated with homonymous hemianopia may be caused by an embolus or a thrombosis in the posterior cerebral artery. **Transient ischemic attack** (TIA) seldom produces substantial headache.

Severe hypertension with diastolic blood pressures of more than 110 mm Hg may be associated with headache, but mild hypertension rarely causes headaches. Severe headache caused by abrupt increases in blood pressure may occur in patients with **acute hypertensive encephalopathy** (often associated with neurologic deficits resulting from cerebral edema, hemorrhage, or vasospasm).

Headache caused by **chronic increased intracranial pressure**, as occurs with cerebral tumor, is often present when the patient awakens in the morning and may be **brought on** with increased Valsalva maneuvers or lowering the head below the level of the heart. In contrast, almost any type of headache may be **worsened** by Valsalva maneuvers, lowering the head below the level of the heart, or excessive stress or tension.

Headache that is caused by **venous circulatory dysfunction** (for example, intracranial venous sinus thrombosis) usually results from increased intracranial pressure and has a tendency to be present when the patient awakens and to be brought on or enhanced by Valsalva maneuvers, supine position, or lowering of the head below the level of the heart. Occasionally, these disorders are associated with central nervous system (CNS) infection and produce fever and headache as a result of meningeal irritation.

The headache of **temporal (cranial) arteritis** is characterized by severe, persistent pain associated with enlarged, beaded, tender, erythematous, or pulseless temporal arteries and jaw claudication. Scalp tenderness is characteristic, and it is often very difficult for patients to comb their hair. Other associated features include general malaise, polyarthralgias, polymyalgias, fever, and unilateral or bilateral loss of vision. This type of headache usually occurs in patients who are older than 55 years but has been reported in patients in their 30s. The diagnosis is suggested by a high sedimentation rate (often >100 mm per hour) and confirmed by temporal artery biopsy. Corticosteroid treatment usually produces a dramatic and rapid improvement in headache.

Migraine headaches usually start in adolescence or early adulthood. There is often a positive family history. The headaches are intermittent, sometimes preceded by 15- to 30-minute prodromes such as scintillating scotomata, usually unilateral, throbbing, and associated with nausea, vomiting, or photophobia. The pain usually builds to a peak in less than 1 hour and persists for hours to 1 or 2 days and is exacerbated by noise and bright light. In some patients, the headaches are precipitated by stress; fasting; menses; and certain foods, such as alcohol, chocolate, cured meats, and monosodium glutamate (often used in Chinese food). Often, the headache is relieved with sleep.

Cluster headaches are characterized by recurrent, nocturnal, unilateral, usually retro-orbital searing pains that last 20 to 60 minutes and typically are accompanied by unilateral lacrimation and nasal and conjunctival congestion. These headaches normally occur in men who are older than 20 years and often include an ipsilateral Horner's syndrome and rhinorrhea during the headache. Episodes are characteristically precipitated by alcohol.

Vascular headaches (Table 2-1) should be distinguished from nonvascular headaches, such as those associated with (1) cerebral trauma (subdural hematoma, posttraumatic headache); (2) infections or tumors of the CNS; (3) contraction, inflammation, or trauma related to cranial or cervical muscles (tension and muscle contraction headache); (4) paranasal sinus disease; (5) glaucoma; (6) benign intracranial hypertension; and (7) nonspecific headaches related to use of various drugs (for example, bromides, indomethacin).

Headache is a very common symptom of subacute (2 to 14 days) or chronic (>14 days) **traumatic subdural hematoma**. The headache often fluctuates in severity, with a deep-seated,

Table 2-1.   Classification of headache

Major Cause of Headache	Clinical Forms of Headache
Migraine	Migraine without aura, migraine with aura, hemiplegic migraine, basilar migraine, ophthalmoplegic migraine, retinal migraine
Tension type	Tension headache, episodic or chronic, caused by excessive stress, anxiety, depression, cervical osteoarthritis, cranial or cervical myalgias
Cluster/chronic paroxysmal hemicrania	Cluster headache, chronic paroxysmal hemicrania
Vascular disorders	Ischemic cerebrovascular disease (TIA, ischemic stroke), intracranial hemorrhage (intracerebral, subdural, epidural, subarachnoid), unruptured aneurysm or arteriovenous malformation, vasculitis, carotidynia, dissection

Table 2-1.   *Continued*

Major Cause of Headache	Clinical Forms of Headache
Nonvascular intracranial disorders	High CSF pressure (primary or metastatic tumor, intracranial hemorrhage, ischemic stroke with edema, abscess, hydrocephalus, pseudotumor cerebri) Low CSF pressure (after lumbar puncture, other CSF leak) Infection (bacterial, viral, fungal, other) Chemical meningitis
Substance use or withdrawal	Acute substance exposure (nitrates, carbon monoxide, alcohol, monosodium glutamate) Chronic substance exposure (ergotamine, analgesic overuse, birth control pills, estrogens) Withdrawal (alcohol, ergotamine, caffeine, narcotics)
Noncephalic infection	Viral, bacterial
Metabolic disorders	Hypoxia, hypercapnia, hypoglycemia, dialysis, other
Trauma	Acute and chronic posttraumatic headache
Facial/cranial structures	Eye (including glaucoma, inflammatory disorders, refractive errors); ears, nose, and sinuses; temporomandibular joint, teeth, cranial bone, neck
Neuralgia/nerve trunk	Compression of upper cranial nerve, demyelination or infarction of cranial nerve, inflammation (herpes zoster, postherpetic neuralgia), Tolosa-Hunt trigeminal neuralgia, glossopharyngeal neuralgia, occipital neuralgia
Other	Benign cough or exertion headache, headache with sexual activity, cold stimulus headache, idiopathic stabbing headache

CSF = cerebrospinal fluid; TIA = transient ischemic attack.
Source: Adapted from Headache Classification Committee of the International Headache Society: Classification and diagnostic criteria for headache disorders, cranial neuralgias and facial pain. *Cephalalgia* 8[Suppl 7]: 1-96,1988, with permission from Scandinavian University Press.

steady, unilateral, or, less common, generalized presentation, often proceeding to involve alterations of consciousness and focal neurologic dysfunction. The diagnosis is established by computed tomography or magnetic resonance imaging (MRI) of the head. **Posttraumatic headaches** may be intermittent, continuous, or chronic (bilateral or, less common, unilateral) and are often asso-ciated with giddiness, vertigo, or tinnitus. Posttraumatic dysau-tonomic cephalalgia is characterized by severe, episodic, throb-bing, unilateral headaches accompanied by ipsilateral mydriasis and excessive facial sweating.

Meningitis or encephalitis often produces intense, deep, con-stant, and increasing headache that is usually generalized and associated with stiff neck, Kernig and Brudzinski signs, and fever. The diagnosis is established by lumbar puncture. Acute persistent headache over a period of hours or days may also occur in systemic infections, such as influenza, without definite CNS involvement.

Headaches that are associated with brain tumors are usu-ally unilateral and slowly progressive in frequency and severity and have a tendency to occur when the patient awakens in the morning. As the tumor grows, the pain is frequently associated with focal neurologic signs or signs of increased intracranial pressure. As with other lesions that cause mass effect, the headaches may be brought on by bending over with the head downward or engaging in Valsalva maneuvers (coughing, sneezing, straining to defecate).

Tension-type headache (muscle contraction headache) is usu-ally steady; deep; generalized; bilateral; and occipital, frontal, or in a bandlike distribution around the head with associated tight-ness and tenderness of the neck muscles. It may persist unremit-tingly for days or weeks and is usually associated with excessive stress or tension, anxiety, insomnia, or depression.

Headache caused by **paranasal sinus disease** is usually local-ized over the affected sinuses, often with associated purulent nasal discharge and fever. The diagnosis is established by tomog-raphy of the sinus or by computed tomography or MRI of the head.

Headache of ocular origin (ocular muscle imbalance, hyper-opia, astigmatism, impaired convergence/accommodation, narrow-angle glaucoma, iridocyclitis) is usually located in the ipsilateral orbit, forehead, or temple and has a steady, aching quality that may follow prolonged, intensive use of the eyes for close work (with glaucoma, the pain is often associated with loss of vision). A care-ful description of the type of headache and a history of its onset, relationship to use of the eyes, duration, and associated symptoms often suggest the diagnosis, which is established from other eye signs. For example, long-lasting, mild to moderate headache that occurs toward the end of a day and is relieved by a few hours of rest or sleep is more likely to be related to an ocular disorder.

Benign intracranial hypertension usually produces inter-mittent mild or severe headache that may be brought on by Valsalva maneuvers or by bending with the head down and is associated with papilledema. Criteria for this diagnosis include evidence of increased intracranial pressure and absence of clini-cal or laboratory evidence of a focal brain lesion, an infection, or hydrocephalus.

Low cerebrospinal fluid pressure headache, sometimes called **spinal headache** (usually occurring after lumbar puncture), is usually generalized and characteristically worsens substantially when the person is sitting or standing. Characteristically, the headache is relieved entirely when the person lies down.

DIZZINESS

It is important to determine whether the patient is describing a sensation of self or environmental movement or spinning (that is, vertigo), a sensation of light-headedness with or without visual graying or postural swaying (that is, faintness or near syncope), or something else (such as an unusual head sensation or gait unsteadiness).

Vertigo

Vertigo indicates dysfunction in the peripheral or central components of the vestibular system. Central vertigo results from disorders that affect brain stem or vestibulocerebellar pathways; peripheral vertigo indicates involvement either of the vestibular end organ (for example, semicircular canals) or of their peripheral neurons, including the vestibular portion of the eighth cranial nerve. A method for categorizing the causes of vertigo is presented in Table 2-2.

Central vertigo is a common part of posterior circulation disturbances such as cerebellar or brain stem infarction, hemorrhage, or vertebrobasilar TIA. In the context of vascular disease, vertigo is almost always associated with other symptoms of brain stem or cerebellar dysfunction. Central vertigo also may be caused by neoplasms of the posterior fossa (often associated with headache or gait or limb ataxia), demyelinating disease, arteriovenous malformation, brain stem encephalitis, and vertiginous epilepsy (tornado epilepsy) originating in the temporal lobe. Medications such as analgesics, antiarrhythmics,

Table 2-2.   Causes of vertigo

Degenerative	Toxic	Neoplastic
Cerebellar degeneration	Phenytoin	Acoustic neuroma, other cerebellopontine angle tumors
Syringobulbia	Aminoglycosides	
Arnold-Chiari malformation	Alcohol	Meningioma
Platybasia	Quinine	Cholesteatoma
	Metabolic	Cerebellar astrocytoma, other cerebellar neoplasms
Infectious or inflammatory	Beriberi	Glomus jugulare tumor
	Pellagra	
Labyrinthitis	Hypothyroidism	**Vascular**
Otitis media	Hypoglycemia	
Viral illness		Brainstem ischemia
Cerebellar abscess	**Traumatic**	Cerebellar hemorrhage
Syphilis of CNS	Petrous bone fracture	Inferior auditory artery occlusion
Arachnoiditis	Concussion	Migraine
Meningitis	Other head trauma	
Multiple sclerosis		**Other**
		Ménière's disease
		Seizure

CNS = central nervous system.

anticonvulsants, antibiotics, loop diuretics, and sedatives also may lead to vertigo.

Peripheral vertigo may be caused by unilateral or bilateral labyrinthine dysfunction (infection, trauma, ischemia, or toxins), vestibular neuronitis, lesions of the cerebellopontine angle impinging on the eighth cranial nerve (such as acoustic neuroma), Ménière's disease (recurrent attacks of vertigo associated with hearing loss, tinnitus, and a sensation of ear fullness, which may improve after the attack subsides), or benign positional vertigo (episodic vertigo occurring after changes of head position, which diminishes with repeated attempts to elicit vertigo with the same movement).

Positional vertigo that results from peripheral and central causes may be differentiated on the basis of clinical features, nystagmus characteristics, and findings with Nylen's maneuver (Table 2-3). Nylen's maneuver is performed by having the patient lie down abruptly from a sitting position and orient the head approximately 30 degrees below the horizontal plane. The test is repeated with the head positioned to the left, straight, and to the right, with observation for nystagmus and notation of any clinical symptoms.

Light-Headedness (Faintness)

Light-headedness is analogous to feelings that precede syncope (near syncope) that is caused by generalized cerebral ischemia. True vertigo almost never occurs during the presyncopal state. Presyncopal, stereotyped faintness may be associated with visual graying, heaviness in the lower limbs, and postural swaying. The causes of light-headedness relate to generalized cerebral hypoperfusion and include various causes of postural hypotension, orthostatic hypotension, decreased cardiac output (for example, cardiac arrhythmias), anemia, or other vasovagal disorders.

Other Causes of Nonvertiginous Dizziness

Other causes include hyperventilation syndrome (often associated with shortness of breath, rapid heartbeat, and a feeling of fear); diabetes mellitus (related to hypoglycemia, autonomic neuropathy, or postural hypotension); and various drugs, such as tricyclic antidepressants, antihypertensives, and tranquilizers.

VISUAL DISTURBANCES

Visual disturbances most often involve **visual loss** (including blurriness) or **diplopia**. It is very important to determine whether these symptoms are a result of cerebrovascular disease, a nonvascular neurologic disorder, a primary ocular disturbance, or something else (for example, a psychogenic disorder). Visual disturbances can be caused by defects in the retina, optic nerve, chiasm, optic tract, lateral geniculate nucleus, geniculocalcarine tract (optic radiation), and striate cortex of the occipital lobes.

Many disturbances of vision are caused by primary ocular disease (Table 2-4). For example, astigmatism or macular lesions may produce distortion of the normal shapes of objects (**metamorphopsia**). **Photophobia** is usually caused by corneal inflammation; aphakia; iritis; ocular albinism; or certain drugs, such as chloroquine or acetazolamide. Color change (**chromatopsia**) may result from systemic disturbances (for example, yellow

Table 2-3.   Differentiating features of peripheral and central vertigo

Feature	Peripheral Vertigo	Central Vertigo
Clinical		
Onset	Sudden	Insidious, less often sudden
Pattern	Paroxysmal	Continuous, occasionally paroxysmal
Severity	Intense	Mild
Tinnitus	Common	Rare
Fall on Romberg's test	To side of lesion, away from fast component of nystagmus	To side of lesion, to fast component of nystagmus
Caloric stimulation	Nonreactive	Normal
Nystagmus		
Spontaneous	May be present	May be present
Types	Horizontal or rotatory, no vertical	Horizontal, rotatory, or vertical
Fast component direction	Consistent direction in all directions of gaze	Varies with direction of gaze
Nylen's maneuver		
Latency	3–45 s	None
Fatigability	Yes	No
Visual fixation	Inhibits vertigo	No change
Nystagmus direction	Fixed	Independent
Reproducibility	Inconsistent	Consistent
Intensity	Severe vertigo, nausea	Mild vertigo, rarely nausea

vision accompanying jaundice), drug use (such as yellow and white vision in digitalis toxicity), chorioretinal lesions, or lenticular changes. **Rings** that are seen when viewing lights or bright objects may be caused by lens changes, incipient cataract, glaucoma, or corneal edema. **Spots** or **dots** before the eyes, which move with movement of the eye, are commonly caused by benign vitreous opacities (floaters). Difficulty seeing in the dark (**nyctalopia**) may result from congenital retinitis pigmentosa, hereditary optic atrophy, vitamin A deficiency, glaucoma, optic atrophy, cataract, or retinal degeneration.

Table 2-4.   Visual disturbances caused by primary ocular disorders

Effect on Vision	Ocular Disease
Metamorphopsia	Astigmatism, macular lesion
Photophobia	Corneal inflammation, aphakia, iritis, ocular albinism, drugs
Chromatopsia	Systemic disturbance, drug use, chorioretinal lesions, lenticular changes
Rings seen	Lens changes, incipient cataract, glaucoma, corneal edema
Spots, dots	Vitreous opacities
Nyctalopia	Congenital retinitis pigmentosa, hereditary optic atrophy, vitamin A deficiency, glaucoma, optic atrophy, cataract, retinal degeneration

Visual Field Defects

Symptoms of visual loss include loss of visual acuity, various types of visual field defects (Table 2-5), and unilateral or bilateral visual loss (the clinical approach to evaluating visual acuity and fields is discussed in Chapter 5).

Vascular retinal lesions may cause **arcuate, central, or ceco-central scotomata** corresponding to the area of vascular supply of the arteriole involved (the patient sees them as wedge-shaped dark spots) (Fig. 2-1). **Arcuate scotomata** may also be caused by

Table 2-5.   Causes of visual field defects

Defect	Cause
Scotomata	
Arcuate	Compressive or vascular lesions of optic disk
Cecocentral	Optic neuritis, retrobulbar optic nerve lesions
Symmetric central, cecocentral	Toxic states, nutritional disorders
Scintillating	Migraine, epilepsy
Peripheral constriction of visual field	Papilledema, perioptic sheath meningioma, psychogenic
Hemianopia	
Bitemporal	Lesions of optic chiasm
Incongruous (less often congruous) homonymous	Lesions of lateral geniculate nucleus, optic tract, optic radiation
Congruous homonymous	Lesions of calcarine cortex

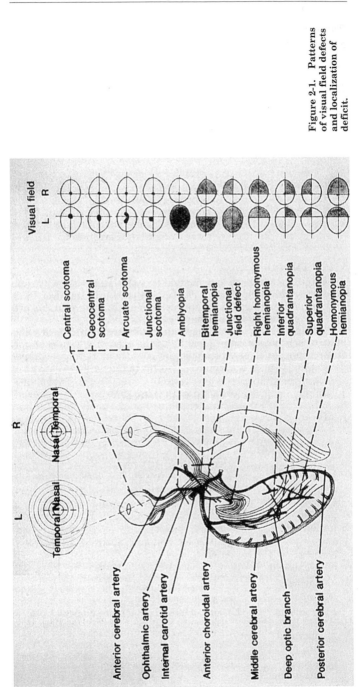

Figure 2-1.   Patterns of visual field defects and localization of deficit.

compressive or vascular lesions of the optic disc as a result of glaucoma or by hyaline bodies (drusen) of the disc. Optic neuritis and retrobulbar optic nerve lesions (demyelinating disease; infiltrative, neoplastic, or infectious diseases; degenerative diseases; aneurysm; tumor) often produce **cecocentral scotomata**. Small, **central scotomata** in macular disease often cause distorted vision for straight lines (metamorphopsia), a trait that aids in the distinction between macular and optic nerve lesions. Toxic states or nutritional disorders (tobacco-alcohol amblyopia) may produce relatively symmetric **central or cecocentral scotomata**. **Scintillating scotoma** (the patient sees bright, colorless or colored lights in the field of vision) usually occurs as a part of migraine or epilepsy with occipital lobe involvement. Progressive **peripheral constriction of the visual field** may be caused by papilledema or perioptic sheath meningioma or may be psychogenic (tunnel vision).

Lesions of the optic chiasm (pituitary tumor, craniopharyngioma, sellar meningioma, suprasellar aneurysm of the circle of Willis) produce **bitemporal hemianopias** (blindness in the temporal half of the visual fields). Pregeniculate optic tract lesions (infection, tumor) produce **homonymous hemianopia** associated with optic atrophy and afferent pupillary defects. Lesions of the lateral geniculate nucleus (infection, tumor, circle of Willis aneurysm) or postgeniculate lesions in the optic radiation (ischemic or hemorrhagic stroke, arteriovenous malformation, glioma) produce **incongruous homonymous hemianopias** (field defects in the two eyes are not identical) with normal pupillary reflexes. **Congruous homonymous hemianopia** (field defects in the two eyes are identical) with normal pupillary reflexes signifies a lesion in the calcarine cortex, usually the result of a cerebrovascular or neoplastic disorder, such as ischemic stroke or glioma.

Unilateral Loss of Vision

Unilateral visual loss may be caused by opticoretinal ischemia, occlusion of the central retinal artery or vein, anterior ischemic optic neuropathy, optic or retrobulbar neuritis, or optic nerve dysfunction resulting from mechanical compression (Table 2-6).

Table 2-6. Causes of unilateral loss of vision

Type of Vision Loss	Cause
Sudden	Ipsilateral carotid system occlusive disease, cardiac valvular abnormalities, blood stasis, cardiac shunts, cranial arteritis, occlusion of central retinal artery or vein, ischemic optic neuropathy
Subacute	Optic neuritis, retrobulbar neuritis, papilledema, migraine
Gradual	Optic nerve dysfunction caused by mechanical compression

Transient monocular blindness from episodic opticoretinal ischemia (**amaurosis fugax**) is frequently caused by ipsilateral carotid system occlusive disease and results in hemodynamic ocular blood flow disturbances or in retinal emboli (cholesterol, fibrin platelet) that originate from proximal carotid system plaque. Alternatively, emboli may reach the eye from the heart in circumstances of valvular abnormalities, blood stasis (arrhythmias, myocardial infarction, congestive heart failure), or right-to-left cardiac shunts with systemic venous thrombosis.

The patient with amaurosis fugax often describes the episode as an acute, transient loss of vision (a perception of a shade being pulled downward from above or upward from below over one eye or, occasionally, proceeding in a circular pattern peripherally to centrally in one eye) that usually lasts seconds or minutes. The clinician must question the patient carefully to determine whether the patient is describing loss of vision in one eye or a homonymous field defect (to localize this field defect, some patients may have alternately closed one eye and then the other at the time of the attack).

The clinical picture of amaurosis fugax may infrequently occur with (1) cranial arteritis (often in patients with associated new-onset, severe, persistent headache; enlarged, beaded, or pulseless temporal arteries; pain or cramping in the jaw during chewing [jaw claudication]; or polyarthralgias and polymyalgias), (2) papilledema (rarely, producing transient unilateral blindness in the form of very brief blurring of vision in one or both eyes, usually during sudden changes of posture), and (3) migraine (although bilateral scotomata are much more common in migraine than are unilateral blindness and visual loss).

Sudden unilateral blindness may also be caused by occlusion of the central retinal artery (typically, complete, long-lasting or permanent visual loss), occlusion of the central retinal vein (usually causing a milder visual loss), ischemic optic neuropathy (sudden mild to moderate visual loss that usually gradually worsens), or optic neuritis (generally in young adults with diminished visual acuity, central or paracentral scotomata, and sometimes painful eye movements, all of which develop subacutely and worsen over a few days). These diagnoses are usually established from characteristic ophthalmoscopic findings.

Gradual onset of unilateral blindness is usually caused by optic nerve dysfunction that results from mechanical compression that is generally associated with neoplasms or inflammatory lesions within the orbit or in the retro-orbital–parasellar areas, such as optic gliomas, meningiomas, hamartomas, hemangiomas, lymphomas, multiple myeloma, sarcoid, paranasal sinus infections or inflammatory disease, pituitary adenomas, and medial sphenoid wing meningiomas. As the compression progresses, acuity becomes impaired further, along with impaired color vision, afferent pupil reflex abnormalities, and, eventually, optic atrophy. The diagnosis is often established with computed tomography or MRI of orbital, retro-orbital, and sellar areas.

Bilateral Complete Loss of Vision

Diseases that affect both **optic nerves** (bilateral optic neuritis, toxic and nutritional optic neuropathies, demyelinating or degenerative disease, cranial arteritis, ischemic optic neuropathy); the **optic chiasm** (usually large lesions, including pituitary adenomas with or without pituitary apoplexy, craniopharyngiomas, meningiomas, and suprasellar aneurysms of the circle of Willis); or, rarely, both **optic tracts** (multiple infarcts, intracerebral hemorrhages, or tumors), both **optic radiations** (multiple infarcts, intracerebral hemorrhages, or tumors), or both **calcarine cortices** (hypertensive encephalopathy, tumors, bilateral infarcts, or intracerebral hemorrhages) may produce bilateral complete visual loss (Table 2-7). Often, a partial bilateral visual loss progresses over time before becoming complete. Characteristic visual field defects (see above) and visual acuity or pupillary reflex abnormalities help to establish the diagnosis.

Occasionally, brief episodes of bilateral darkening of vision that lasts seconds to a few minutes may precede a basilar territory infarction. Demyelinating or degenerative diseases usually produce intermittent bilateral loss of vision associated with bitemporal optic atrophy and early impairment of color vision. Tumors (for example, meningiomas) or aneurysms that affect the above-mentioned structures often lead to gradual, progressive (usually asymmetric) losses of vision.

Simultaneous bilateral impairment of vision with relatively symmetric central or cecocentral scotomata that develop during a period of days to weeks may occur with toxic or nutritional optic neuropathy associated with such agents as methyl alcohol, isoniazid, ethambutol, penicillamine, chloroquine, or phenylbutazone; with tobacco-alcohol abuse; or with deficiencies of thiamine, riboflavin, pyridoxine, niacin, vitamin B_{12}, or folic acid. Drug-induced alterations in color vision may be caused by trimethadione, sulfonamides, streptomycin, methaqualone, barbiturates, digitalis, or thiazides.

Nonorganic (functional) bitemporal sudden visual loss is characterized by no objective evidence of ocular pathology or disease of the optic pathways (including negative results of computed tomography or MRI of the head). Some patients may have tunnel vision (the remaining tunnel of vision does not change, regardless of the size of the target or the testing distance) or variable visual field defects with anatomic inconsistencies.

Table 2-7. Causes of bilateral complete loss of vision

Type of Vision Loss	Cause
Complete	Diseases or lesions of both optic nerves, optic chiasm, both optic tracts, both calcarine cortices
Episodic, bilateral darkening	Basilar territory transient ischemia
Intermittent	Demyelinating or degenerative
Gradual, progressive	Tumors, aneurysms
Impairment simultaneous with scotomata	Toxic or nutritional optic neuropathy

Diplopia

Diplopia may be caused by a wide variety of disorders. A careful history is very helpful for determining the diagnosis and the origin of diplopia and may even provide information about the most likely location of the lesion. The clinician should clarify several issues (Table 2-8). **Did the diplopia develop suddenly or gradually?** Sudden onset is typical for acute brainstem ischemia or hemorrhage, and gradual onset with slow progression is typical for growing aneurysms or tumors. **Has the diplopia been associated with orbital or periorbital pain?** Pain around the eye and the frontal area may be caused by cavernous sinus thrombosis, by aneurysms of the internal carotid artery at the infraclinoid-intracavernous or middle cranial fossa level, or by inflammatory disease of the orbit. Bleeding from the aneurysms usually causes generalized severe headache. **Does closing one eye change the diplopia in any way?** If the diplopia is caused by misalignment of the eyes, then closing either eye will correct it; if not (monocular diplopia), then either an ocular problem (a dislocated lens, cataract, retinal or macular lesion) or a functional disorder should be suspected. **Are the two objects seen horizontally, vertically, or as a combination of both?** Horizontal displacement of the

Table 2-8.   Questions to answer in evaluation of diplopia

Question	Significance
Was onset sudden or gradual?	Sudden: brainstem ischemia or hemorrhage Gradual: aneurysm, tumor
Is diplopia associated with orbital or periorbital pain?	Pain may be caused by cavernous sinus thrombosis, aneurysm of ICA, inflammatory orbital disease
Does diplopia change with eye closing?	If corrected with closing: misalignment If not corrected: ocular problem or functional disorder
Are the objects horizontal, vertical, or both?	Horizontal: possible dysfunction of abducens nerve or lateral rectus muscle Vertical: possible involvement of oculomotor nerve or trochlear nerve Horizontal and vertical: possible dysfunction of oculomotor nerve or trochlear nerve
Does a direction of gaze widen or narrow distance between images?	Images farthest apart when looking in direction of action of weak muscle: dysfunction of cranial nerves III, IV, VI
Is the diplopia intermittent or constant?	Constant: tumor, inflammation, infarction, infection Intermittent: TIA, aneurysm, neuromuscular junction defect, extraocular muscle dysfunction

ICA = internal carotid artery; TIA = transient ischemic attack.

objects may be a sign of dysfunction of the abducens nerve or lateral rectus muscle, vertical displacement of the images may indicate involvement of the oculomotor nerve or trochlear nerve, and combined horizontal/vertical diplopia also may occur with dysfunction of the oculomotor nerve or trochlear nerve.

Is there a direction of gaze that widens or narrows the distance between the images? The images are displaced farthest apart when the patient is looking maximally in the direction of action of the weak muscle in cases of dysfunction of the third, fourth, or sixth cranial nerve, but this test cannot be used easily in assessing weakness of multiple extraocular muscles, such as in myasthenia gravis or ocular myopathies. Also, the eye may be displaced forward (exophthalmos) or in other directions as a result of an orbital mass lesion with or without diplopia.

Is the diplopia intermittent or constant? It is important to know the time and the mode of onset of the diplopia and whether it is constant or intermittent. Constant or slowly changing diplopia may result from tumor, inflammation, infarction, or infection; intermittent diplopia is more suggestive of TIA, aneurysms, and disorders of the neuromuscular junction or ocular muscles.

Lesions of the third, fourth, and sixth cranial nerves may occur at the level of their nuclei, along their course from the brainstem through the subarachnoid space, cavernous sinus, or superior orbital fissure. Isolated horizontal or vertical diplopia that results from oculomotor nerve palsy is commonly caused by head trauma; diabetic vasculopathy; intracranial aneurysm of the internal carotid or posterior communicating artery; herniation of the uncus; or other rare conditions, such as a tumor at the base of the brain, infarction of the nerve, inflammation, mass lesions or thrombosis of the cavernous sinus, syphilis, vasculitis, demyelinating disease, or complicated migraine (ophthalmoplegic migraine).

Common causes of vertical or vertical/horizontal diplopia that results from trochlear nerve palsy include brainstem ischemic stroke, entrapment against the tentorium in herniation and trauma, cavernous sinus thrombosis, and inflammation or mass lesion. Isolated trochlear nerve palsy may be caused by aneurysms or neoplasms of the posterior fossa, trauma, sphenoid sinusitis, diabetic angiopathy, complicated migraine, nerve infarction, and syphilitic or tuberculous meningitis.

Isolated, unilateral, horizontal diplopia that results from abducens nerve palsy may be caused by diabetic angiopathy; aneurysms of the circle of Willis; increased intracranial pressure with or without downward herniation; or, less common, sixth cranial nerve infarction, mass lesions in the orbit, and pontine glioma in children or metastatic nasopharyngeal tumor in adults.

MUSCLE WEAKNESS

When a patient experiences weakness, heaviness, or difficulty in performing some activity, several historical features must be considered. The clinician should clarify the precise area of the body that is involved: Is the process focal, multifocal, or generalized? One must also inquire about onset: Was the problem acute or insidious in onset, and was there progression after the symptoms started? Are the symptoms episodic or continuous? Does anything seem to bring on the symptoms, and what leads to worsening? What is the pattern of weakness? Are there any symptoms other than weakness? After these questions are answered and a comprehensive examination is performed, the location of the neurologic abnormality that is leading to the weakness may be determined and a differential diagnosis may be outlined.

Important aspects of the neurologic examination are the pattern of muscle weakness; the appearance of the muscles; and the presence of fasciculations, atrophy, or hypertrophy. Deep tendon reflexes and muscle tone also should be evaluated. Other aspects of the neurologic examination should delineate the presence of abnormalities in other areas of the nervous system. Symptoms and signs associated with muscle weakness that is caused by lesions at various sites are reviewed in Table 2-9 and Figure 2-2.

SENSORY DISTURBANCES

When patients with ischemic or hemorrhagic cerebrovascular events have a sensory abnormality, it is usually in the form of numbness. It is important to clarify that the numbness nearly always reflects deadness or a loss of sensation (negative phenomenon), in contrast, for example, to sensory seizures, which characteristically involve a tingling or too much feeling (positive phenomenon). Occasionally, the patient with a thalamic or spinothalamic tract lesion may have a burning discomfort or pain after hemianesthesia or subjective numb feelings in the contralateral limbs. Lacunar stroke that affects the thalamus may also cause **pure sensory stroke**, manifested by loss of sensation over the contralateral side of the body and face, without motor deficit.

In a patient with isolated unilateral or bilateral facial numbness, it is important to analyze carefully the distribution of the numbness. An "onionskin" distribution is diagnostic for a lesion in the descending trigeminal nucleus at the level of the lower pons, medulla, or upper cervical cord, which may be caused by infarction (such as Wallenberg's syndrome of lateral medullary infarction), demyelinating disease, or syringobulbia. Mandibular, maxillary, ophthalmic, or hemifacial numbness may result from lesions involving the extramedullary part of the trigeminal nerve, often a result of tumor or trigeminal sensory neuropathy.

Information also should be sought about the **type of onset, temporal pattern** (intermittent numbness, especially with sudden onset, may occur with a vascular lesion or as a part of epilepsy; gradual onset is more typical of neoplastic lesions), and **association with other neurologic signs** (isolated facial numbness is seldom caused by a cerebrovascular lesion). As mentioned above, a sensory seizure that originates in or near the sensory cortex may produce transient, unilateral numbness (tingling or positive phenomenon) of the face, arm, or leg, which usually advances quickly (within a few minutes) from one area to another and may be accompanied by clonic jerks of the involved extremity. Migraine may also produce a sensory spell and involve deadness or tingling, characteristically beginning in one hand and marching up the arm before involving the ipsilateral face and, sometimes, the ipsilateral leg. This type of spell usually lasts 15 to 30 minutes and is often followed by a unilateral, throbbing headache.

Table 2-9.   Localization of muscle weakness

Location	Symptoms	Signs (Side, Relevant to Lesion Site)
Cortical/hemispheric	Weakness: in a single limb or in the face, may involve combinations of weakness on single side Other: associated sensory loss ipsilateral to weakness, visual loss, speech difficulty	Contralateral limb, face, or tongue weakness Spasticity Increased reflexes Extensor plantar response Aphasia Apraxia Hemianopia
Subcortical/internal capsule	Weakness: more likely to involve entire side, including face, arm, and leg Other: sensory loss may involve same areas as weakness; no aphasia, apraxia, hemianopia	Contralateral limb, face, or tongue weakness Spasticity Increased reflexes Extensor plantar response Sensory loss
Brain stem	Weakness: in arm and leg, may involve only face or tongue, may be bilateral Other: diplopia, vertigo, dysphagia, hoarseness, numbness in face or limbs	Same as for subcortical site Ipsilateral cranial nerve deficits, including face or tongue weakness Ipsilateral (middle to low brainstem) or contralateral (high brainstem) facial pain and temperature loss Contralateral limb pain, trunk pain, and temperature loss

(Continued)

Table 2-9. *Continued*

Location	Symptoms	Signs (Side, Relevant to Lesion Site)
Spinal cord (segment)	Weakness: in arm and leg, often bilateral Other: bowel and bladder problems, numbness	Limb weakness Spasticity Increased reflexes below lesion Decreased reflexes at level of lesion Extensor plantar response Contralateral pain and temperature loss Ipsilateral proprioception loss
Anterior horn cell	Weakness: confined to involved segment(s) Other: cramps, fasciculations	Weakness: confined to involved segment(s) Atrophy Fasciculations Decreased reflexes No extensor plantar response
Nerve root	Weakness: in nerve root distribution Other: local pain, paresthesias, numbness	Weakness in nerve root distribution Decreased reflexes in root distribution Segmental atrophy Segmental sensory loss Segmental fasciculations (uncommon)
Plexus	Weakness: in single limb Other: local pain, paresthesias, numbness	All signs may incompletely involve plexus Weakness in single limb Decreased reflexes in single limb Limb atrophy Sensory loss in single limb Fasciculations in single limb

Peripheral nerve	Distal weakness: footdrop, clumsy gait Other: distal numbness, distal paresthesias	Distal weakness Distal sensory loss Distal atrophy Distal fasciculations (uncommon) Decreased reflexes
Muscle	Weakness: proximal greater than distal, with difficulty arising from chair or elevating arms over head	Proximal weakness Normal sensation and tone Reflexes may be affected late
Neuromuscular junction	Weakness: fluctuating Other: fluctuating ptosis, dysarthria, dysphagia, diplopia	Worsening weakness with repetitive or persistent effort Normal sensation and tone Reflexes usually normal

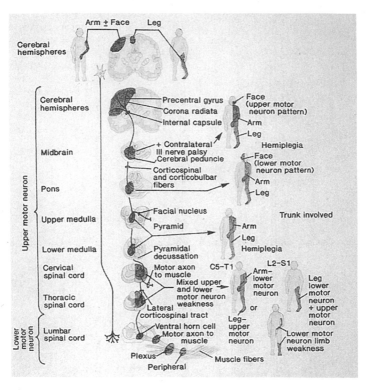

Figure 2-2.   Clinical features of motor system lesions at different levels.

SPEECH AND SWALLOWING DISTURBANCES

Dysarthria, as defined neurologically, is a specific difficulty with articulation caused by a cortical (associated contralateral limb weakness or dysphasia), corticobulbar (accompanying other signs of pseudobulbar palsy), subcortical extrapyramidal (associated with bradykinesia, rigidity, and rest tremor in the extremities), cerebellar (other signs of gait or appendicular ataxia may be noted), or brainstem (often with associated cranial nerve deficits) lesion.

Dysphonia is an impaired ability to produce sound because of respiratory disease or vocal cord paralysis (medullary involvement or a result of a carotid or thyroid surgical procedure, bronchial neoplasm, or aortic aneurysm). In middle-aged or elderly patients, spastic dysphonia may occur. This disorder of unknown nature is characterized by nonprogressive, isolated spasm of all of the throat muscles on attempted speech. **Dysphasia** is a loss of production or comprehension of spoken or written language, often as a result of a cortical lesion, such as an ischemic or hemorrhagic stroke.

In a patient with speech and swallowing abnormalities, the physician must determine whether the symptoms are caused by pseudobulbar palsy (bilateral corticobulbar tract involvement) or by true bulbar palsy (including the nuclei of cranial nerves IX, X, and XII; the neuromuscular junction; or muscle involvement) (Table 2-10).

In a patient with acute bulbar palsy, the differential diagnosis should include stroke (often associated with other symptoms of a brainstem lesion), myasthenia gravis (usually with accompanying weakness of extraocular, pharyngeal, or extremity muscles), botulism (often with accompanying dilated, sluggishly reactive pupils and extraocular muscle weakness), Guillain-Barré syndrome (often preceded by ascending symmetric limb weakness), tick paralysis (commonly preceded by tick bite, muscle pain, and fever), and bulbar poliomyelitis (often with asymmetric limb weakness and fever).

MOVEMENT AND GAIT ABNORMALITIES

In a patient with movement or gait disturbances, a carefully obtained history may indicate the likely origin and site of the causative lesion. The physician should ask the patient whether the disturbance occurs more in the dark than in the light, whether there is any accompanying vertigo (brainstem involvement) or other symptoms, whether there is difficulty in the initiation or termination of walking, and whether there is a family history of movement or gait abnormalities.

A patient with unsteadiness and gait disturbances that do not change much in the dark from what they are in the light usually has cerebellar (or cerebellar connection) dysfunction involving either the anterior lobe or the midline vermis. The acute onset of such disturbances suggests a cerebrovascular lesion, most commonly a cerebellar infarct. More gradual onset of isolated gait ataxia is most often caused by aging or by chronic alcohol consumption. Other causes of cerebellar gait ataxia include cerebellar hemorrhage; tumor; infection; developmental lesions (agenesis, Dandy-Walker deformity, Arnold-Chiari malformation, von Hippel-Lindau disease); degenerative disorders (ataxia-telangiectasia, Friedreich's ataxia); metabolic, drug, paraneoplastic, or toxic disorders (myxedema, malignancy, inborn disorders of metabolism, use of alcohol, phenytoin); or hydrocephalus.

Unsteadiness on standing, walking, or sitting that markedly increases in the dark or when the patient's eyes are closed but without substantial impairment of limb coordination or nystagmus is suspicious for sensory ataxia caused by peripheral nerve or spinal cord posterior column lesions (tabes dorsalis, vitamin B_{12} deficiency, pernicious anemia, paraneoplastic disorders, Sjögren's syndrome, excess vitamin B_6). In contrast, diseases of the cerebellar hemisphere (infarction, hemorrhage, neoplastic or demyelinating disease) often cause prominent impairment of ipsilateral limb coordination.

TRANSIENT LOSS OF CONSCIOUSNESS AND SEIZURES

Because the physician usually has not witnessed these disorders, a detailed history, including the time just preceding a spell and the time after it, is very important in the evaluation. The

Table 2-10.   Differentiating features of bulbar and pseudobulbar palsies

Syndrome	Structures Involved	Major Causes	Characteristic Clinical Features
Bulbar palsy	Nuclei of cranial nerves IX, X, XII Neuromuscular junction or muscles	Brainstem infarction, demyelinating disease, syringobulbia, botulism, Guillain-Barré syndrome, tick paralysis, bulbar poliomyelitis, diphtheria, myasthenia gravis	Nasal regurgitation of fluids is common; speech tends to be nasal and breathy; flaccid weakness (atrophy may also be present) of the muscles associated with talking, chewing, swallowing, and movement of the tongue and lips
Pseudobulbar palsy	Bilateral corticobulbar tract	Bilateral hemispheric stroke, bilateral lacunar infarction, encephalopathy, demyelinating disease, encephalitis, trauma, amyotrophic lateral sclerosis	Speech tends to be slow, strangulated, low pitched, and harsh; nasal regurgitation of fluids is rare; emotional incontinence, dementia, bilateral pyramidal tract signs, an active jaw jerk, snout reflex, or grasp reflex

clinician should inquire whether the disturbances occurred with prodromal features (pallor, nausea, and sweating often precede vasovagal **syncopal or presyncopal attacks**; palpitation, sweating, behavioral disturbances, or seizures may precede **hypoglycemic syncope**; vertigo and scintillating scotomata often precede transient loss of consciousness [LOC] caused by **basilar migraine**; and abnormal stereotyped movements, sensations, or experiences just before the LOC may suggest **seizure**); whether the disturbances occurred suddenly or gradually when the patient was standing (disturbances with standing associated with gradual onset of LOC are typical of **syncope** or of **functional disturbances**), sitting, or lying (disturbances with lying that are associated with abrupt onset of LOC are more suggestive of **seizure**); whether the patient had been using alcohol or other drugs (**drug-induced syncope or seizure**); whether the patient had been ill or febrile at the time the incident occurred (suggestive of **syncope or febrile seizure**); whether there were any focal motor or sensory manifestations such as speech disturbances, localized sensory abnormalities, or hemiparesis or monoparesis preceding or following the event (suggestive of a **localized structural cerebral lesion**); and whether there was tongue laceration, bruising, or urinary or fecal incontinence noted after the LOC (suggestive of **seizure** rather than simple syncope).

The stereotyped and uncontrollable nature of the focal (partial seizures with or without LOC and secondary generalization) or generalized (absence, myoclonic, clonic, tonic, tonic-clonic, or atonic) seizures is characteristic of epilepsy. Differentiating features of seizures and syncope are reviewed in Table 2-11.

Transient Loss of Consciousness

Transient LOC most often results from syncope caused by reduced cardiac output or mechanical reduction of venous return or from concussion caused by trauma (Table 2-12). Metabolic disorders, such as hypoglycemia, may cause transient LOC, and basilar migraine may cause such LOC, particularly in young women. Primary cerebrovascular insufficiency almost never causes transient LOC.

Reduced cardiac output (cardiac syncope) most often results from cardiac arrhythmias (especially atrioventricular block with Stokes-Adams attacks, ventricular asystole, sinus bradycardia, episodic ventricular fibrillation, ventricular tachycardia, and supraventricular tachycardia without atrioventricular block), massive myocardial infarction with pump failure, obstruction of left ventricular outflow (aortic stenosis, hypertrophic subaortic stenosis), obstruction of pulmonary flow (pulmonic stenosis, primary pulmonary hypertension, pulmonary embolism), and cardiac tamponade. For patients with suspected cardiac syncope, electrocardiography is mandatory (in many cases, prolonged monitoring, tilt-table testing, or cardiac electrophysiology studies also are needed).

Vasovagal (vasodepressor) syncope is characterized by a generalized weakness with loss of postural tone, inability to stand upright, and a LOC caused by global reduction of cerebral blood flow. A short prodromal phase usually includes various combinations of pallor, nausea, yawning, epigastric distress, hyperpnea or

Table 2-11.   Transient loss of consciousness: seizure compared with syncope

Symptoms	Seizure	Syncope

Prodromal	None: sudden LOC
	Aura
	   Epigastric discomfort
	   Déjà vu
	   Sensation of fear
	   Focal sensory or motor
	     phenomena
		Nausea
		Diaphoresis
		Light-headedness
		Visual darkening

During
  the spell
	Convulsive
	  Tonic-clonic
	   movements
	  Bowel or bladder
	   incontinence
	  Tongue biting
	Nonconvulsive
	  Stare
	  Automatistic
	   movements of limbs
		Unresponsive
		Flaccidity
		Occasional
		  stiffness with
		  jerking movements
		Occasional bladder
		  incontinence

After the
  spell
	Confusion lasting
	  minutes
	Agitation lasting
	  minutes
		Prompt recovery

Activity	Sleep Standing, sitting, or lying Alcohol use	Standing or sitting Lying (less common) Exertion Alcohol use
Cause	See Table 2-13	Table 2-12

LOC = loss of consciousness.

tachypnea, weakness, confusion, tachycardia, pupillary dilation, and sweating. The patient is pale and has bradycardia and hypotension. This syncope may be experienced by people without significant medical or neurologic disease and tends to take place during emotional stress (especially in a warm, crowded room) and often when the patient is standing (silting may alleviate or minimize the spell). Circumstances that precipitate this type of syncope include Valsalva maneuver, cough, or micturition. Occasionally, paroxysms of coughing in patients (especially men) with chronic bronchitis produce a **tussive syncope**. After hard coughing, the patient suddenly becomes weak and loses consciousness momentarily. The mechanism is thought to be decreased cardiac venous return associated with the Valsalva maneuver. Defecation syncope has a similar underlying mechanism. In all vasovagal syncope subtypes, LOC is generally short-lived, but tonic or clonic movements may develop if impaired cerebral blood flow is prolonged (anoxic seizures).

    Postural (orthostatic) hypotension with syncope is a fairly common cause of LOC in middle-aged or elderly patients who

Table 2-12.   Classification of causes of syncope

Category	Causes
Cardiopulmonary	
Dysrhythmias	
Tachycardia	Supraventricular
	Atrial fibrillation
	Atrial flutter
	Other
	Ventricular
	Ventricular tachycardia
	Ventricular fibrillation
Bradycardia	Sinus bradycardia
	Second- or third-degree heart block
	Pacemaker failure
Sick sinus syndrome	
Drug toxicity	
Outflow obstruction/	Pulmonary stenosis
cardiac failure	Aortic stenosis
	Pulmonary embolus
	Myocardial infarction
	Hypertrophic obstructive
	cardiomyopathy
Inflow obstruction	Pericardial tamponade
	Mitral stenosis
	Atrial myxoma
	Cardiomyopathies (restrictive)
Cerebrovascular	
(unusual cause)	
Stenosis/occlusion of	Multiple causes (see Table 8-1,
bilateral carotid	large vessel diseases)
and/or vertebrobasilar	
arteries	
Other neurologic	
Neurologically mediated	Vasovagal syncope
	Cardiac sinus syncope
	Glossopharyngeal neuralgia
	Micturition syncope
Orthostatic hypotension	Autonomic neuropathy
	Multisystem atrophy
	Prolonged recumbency
Metabolic/hematologic	Hypoglycemia, hypoxia, anemia
Psychological	Anxiety

have instability of vasomotor reflexes. The blood pressure should be measured when the patient is supine, immediately on standing, and 1 to 2 minutes after standing. A decrease in systolic blood pressure of more than 25 mm Hg on standing and associated with near syncope or syncope is highly suggestive of the diagnosis. This syndrome may be caused by medications (antihypertensive agents, beta-adrenergic blockers, tricyclic antidepressants, nitrates, dopaminergics, or dopamine agonists) or concomitant disease (Addison's disease, parainfectious or paraneoplastic autonomic neuropathy, amyloidosis with associated neuropathy, Shy-Drager syndrome, familial dysautonomia), or it may be idiopathic with no evident cause. Although the character of the syncopal attack differs little from that of the vasovagal type, the effect of posture (occurring when the patient arises suddenly from a recumbent position) is its cardinal feature.

Carotid sinus syncope may be initiated by direct palpation over the carotid bifurcation area, by turning of the head to one side, by a tight collar, or by shaving over the region of the sinus, particularly in elderly individuals. Carotid sinus palpation and massage should be avoided in patients in whom this diagnosis is suspected. Auscultation of the carotid arteries should be performed carefully, and, in selected patients, neurovascular noninvasive investigations may be useful to look for evidence of carotid occlusive disease.

Seizures

Seizure is a generic term that can be defined as a transient disturbance in neurologic function related to an abnormal and excessive electrical discharge of a population of neurons in the brain. The clinical manifestations of seizures are many and varied. Spells are generally categorized as generalized (convulsive or nonconvulsive, primary or secondary) or partial (simple or complex) seizures and may be isolated, cyclic, prolonged, or repetitive.

A **jacksonian clonic convulsion** or transient hemiparesis or monoparesis after a motor seizure (**Todd's paralysis**) is indicative of a frontal motor cortex lesion. **Simple sensory seizures** (paresthesia or tingling in a limb or on the face, with or without sensation of body image distortion, or other strange, localized, or stereotyped feelings such as olfactory or visual hallucinations, feeling of familiarity or strangeness, ecstasy, fear, dreamy states, or illusions) are suggestive of a contralateral sensory cortex lesion. The clinical picture of **complex partial seizures** or psychomotor epilepsy (originating usually in the temporal or frontal lobe) usually includes complex aura (stereotyped visceral, memory, movement, or affective disturbances) and LOC in the form of loss of responsiveness without falling, with or without automatisms (involuntary, often repetitive, and seemingly forced complex motor activity), commonly followed by a confusional state that lasts a few minutes or longer. The type of aura before secondary **generalized tonic-clonic seizures** (grand mal) provides information about the site of the lesion.

Once a seizure disorder has been diagnosed, the physician should establish its cause (Table 2-13). Idiopathic epilepsy usually develops when a person is young and is commonly characterized by generalized seizures. The most common causes of seizures in early adulthood include trauma (with or without subdural hematoma), withdrawal from drugs or alcohol (usually within 48 hours after cessation of heavy drinking), CNS infection, tumor, and arteriovenous malformation.

The onset of seizures in late adulthood may be associated with cerebrovascular disease (previous cerebral infarction, acute cerebral infarction [especially embolic], arteriovenous malformation,

Table 2-13. Classification of causes of seizures

Hereditary/ Degenerative	Infectious/ Inflammatory	Toxic/Metabolic	Neoplastic	Vascular	Other
von Recklinghausen's disease	Meningitis and encephalitis	Severe electrolyte disturbances, hypocalcemia, hyponatremia, vitamin B_6 deficiency, phenylketonuria	Primary brain tumor, brain metastasis	Cerebral infarction	Traumatic hematoma
Tuberous sclerosis	Bacterial			Intracerebral hemorrhage	Subdural
Sturge-Weber syndrome	Fungal			Subarachnoid hemorrhage	Epidural
Inborn errors of metabolism	Viral	Hypoglycemia		Sinus thrombosis	Penetrating brain injury
	Syphilitic	Hypothyroidism		Hypertensive encephalopathy	Fever
	HIV	Drug-induced		Cerebral vasculitis	Infantile spasms
	Lyme disease	Alcohol or other drug withdrawal		Arteriovenous malformation	Idiopathic
	Tuberculosis	Liver or kidney failure		Cavernous malformation	Global hypoxia/ anoxia
	Parasitic			Large unruptured intracranial aneurysm	
	Brain abscess				
	Collagen vascular diseases				

HIV = human immunodeficiency virus.

acute subarachnoid hemorrhage, intracerebral hemorrhage), trauma, drug or alcohol withdrawal, tumor, degenerative disease, CNS infection, toxic or metabolic encephalopathy (tricyclic antidepressants, phenothiazines, theophylline, hyponatremia, hypoglycemia, nonketotic hyperglycemia, magnesium deficiency, hypocalcemia, hepatic or renal failure), and collagen vascular disorders.

COGNITIVE ABNORMALITIES

When cognitive function is impaired, the clinician needs to distinguish **dementia** (progressive deterioration of intellect, behavior, and personality caused by diffuse disease processes that affect the cerebral hemispheres) from several **pseudodementias**, including

1. psychiatric illnesses
2. isolated dominant hemisphere lesions
3. isolated nondominant hemisphere lesions
4. isolated memory disturbances
5. acute confusional state (delirium)

Depressed patients and patients with psychosis and other **psychiatric disorders** (such as anxiety) that cause reduced concentration often complain of memory difficulties. In these situations, a careful search for an organic cause should be undertaken.

Dominant hemisphere lesions are often accompanied by abnormalities of language function (aphasia or dysphasia). Gerstmann's syndrome, agraphia, acalculia, right-left confusion, and finger agnosia all can occur with left hemisphere lesions. Apraxia of speech may also occur in patients with dominant hemisphere lesions.

Most patients with **lesions of the nondominant hemisphere** show more dramatic constructional impairment, such as constructional apraxia and dressing apraxia, than do patients with dominant hemisphere lesions. Prosopagnosia (difficulty in recognizing faces), impairment of spatial orientation, anosognosia (ignorance of the presence of disease), motor impersistence, and aprosody may also occur in these patients.

Isolated memory disturbances include **transient global amnesia**, a syndrome that usually occurs as a single event in middle-aged to elderly individuals and is characterized by the inability to form new memories (anterograde amnesia) along with some degree of loss of memory of the events that preceded the onset of the episode (retrograde amnesia). The condition usually resolves during a period of minutes to hours, and the person has complete recovery. Approximately 10% of patients have recurrent events. The cause of transient global amnesia is probably multifactorial, but, in at least some cases, it seems to involve posterior circulation cerebral ischemia. A migrainous cause has also been suggested but should be considered only when no other neurologic deficit is associated with the amnestic symptoms.

Patients with **acute confusional state** (acute brain syndrome, toxic encephalopathy, organic brain syndrome with psychosis) are inattentive, incoherent, agitated, and inconsistent in reporting recent events. In addition, they often demonstrate hallucinations (visual hallucinations are more typical in patients with neurologic disorders, whereas auditory hallucinations are more common in patients with primary psychiatric disease) and fluctuation in their level of consciousness. At night, when environmental stimuli are reduced, the confusion and agitation become accentuated. The most common causes of acute confusional state are (1) toxic-metabolic disturbances, including drug and drug withdrawal reactions; (2) sepsis; and (3) increased intracranial pressure.

When obtaining a history from a patient with **dementia** and from the patient's relative or friend, the physician should obtain details of the **patient's previous mental status** and of the **onset and the rapidity of mental deterioration** (acute or stepwise deterioration of the intellectual function may be associated with multi-infarct dementia; subacute progression during a period of days or weeks may be caused by encephalitis; progression during a period of months may result from Jakob-Creutzfeldt disease; and chronic progression during several months to years may be associated with Alzheimer's disease, normal-pressure hydrocephalus, or metabolic encephalopathies). Evaluation of the patient's **drug history** enables one to determine dementia that is caused by taking barbiturates, bromides, tranquilizers, tricyclic antidepressants, lithium, anticonvulsants, steroids, anticholinergic drugs, dopaminergic agents, methyldopa, clonidine, or propranolol.

Questions about **nutritional status** may reveal dementia that results from thiamine deficiency (chronic alcoholic dementia or Wernicke-Korsakoff syndrome); vitamin B_{12} or folate deficiency; pellagra; alcohol abuse; or toxicity of heavy metals such as arsenic, lead, thallium, or mercury. Questions about **general health and relevant disorders** help to determine the probable cause of a dementing process (Table 2-14).

The physician also should inquire about a **family history of dementia** (suggestive of Huntington's disease and, possibly, Alzheimer's disease). Alzheimer's disease causes approximately 60% of all dementias; cerebrovascular diseases (multi-infarct dementia, progressive subcortical encephalopathy, or Binswanger's disease) cause 20% of dementias.

Table 2-14.   Classification of common causes of dementia

Hereditary/ Degenerative	Infectious/ Inflammatory	Toxic/ Metabolic	Neoplastic	Vascular	Other
Alzheimer's disease	Meningitis and encephalitis	Uremia	Bilateral tumors Primary	Multi-infarct	Multiple head injuries
Lewy body disease	Bacterial	Liver failure	Metastatic	Binswanger's disease	Chronic SDH
Pick's disease	Fungal	Hypopituitarism	Meningeal carcinomatosis	Vasculitis	Hydrocephalus
Huntington's disease	Viral	Hypothyroidism	Paraneoplastic syndromes		Communicating
Parkinson's disease	Syphilitic	Parathyroid disease	(e.g., limbic encephalitis)		Noncommunicating
Progressive supranuclear palsy	HIV	Hyponatremia			
Wilson's disease	Lyme disease	Vitamin deficiencies			
	Brain abscess	Pernicious anemia			
	Jakob-Creutzfeldt disease	B_{12}			
	Collagen vascular diseases	Folate			
		Toxins			
		Medication			
		Heavy metals			

HIV = human immunodeficiency virus; SDH = subdural hematoma.

General Medical Review

The patient's family history, medical history, and social and environmental history may provide information that clarifies the cause of an ischemic or hemorrhagic cerebrovascular event (Table 3-1). Familial risk factors for ischemic stroke have been difficult to define with certainty, although hypertension, atherosclerosis, diabetes mellitus, and hyperlipidemia seem to have at least some hereditary predisposition in many patients. A family history of ischemic stroke and formation of arterial or venous thromboses should be noted (see Chapter 23 regarding inherited stroke syndromes). In patients with subarachnoid hemorrhage or intracerebral hemorrhage, one should ask about a family history of intracranial hemorrhage, saccular aneurysm, arteriovenous malformation, cavernous malformations, polycystic kidney disease, connective tissue disorders, and bleeding disorders.

A comprehensive medical history also should be obtained. Previous cerebrovascular events of either ischemic or hemorrhagic type should be recorded. Because the presence of systemic atherosclerosis is a risk factor for cerebrovascular atherosclerosis, one should ask about previous myocardial infarction, angina, and claudication of extremities. A history of hypertension, diabetes mellitus, or hyperlipidemia is also an important risk factor for atherosclerosis. Other medical disorders that may be relevant for ischemic stroke are cardiac arrhythmias, valvular heart disease, connective tissue disorders, and coagulopathy of both thrombotic and hemorrhagic subtypes. Previous head or neck trauma or radiation therapy also should be noted. For ischemic or hemorrhagic strokes, use of antiplatelet agents, anticoagulants, fibrinolytic therapies, estrogen supplements, dietary aids or appetite suppressants, decongestants, and herbal medications should be recorded.

The social and environmental history should include clarification of the quantity and the duration of tobacco use, alcohol consumption, and recreational drug use. Because sedentary life style is a risk factor for ischemic stroke, the nature and the duration of the patient's physical activity should be defined. A dietary history is also useful with emphasis on intake of cholesterol, saturated fat, and trans-fatty acids as well as daily intake of fruits and vegetables.

Table 3-1. General medical history for patients with stroke

Risk Factors for Cerebral Ischemia	Risk Factors for Cerebral Hemorrhage	Risk Factors for Subarachnoid Hemorrhage
Family history		
Ischemic stroke, arterial or venous thromboses	Intracerebral hemorrhage, saccular aneurysm, AVM, cavernous malformation, bleeding disorders	Subarachnoid hemorrhage, saccular aneurysm, AVM, polycystic kidney disease, Ehlers-Danlos syndrome, Marfan's syndrome, neurofibromatosis, pseudoxanthoma elasticum, bleeding disorders
Previous diseases		
Ischemic stroke(s) or TIA; ischemic cardiac disease; hypertension; diabetes mellitus; hyperlipidemia; systemic atherosclerosis; cardiac arrhythmias; valvular heart disease; arterial or venous thromboses; hematologic disorders such as lupus anticoagulant positivity (history of multiple miscarriages), anticardiolipin antibody positivity (history of livedo reticularis), polycythemia, thrombocythemia, thrombocytopenic purpura, sickle cell disease, leukemia; connective tissue diseases; recent operation; head or	Intracerebral hemorrhage; head trauma; hypertension (particularly severe or poorly treated); intracranial aneurysm; embolic stroke; CNS infection; SBE; systemic vasculitides; primary CNS angiitis; intracranial neoplasm; hematologic disorders such as thrombocytopenic purpura, sickle cell anemia, leukemia, hypercoagulable states (venous thrombosis); moyamoya disease	Subarachnoid hemorrhage(s), head trauma, unruptured aneurysm(s), unruptured AVM(s), other disorders listed under "family history" (above), coarctation of the aorta, tuberous sclerosis, fibromuscular disease, bleeding disorders, SBE, primary CNS angiitis, head trauma

neck trauma; head or neck radiation therapy

Social and environmental history

Cigarette smoking; dietary (excessive cholesterol/saturated fat/trans-fatty acid intake or deficient intake of fruits and vegetables); use of oral contraceptives or estrogen replacement; use of recreational drugs, diet aids or appetite suppressants, decongestants, herbal medications

Anticoagulant or fibrinolytic therapy, heavy alcohol consumption, recreational drug use, diet aids or appetite suppressants, decongestants, herbal medications

Anticoagulant or fibrinolytic therapy, heavy alcohol consumption, recreational drug use, diet aids or appetite suppressants, decongestants, herbal medications

AVM = arteriovenous malformation; CNS = central nervous system; SBE = subacute bacterial endocarditis; TIA = transient ischemic attack.

General Examination

A systematic general examination of the patient with cerebrovascular disease is directed at finding evidence of disease of the cardiovascular system and at evaluation of the functional status of other vital internal organs (lungs, kidneys, liver). The examination of a patient with neurologic symptoms should begin with brief observation and proceed with comprehensive general and neurologic examinations.

OBSERVATION

Body and Limb Position and Spontaneous Movements

Patients with acute monoparesis or hemiparesis have variable spontaneous movements of the affected limb(s). Often, comatose patients with acute hemiplegia lie with the affected leg externally rotated and occasionally have unilateral twitching, unilateral myoclonic jerks, or spontaneous unilateral or asymmetric bilateral decerebrate or decorticate movements (see Chapter 6). Various metabolic disturbances may produce bilateral myoclonic jerks (seen with uremia) and asterixis (irregular flapping movements of the hands with the arms out straight and the wrists extended) in association with tremor and diffuse twitching (seen with hepatic failure, hypoglycemia, or hyponatremia).

General Appearance and Hygiene

These traits usually reflect the patient's self-image and may provide information about underlying preexisting medical or neurologic conditions.

Specific Signs of Chronic Illness

Observation of some specific signs of chronic illness may provide information about the underlying pathophysiology for various neurologic signs and symptoms, including altered levels of consciousness. Although the odor of alcohol on a patient's breath usually indicates alcohol intoxication, one must also consider superimposed subdural hematoma, other intracranial hemorrhage, trauma, seizure, Wernicke's encephalopathy, or infection. Other examples are the smell of ketones, which often indicates diabetic ketoacidosis, and fetor hepaticus, which suggests liver failure. Gingival hypertrophy is common in patients who are taking phenytoin for epilepsy. Lacerations on the lateral borders of the tongue (recent seizure), needle marks on the arms (drug intoxication), and skin ecchymoses and petechiae (recent trauma or bleeding disorder) may also be very helpful signs.

Dermatologic Examination

Among patients with trauma, "raccoon eyes" may indicate the presence of orbital fracture, Battle's sign may signify underlying mastoid fracture, and other **bruises or abrasions** on the head or the body may indicate trauma as the underlying cause. One should also characterize skin color changes by the nature of the pigmentation (hypo- or hyperpigmentation), localization (focal or generalized), presence of erythema, and specific pattern of the changes. The features may allow consideration of the presence of an underlying medical or neurologic disorder (Table 4-1).

Cyanosis in the distal extremities associated with cool skin may indicate vasoconstriction in patients with severe heart failure. Venous obstruction or venous hypertension usually results in localized or generalized cyanosis. Arterial obstruction in an extremity caused by embolism, arteriolar constriction, or cold-induced vasospasm usually results in localized pallor and coldness.

Various conditions may be associated with **localized** or **generalized edema**. Possible causes of localized edema include deep venous thrombosis, lymphatic obstruction caused by tumor, primary lymphedema, stasis edema of a paralyzed leg, and facial edema caused by obstruction of the superior vena cava or limited effect from an allergic reaction. Bilateral leg swelling is seen in

Table 4-1.   Differentiating features of some abnormalities of skin color

Skin Color Abnormality	Most Common Cause(s)
"Butterfly" rash on the face	Systemic lupus erythematosus
Erythematous rash on the elbows and knees	Dermatomyositis
Livedo reticularis	Idiopathic, collagen vascular diseases, hematologic disorders, Sneddon's syndrome, drug ingestion, cholesterol emboli, prolonged immobility
White macules on the trunk or limbs	Diabetes mellitus, vitiligo, hypothyroidism, thyrotoxicosis, pernicious anemia, adrenal insufficiency, sarcoidosis, leprosy, tuberous sclerosis
Generalized diffuse brown hypermelanosis	Addison's disease, ACTH-producing tumors, hemochromatosis, systemic scleroderma, porphyria cutanea tarda
Circumscribed brown macules	von Recklinghausen's neurofibromatosis, malignant melanoma, Peutz-Jeghers syndrome
Localized pallor or coldness	Arterial obstruction (embolism, arteriolar constriction, cold-induced vasospasm)
Cyanosis of the nail beds, lips, or mucous membranes	Chronic pulmonary insufficiency, pulmonary arteriovenous fistula, congenital heart disease with right-to-left shunting, severe heart failure, venous obstruction, venous hypertension

ACTH = adrenocorticotropic hormone.

cardiac failure, inferior vena cava obstructions, or cirrhosis. Hypothyroidism may be associated with periorbital puffiness. Drugs, such as steroids, estrogens, and vasodilators, and pregnancy and refeeding after starvation may also cause edema.

Varicose veins may indicate increased intra-abdominal pressure or, in rare instances, arteriovenous fistulas. **Thrombophlebitis** that leads to deep venous thrombosis may result in pulmonary thromboembolism.

CARDIAC EVALUATION

During the general examination, special attention should be given to the patient's heart, including cardiac auscultation, precordial palpation, and evaluation of heart rate and rhythm. **Cardiac auscultation** may reveal abnormalities of the cardiac valves, the presence of pulmonary hypertension, ventricular septal or atrial septal defect, cardiac wall abnormalities, or constrictive pericarditis (Table 4-2). Precordial palpation will clarify cardiac size and may also suggest the presence of valvular disease (Table 4-3).

Table 4-2.   Cardiac evaluation: auscultation

Auscultation Feature	Common Cause
Accentuated first heart sound	Mitral stenosis, hyperkinetic heart, thin chest wall
Diminished first heart sound	Heart failure, mitral regurgitation, thick chest wall, pulmonary emphysema
Abnormal splitting of second heart sound	Pulmonary hypertension, pulmonic stenosis, right bundle-branch block, mitral regurgitation, atrial septal defect, aortic stenosis
Low-pitched third heart sound	Left ventricular failure or volume overload
High-pitched third heart sound	Constrictive pericarditis
Low-pitched fourth heart sound	Aortic stenosis, systemic hypertension, hypertrophic cardiomyopathy, coronary artery disease
High-pitched opening snap after second heart sound	Mitral stenosis
High-pitched ejection clicks after first heart sound	Dilation of aortic root or pulmonary artery, congenital aortic stenosis or pulmonary stenosis
Systolic murmurs	Mitral or tricuspid regurgitation, ventricular septal defect, aortic stenosis, aortopulmonary shunt
Diastolic murmurs	Aortic or pulmonary regurgitation, mitral stenosis, patent ductus arteriosus, coarctation of aorta, pulmonary arteriovenous fistula

Table 4-3.   Cardiac evaluation: precordial palpation

Examination Finding	Common Cause
Exaggerated amplitude, duration, and lateral displacement of left ventricular apex impulse	Left ventricular hypertrophy
Presystolic distention of left ventricle	Excess left ventricular pressure, myocardial ischemia
Double systolic impulse	Hypertrophic cardiomyopathy
Low-frequency vibrations	Mitral or aortic valve disease
Pulsation of right sternoclavicular joint	Aneurysmal dilation of ascending aorta, right-sided aortic arch

PERIPHERAL VASCULAR EXAMINATION

Absence or reduction of the peripheral arterial pulses in the upper and lower limbs is indicative of primary arterial stenotic or occlusive lesions or lesions that result from proximal emboli. The **time of arrival** of the radial pulse at the wrist may also be helpful. A tardy radial pulse may result from an occlusive lesion in a proximal vessel, usually the subclavian artery. Simultaneous palpation of the radial and femoral arterial pulses, which normally are virtually coincident, allows one to detect the **weaker and delayed pulse**, which is suggestive of aortic coarctation. A **decreased or thready pulse** may occur in patients with myocardial infarction, restrictive pericardial disease, and other conditions associated with decreased cardiac output or in patients with increased peripheral vascular resistance. An **increased, bounding pulse** occurs characteristically in patients with anemia, fever, mitral regurgitation, aortic regurgitation, or peripheral arteriovenous fistula. **Alterations of the pulse amplitude** may result from severe left ventricular decompensation, paroxysmal tachycardia, premature ventricular contraction, pericardial tamponade, airway obstruction, or obstruction of the superior vena cava.

Blood pressure (BP) should be measured in both arms with the patient supine and, if possible, sitting and standing to detect significant asymmetry in BP and to document postural hypotension. One must be certain that the cuff size is appropriate for the arm size of the patient. A difference of 20 mm Hg or more in either systolic or diastolic BP between two arms may be caused by occlusive disease in or distal to the subclavian artery on the side of the lower systolic or diastolic BP or more proximally in the innominate artery or aorta between the innominate and left subclavian arteries. A significant decrease in the brachial BP when the patient assumes the upright position indicates postural hypotension, which may be symptomatic. The absence of compensatory tachycardia may signify central (such as Shy-Drager syndrome) or peripheral (such as autonomic neuropathy) autonomic dysfunction. The latest BP criteria suggest that normal BP is considered <120 mm Hg systolic and <80 mm Hg diastolic, prehypertension 120 to 139 mm Hg systolic or 80 to 89 mm Hg diastolic, stage 1 hypertension 140 to 159 mm Hg systolic or 90 to 99 mm Hg diastolic, and stage 2 hypertension ≥160 mm Hg systolic or ≥100 mm Hg diastolic.

Although as much as 90% of all patients with hypertension have so-called idiopathic or essential hypertension, the physician should try to determine a specific cause for the elevated BP (Table 4-4). The essential components of evaluation are (1) the medical history (including salt intake, use of oral contraceptives or hormones, presence of diabetes mellitus, smoking history, lipid abnormalities, and cardiac or renal disease) and family history of hypertension; (2) physical examination—ophthalmoscopy, assessment of thyroid size, auscultation for neck and abdominal bruits, palpation of peripheral pulses, determination of heart and kidney size, auscultation of the heart and lungs; and (3) laboratory evaluation—determination of hematocrit, blood urea nitrogen or creatinine, serum potassium, leukocyte count, blood glucose, cholesterol, triglycerides, serum calcium, phosphate, and uric acid; urinalysis; electrocardiography; and chest radiography. In certain circumstances, special studies, such as determination of creatinine clearance, renal ultrasonography, renal angiography, and 24-hour urine study for metanephrine, catecholamine, or cortisol levels, may be indicated.

HEAD, CHEST, AND ABDOMEN EXAMINATION

The clinical examination of the head (scalp and face), chest (lungs), and abdomen (liver, spleen, and gastroenteric and urogenital systems) may provide additional important findings.

Palpation and examination of the patient's **scalp, mastoid area**, and **zygomatic arches** may reveal a depressed fracture or laceration. Examination of the **auditory meatus and nose** to detect the presence of a cerebrospinal fluid leak or hemorrhage may indicate fracture of the cribriform plate or of the petrous portion of the temporal bone. The ocular sclerae also should be examined for hemorrhage because a hemorrhage of the lateral aspect of the eye, which is not bordered posteriorly by normal sclera, is somewhat characteristic of fracture of the anterior cranial fossa.

The **neck** (cervical vertebral bodies), **chest** (clavicles, ribs, trunk, and vertebral bodies), and **limbs** (long bones) must be examined for the presence of fracture, particularly in comatose patients who have uncertain histories or evidence of possible injury. **Lymph node enlargement** is most frequently indicative of infectious, immunologic, or malignant disease.

Pulmonary examination may reveal unsuspected lung or heart disease, including pneumonia, chronic obstructive pulmonary disease, and congestive heart failure.

The patient's abdomen should be palpated for the presence of muscle rigidity as evidence of possible abdominal hemorrhage or infection. **Hepatomegaly** may indicate tumor, hepatitis, cirrhosis, right-sided heart failure, Budd-Chiari syndrome, or hepatic infiltrative disorders. **Splenomegaly** occurs in a wide variety of

Table 4-4.   Common clinical forms of arterial hypertension

Form of Hypertension	Clinical Feature	Common Causes
Essential (primary) hypertension	Varies	Unknown
Secondary hypertension	Primarily systolic hypertension	Aortic atherosclerosis, aortic regurgitation, thyrotoxicosis, hyperkinetic heart syndrome, fever, arteriovenous fistula, patent ductus arteriosus
	Systolic and diastolic hypertension	Renal causes: stenosis of a main or branch renal artery, renal infarction, arteriolar nephrosclerosis, preeclampsia, eclampsia, chronic pyelonephritis, acute or chronic glomerulonephritis, polycystic renal disease, diabetic nephropathy, renin-producing tumors
		Endocrine causes: primary hyperaldosteronism, Cushing's syndrome, pheochromocytoma, congenital adrenogenital syndromes, acromegaly, hypercalcemia, myxedema, oral contraceptives
		Neurogenic causes: diencephalic syndrome, familial dysautonomia (Riley-Day), bulbar poliomyelitis, acute increased intracranial pressure, acute spinal cord transection
		Other causes: coarctation of aorta, toxemia of pregnancy, acute intermittent porphyria, excessive transfusion

hematologic, infectious, hepatic, and connective tissue disorders, such as sickle cell disease, thalassemia, hemolytic anemias, thrombocytopenias, neutropenias, infectious mononucleosis, septicemia, endocarditis, tuberculosis, parasitic infection, acquired immunodeficiency syndrome, histoplasmosis, and rheumatoid arthritis. Splenomegaly may also be associated with various forms of portal or splenic venous hypertension or with primary splenic tumor or abscess.

Neurologic Examination

Neurologic examination of the patient with cerebrovascular disease is similar to any other formal neurologic examination. However, certain combinations of neurologic signs may establish the location of the disease. A complete neurologic examination is necessary to determine current neurologic status, and serial assessments are often desirable to determine whether there is any improvement or worsening of the condition. Some elements of the neurologic examination relating to preliminary evaluation of the level of consciousness, mental status, speech, vision, and focal weakness of the limbs are completed when the history is taken and also during the general examination.

Other elements of the neurologic examination provide further detail about whether the patient's current illness is caused by cerebrovascular disease and, if so, the location and sometimes the type and the origin of the lesion(s). With the data from the history and the general and neurologic examinations, a logical differential diagnosis and evaluation strategy can be proposed. Further evaluation of laboratory study results usually helps to clarify the diagnosis and define an appropriate treatment plan.

NEUROVASCULAR EXAMINATION

Auscultation

Auscultation of the proximal great vessels (Fig. 5-1) arising from the aortic arch (over the supraclavicular fossa), the carotid arteries (particularly over the carotid bifurcation below the angle of the mandible), the orbits (while closing the eye being auscultated), and the cranial vault is performed to listen for bruits. With the patient lying or sitting, the bell of the stethoscope should be applied over the area being examined without using pressure, which may produce artificial noise. First, the cardiac sounds should be auscultated over the base of the heart, and then the stethoscope should be moved superiorly to distinguish transmitted cardiac sounds from sounds arising in brachiocephalic, subclavian, vertebral, or carotid arteries. Bruits that are heard proximally over the aortic arch vessels may be associated with transmitted cardiac murmurs, underlying large vessel stenosis or tortuosity, or no identifiable underlying abnormality.

All bruits should be graded on a scale of 1 to 6 according to their intensity (1, barely audible with stethoscope; 6, audible without a stethoscope). The quality of a carotid bruit is a poor predictor of the severity of the underlying stenosis, although high-pitched bruits may be more predictive of an underlying significant stenosis. A bruit is a reflection of turbulence in the underlying artery. A carotid bruit, without regard to its quality or duration, is a relatively poor predictor of stenosis of the internal carotid artery in asymptomatic patients. It is noted in approximately 40% of patients with stenosis of more than 90% of the diameter of the artery, but 10% of patients with stenosis of less than 50% of the artery's diameter may have an audible

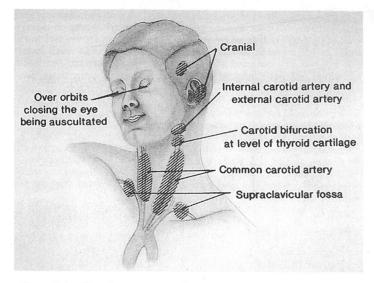

Figure 5-1.   Sites for neurovascular auscultation.

bruit. In patients with symptoms of cerebral ischemia, however, a diffuse or localized bruit is 85% predictive of a moderate or high-grade stenosis. Soft, continuous cervical bruits that vary with changes in neck position or that can be obliterated by jugular compression are suggestive of a benign venous hum.

Most **arterial bruits** begin in systole, but **systolic-diastolic bruits** strongly suggest high-grade arterial stenosis (>90% cross-sectional area stenosis). While listening over the carotid arteries, the physician should distinguish **diffuse** bruits (relatively constant magnitude and pitch along the carotid arteries in the neck or mildly decreasing distal intensity) from **localized** carotid bruits, although either may or may not be associated with underlying carotid stenosis. Diffuse bruits, especially if bilateral, often reflect a transmitted heart murmur; an aortic arch lesion; or a condition of diffuse, increased flow and turbulence without an underlying structural lesion. It may be difficult or impossible to distinguish lesions of the internal carotid artery from stenoses of the common carotid or external carotid arteries or to distinguish lesions of the vertebral artery from those of the subclavian or brachiocephalic arteries on the basis of the location or sound characteristics of a bruit.

Orbital bruits, particularly continuous, machinery-like bruits, are encountered with occlusive lesions of the carotid siphon, ipsilateral internal carotid artery occlusion with increased ophthalmic collateral backflow in the external carotid system, and other lesions that produce intracranial turbulent flow, such as arteriovenous malformations (AVMs). **Cephalic bruits** are commonly found in otherwise normal children but may also be found in 10% to 25% of patients with intracranial AVMs (usually associated with a rhythmic, localized head noise referred to as "pulsatile tinnitus").

Palpation

Palpation of the carotid pulses in the neck is generally unreliable (minor differences in the pulses of the left and right carotid arteries are unlikely to be important) and may even be dangerous, particularly at the level of the carotid bifurcation or over carotid arteries with associated bruit. Material from atheromatous plaques may be dislodged and cause cerebral infarction distally in the carotid system. Direct pressure applied to the carotid sinus may also cause cardiac arrhythmias.

Palpation of the superficial temporal, facial, infraorbital, and occipital arteries provides an estimate of flow in the external carotid system (Fig. 5-2). This flow may be reduced in the cranial arteries or with an ipsilateral common carotid or external carotid artery occlusion. Increased external carotid flow may reflect an occlusive lesion of the internal carotid artery with increased compensatory collateral flow. In addition, palpation of the superficial temporal arteries may be helpful in the diagnosis of cranial

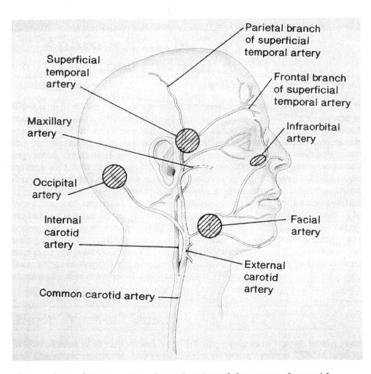

Figure 5-2.   Common sites for palpation of the external carotid artery system.

arteritis, which is indicated by a decreased pulse, increased arterial tenderness or beading, and erythema of the overlying skin. Palpation of the radial arteries may provide information about the status of the subclavian systems: A weaker pulse in one radial artery or one pulse that follows the other asynchronously (delayed) suggests proximal stenosis in the subclavian system on that side.

Ophthalmic Ocular Examination

Ophthalmic examination consists of a careful evaluation of the patient's history (see Chapter 2, Visual Disturbances), a general ocular examination, and special ophthalmic examinations.

General Ocular Examination

General examination includes inspection of external ocular structures (lids, conjunctivae, corneas, sclerae, and lacrimal apparatus), irides, pupils, and position of the eyes; determination of visual acuity; and confrontational visual field testing.

Inspection of the **external ocular structures** allows detection of various disturbances, such as pupillary abnormalities, ptosis, exophthalmos, foreign bodies, inflammation, dryness, corneal clouding, and iridic color abnormalities. Both upper eyelids normally cover 1 to 2 mm of the irides. Unilateral ptosis of 1 to 2 mm associated with miosis is usually caused by Horner's syndrome. Ptosis also may be caused by a lesion of the third cranial nerve (accompanied by convergent strabismus and pupillary dilation) or by muscle (such as muscular dystrophy) or neuromuscular junction abnormalities (such as myasthenia gravis—often fluctuating, gradually worsening, unilateral or bilateral ptosis with fatigability and associated diplopia). Other varieties are congenital ptosis, ptosis associated with aging (usually with redundant eyelid[s]), and ptosis associated with other mechanical factors (lid swelling, tumor, or xanthelasma). Erythema or congestion of the lids, conjunctivae, or sclerae may be caused by infection, trauma, allergy, or acute glaucoma.

Unilateral subconjunctival hemorrhage is commonly caused by trauma or rupture of a small conjunctival vessel; bilateral and recurrent subconjunctival hemorrhages may be caused by blood dyscrasias. The corneal reflex is tested by touching the lateral edge of the cornea with a wisp of cotton. The normal response is a bilateral equal and prompt blink and may be diminished or lost as a result of abnormality in the afferent portion of the fifth cranial nerve, the efferent portion of the seventh cranial nerve, or damage to their reflex connections within the pons.

Both **irides** are normally the same color (a lack of melanin pigment within the iris may cause a unilateral blue iris resulting from Horner's syndrome that occurs congenitally or during the first 2 years of life; differences in iris color may also be inherited without Horner's syndrome). Holes on the iris usually indicate atrophy; capillaries on the surface (rubeosis) usually indicate anterior segment ischemia.

Extraocular Muscle Movements

Movement of the eyes is normally smooth, in the same direction, and at the same speed, except for convergence, when both eyes move mediad. Ocular movements are normally tested by having the patient direct gaze to follow the examiner's finger to the extreme right and left in the horizontal plane, upward and downward in the vertical plane, and within a few inches of the face in the midline to test convergence.

Reflex ("doll's eyes") ocular movements are occasionally tested to differentiate supranuclear from nuclear palsies; the patient fixes gaze on a central point straight ahead, and the examiner then moves the patient's head from side to side and up and down. Gaze palsies may result from supratentorial and infratentorial lesions. **Destructive cerebral lesions**, such as cerebral infarcts, often cause conjugate ocular deviations toward the side of the lesion, with the head turned in the direction of deviation, whereas **activating lesions**, such as seizures, cause deviation of the eyes and head away from the lesion. **Destructive cerebral lesions** typically cause a contralateral hemiparesis in which the eyes look **at** the lesion and **away** from the hemiparesis. Lesions in the **brainstem** may also cause lateral gaze palsies. **Destructive lesions** may cause conjugate or dysconjugate ocular deviation, usually away from the side of the lesion. These brainstem lesions are often accompanied by diplopia and also may produce a contralateral hemiparesis. A lateral gaze deviation with a **lesion at a brainstem site** has the eyes looking **away** from the lesion and **at** the hemiparesis. Supratentorial gaze palsies may occur with both frontal and occipital lobe lesions. In **frontal lobe lesions**, voluntary eye movement to command (without following the examiner's finger) away from the side of the lesion is lost; in **occipital lobe lesions**, however, such eye movement to command is spared (Table 5-1).

Table 5-1. Localization of eye movement disorders

Localization of Lesion	Clinical Features
Supranuclear palsies	
Activating lesions in frontal lobe	Jerk-like conjugate deviation of the eyes toward the affected limbs away from the lesion
Destructive lesions in frontal lobe	Conjugate deviation of the eyes toward the side of the lesion away from the hemiparetic limb(s); voluntary eye movement to command away from the side of the lesion is lost
Destructive lesions in occipital lobe	Conjugate deviation of the eyes toward the side of the lesion away from the hemiparetic limb(s); voluntary eye movement to command away from the side of the lesion is spared
Destructive lesions in midbrain, pineal gland tumors	Parinaud's syndrome: loss of voluntary upward and convergence gaze, pupils are sluggish in response to light but constrict briskly to near vision or accommodation, convergence-retraction nystagmus, lid retraction

Table 5-1. *Continued*

Localization of Lesion	Clinical Features
Nuclear palsies	
Destructive lesions in pons	Conjugate or dysconjugate ocular deviation away from the side of the lesion toward the hemiparetic limb(s); diplopia is common
	Skew deviation (the higher eye ipsilateral to the side of the lesion)
Rostral midbrain lesions	Impairment or paralysis of convergence, diplopia for near vision, with absence of any individual extraocular muscle palsy
Lesions of uncertain localization (multiple lesions)	Spasm of the near reflex: convergent strabismus, diplopia, miotic pupils, and spasm accommodation

Vertical gaze palsy that affects downgaze may be caused by infarcts in the territory of the paramedian thalamomesencephalic or posterior cerebral arteries. **Ocular apraxia**, inability to move the eyes voluntarily to command, with a full range of random eye movements, occurs with bilateral prefrontal motor cortex damage. In **internuclear ophthalmoplegia**, weakness of adduction on the side of a lesion of the medial longitudinal fasciculus occurs with monocular, horizontal nystagmus of the abducting eye. Typical causes include various disorders involving the brainstem, such as multiple sclerosis, infarction, trauma, encephalitis, and syringobulbia.

Tectal or pretectal lesions in the midbrain, caused by pineal region tumors, infiltrating gliomas, infarction, hemorrhage, trauma, or multiple sclerosis, may produce **Parinaud's syndrome**. This syndrome is characterized by loss of voluntary upward gaze; light-near reflex dissociation of the pupils (sluggish in response to light but brisk constriction to near gaze or accommodation); and, occasionally, retraction nystagmus, paralysis of convergence, ptosis, papilledema, or third cranial nerve palsy. **Spasm of the near reflex** (convergent strabismus, diplopia, miotic pupils, and spasm of accommodation) is usually caused by encephalitis, tabes dorsalis, meningitis, or functional disturbances. **Skew deviation** (a vertical misalignment of the eyes) usually signifies a structural brainstem lesion with the higher eye ipsilateral to the side of the lesion. **Impairment or paralysis of convergence** (sudden onset of diplopia for near vision, with absence of any individual extraocular muscle palsy) may be caused by rostral midbrain lesions (such as infarction, multiple sclerosis, encephalitis, tabes dorsalis, tumors, Parkinson's disease) or may be functional. Limitation of ocular movements may also result from paresis of the third, fourth, or sixth cranial nerve (see Oculomotor [III], Trochlear [IV], and Abducens [VI] Nerves, page 68).

Nystagmus

Nystagmus is an involuntary, rapid to-and-fro eye movement that may be either pendular in type, with smooth movements, or jerk nystagmus, with a slow drift and quick corrective movement. When classifying nystagmus, one must consider the type of movement (horizontal, vertical, rotatory, or mixed), whether it is pendular or has quick and slow components, the direction of the fast component, whether the nystagmus direction changes with gaze direction, and whether the nystagmus is similar in both eyes. Nystagmus subtypes are classified in Table 5-2.

Pupils

The **pupils** should be inspected for (1) size, (2) shape (they should be approximately equal in size and round), (3) reaction to light (bright light directed into the pupil of one eye normally causes equal and quick constriction of both pupils; the contralateral response is called the consensual response), and (4) accommodation/convergence (the pupils normally constrict equally under the stimuli of accommodation and convergence). Pupillary constriction on near gaze is tested by asking the patient to look first at a distant object and then at a close object.

The pupils may be markedly **constricted** from the effect of narcotics, parasympathomimetic drugs, central nervous system (CNS) syphilis, or pontine disorders such as pontine hemorrhage, in which the reaction to light is difficult to observe but should be present. **Argyll Robertson pupils** caused by CNS syphilis are commonly irregular, eccentric, and small (<3 mm in diameter). They react promptly on convergence and accommodation for near objects but do not contract to light and dilate poorly with mydriatics. This type of light-near dissociation of pupillary response, with greater response to convergence than to light, may also occur in patients with tumors of the midbrain, diabetes mellitus, encephalitis, multiple sclerosis, CNS degenerative disease, meningitis, and chronic alcoholism. The pupils may be relatively fixed and equally **dilated** as a result of diffuse cerebral swelling or sympathomimetic or anticholinergic drugs (epinephrine, ephedrine, amphetamine, cocaine, atropine, homatropine, scopolamine, pilocarpine, acetylcholine).

Adie's pupil is typically a unilaterally dilated pupil that has slow reaction to light and that may respond to accommodation. This is a benign condition that usually affects young women and may be related to dysfunction of the ciliary ganglion or postganglionic neuron. The pupil characteristically promptly constricts with administration of low-dose pilocarpine. When the pupil is completely unreactive to both light and accommodation, with depressed or absent deep tendon reflexes, the condition is called **Holmes-Adie syndrome**.

Nonreactive pupils 3 to 5 mm in diameter may accompany a midbrain lesion. A unilaterally dilated, fixed, and unreactive pupil may be a sign of third cranial nerve compression caused by temporal lobe herniation. **Unequal pupils (anisocoria)** may be a normal finding, especially when associated with a normal reaction to light. However, if one or both pupils do not react well to light, then a pathologic process is strongly suggested. For example, pathologic anisocoria may result from third cranial nerve

Table 5-2.   Classification of nystagmus

Subtype	Characteristic
Voluntary or functional	Horizontal, rapid movements, nonsustained
End position	Nonsustained, at end of horizontal gaze; normal; not noted with vertical gaze
Retinal disease	Conjugate and horizontal, persisting throughout life, caused by congenital macular defect or albinism
Congenital defects	Conjugate, horizontal jerk; occurs from birth, often with impairment of vision or strabismus
Labyrinthine disease (Ménière's disease labyrinthitis, vascular lesions of vestibular apparatus or vestibular nerve)	Jerk nystagmus, fast component toward lesion in all directions gaze; generally has rotatory component
Cerebellar-brainstem (vascular disease, multiple sclerosis, tumor, alcohol intoxication, Wernicke's encephalopathy, phenytoin toxicity)	Multidirectional nystagmus with fast component in direction of gaze; other nuclear or tract involvement; may be pendular, jerky horizontal, or vertical nystagmus in brainstem lesions
Retraction nystagmus (midbrain tectum, pretectal lesions, pineal lesions)	Best seen with optokinetic testing in downgoing direction; convergence and retraction movements, especially with convergence or upgaze
Downbeating (cervicomedullary junction)	Fast component downbeating nystagmus in primary or lateral gaze
Upbeating (medulla, cerebellum)	Fast component upbeating nystagmus in primary or lateral gaze
Cyclic rotatory or seesaw (lesions in region of optic chiasm and diencephalon)	Regular reciprocating oscillations in which one eye rises and the other falls; bitemporal hemianopia may be associated
Dissociated nystagmus (posterior fossa disease)	Direction of nystagmus differs when eyes are compared
Periodic alternating (cerebellum)	Primary gaze nystagmus with 60- to 120-s episodes of jerk nystagmus, then brief period with no nystagmus, followed by similar episode of nystagmus in contralateral direction

involvement at the level of the midbrain (infarction, basilar aneurysm, demyelination, tumor), interpeduncular cistern (aneurysm of the posterior communicating or basilar artery, transtentorial herniation, basal meningitis, oculomotor nerve trunk infarction.), cavernous sinus (intracavernous aneurysm, cavernous sinus thrombosis, pituitary adenoma, meningioma, metastasis, nasopharyngeal carcinoma), or orbit or orbital fissure (tumor, periostitis, sphenocavernous lesion).

Horner's syndrome, with unilateral miosis, ptosis, lower eyelid elevation, and loss of sweating on the same side of the face, may result from an ipsilateral lesion that causes sympathetic nervous system damage at various levels: **hypothalamus** (tumor, vascular lesion), **brainstem** (tumor, vascular lesion, syringobulbia), **middle fossa** (tumor, granuloma), **carotid artery in the neck** (dissection, occlusion, aneurysm, trauma), **cervical sympathetic chain** (enlarged cervical lymph node, goiter, aneurysm of the subclavian artery, carcinoma of the lung apex, apical tuberculosis, or mediastinal tumor), **anterior C-8, T-1, T-2,** or **T-3 roots** (neurofibroma, lower brachial plexus palsy, Pancoast tumor), or **other cervical lesions** (vertebral fractures, tabes dorsalis, syringomyelia, tumor).

Visual Acuity

Visual acuity is usually tested for each eye separately at a near point (approximately 14 cm) with a handheld card (patients who wear glasses for reading should wear them during the test). To overcome hypermetropia or myopia refractory errors without glasses, the patient may look at the card through a pinhole to restrict vision to the central beam of light, which is undisturbed by abnormal ocular distances or transparent media. Once refractory defects have been excluded, **acute impairment of visual acuity** in one eye usually suggests a vascular lesion such as acute occlusion of the ophthalmic or central retinal artery, a lesion that affects the macular region of the retina (for instance, a hemorrhage in the macular area), or ischemic optic neuropathy. **Gradual impairment of vision** may be caused by optic atrophy that results from compression, toxins, ischemia, neuritis, retinitis pigmentosa, macular degeneration, choroiditis, diabetic retinopathy, or retinoblastoma (Table 5-3). Unilateral lesions of the optic tract, lateral geniculate body, optic radiation, or striate cortex usually do not impair optic acuity, but bilateral occipital cortex lesions can cause complete blindness.

Visual Fields

Visual fields are assessed clinically to detect areas of partial or complete loss of vision by confrontation testing. The examiner covers one of the patient's eyes at a time. The examiner then holds up one or two fingers in the six primary visual quadrants, and the patient identifies whether the examiner is holding up one or two fingers while looking straight ahead at the examiner's nose. Alternatively, the examiner may move his or her finger or, for a more precise determination, move a red 5-mm pin from the extreme periphery toward the center. The patient reports when he or she first sees the object while looking straight ahead

Table 5-3.   Causes of unilateral visual loss

Acute Unilateral Visual Loss	Subacute or Chronic Unilateral Visual Loss
Central retinal artery occlusion (embolism, vasospasm, hypercoagulable state, vasculitis)	Primary optic atrophy caused by: Compression resulting from orbital lesions (tumor, granuloma); lesions within optic canal (meningioma, granuloma, hyperostosis); intracranial lesions (aneurysms of internal carotid, anterior cerebral, or anterior communicating artery, prechiasmal neoplasms, e.g., meningioma of sphenoid wing or olfactory groove, granuloma, optic nerve glioma, craniopharyngioma, neoplasm of frontal lobe or pituitary, osteosarcoma, prechiasmal arachnoiditis, third ventricle dilation). Central scotoma is common early in the course of the compression.
Papillitis (retrobulbar neuritis)	
Retinal detachment (traumatic or spontaneous)	
Optic nerve trauma	

Toxins (alcohol or tobacco amblyopia).
Centrocecal scotoma is common.
Ischemia (often associated with diabetes
mellitus, hypertension, glaucoma, or
vasculitis, e.g., temporal arteritis, or
syphilis)
Optic neuritis (viral, parasitic, fungal,
postinoculation syphilis, polyneuritis,
bacterial or tuberculous meningitis)
Metabolic (Addison's disease, uremia,
pernicious anemia, hyperthyroidism,
toxemia)
Degenerative (multiple sclerosis, vitamin
deficiency or starvation, Paget's disease of bone, Hand-Schüller-Christian
disease, Tay-Sachs disease, Niemann-
Pick disease, Laurence-Moon-Biedl
syndrome, fibrous dysplasia)
Congenital/hereditary (Leber's
hereditary optic atrophy, oxycephaly)
Secondary optic atrophy after
papilledema (enlarged blind spot is
common with or without contraction
of the fields)
Retinitis pigmentosa
Glaucoma or choroiditis (toxoplasmosis,
cytomegalovirus infection). Arcuate
scotoma is common.
Diabetic or hypertensive retinopathy
Malignant melanoma, macular
degeneration
Cataract

at the examiner's nose. Repeated testing from multiple directions provides a record of affected or spared visual fields.

For detection of **visual neglect** (in which the patient ignores one half the visual field), both eyes are uncovered, and the patient looks at the examiner's nose. The examiner then asks the patient to identify which finger(s) is wiggling while wiggling fingers in one of the primary peripheral quadrants, either unilaterally or bilaterally. Patients with neglect often ignore fingers to one side when the examiner is wiggling fingers simultaneously on each side. In addition, the patient with left visual neglect, when drawing a clock face, will write all of the numbers on the right-hand side of the clock or, when trying to mark the center of a line, will place the mark far to the right of the real midpoint of the line.

Monocular visual field defects are usually caused by retinal or optic nerve lesions; binocular defects usually reflect a lesion localized at or behind the optic chiasm. The precise determination of visual field defects has an important role in the localization of vascular lesions. Some of the most common variants of visual-spatial disorders are depicted in Figure 2-1. **Central scotoma** may result from retrobulbar neuritis (sometimes as the first sign of multiple sclerosis) or optic nerve compression (anterior communicating artery aneurysm, meningioma, granuloma, or hyperostosis of the optic canal from Paget's disease). **Cecocentral scotoma** is characteristic of toxic (alcohol, tobacco) amblyopia. An **arcuate scotoma** often reflects underlying glaucoma, and a **junctional scotoma** indicates the presence of an optic nerve lesion immediately anterior to the optic chiasm.

Bitemporal hemianopia with involvement of the upper quadrants first indicates compression of the optic chiasm from below by lesions such as a pituitary adenoma, nasopharyngeal carcinoma, or sphenoid sinus mucocele; involvement of the lower quadrants first indicates compression of the optic chiasm from above, such as a craniopharyngioma or third ventricular tumor. **Homonymous hemianopia** may have sudden onset, typically of vascular cause, or gradual onset, caused by neoplastic, infectious, or inflammatory conditions. Lesions may involve the contralateral geniculate body (homonymous defect in the upper and lower quadrants with sparing of a horizontal sector), optic radiations, or occipital lobe. **Inferior quadrantanopia** is more often caused by lesions of the optic radiations deep in the parietal lobe or cuneus of the occipital lobe; **superior quadrantanopia** arises from lesions involving the temporal loop of the optic radiations or inferior bank of the calcarine fissure.

Bilateral homonymous hemianopia results in complete visual loss (**cortical blindness**) with or without sparing of a small central visual field (macular sparing) and the pupillary response. In **Anton's syndrome**, the patient denies the visual defect and confabulates about what is being seen because of bilateral visual association cortex damage that results from occlusion of either the basilar or both posterior cerebral arteries.

Ophthalmoscopy

Use of ophthalmoscopy is important in evaluating patients with suspected cerebrovascular disease. The normal optic disc is a yellowish red, round or oval, platelike structure; is typically flat with a white central depression (physiologic cup); and has an average diameter approximately one third the disc diameter. Margins are clearly defined, although the nasal edge is often slightly less distinct than the temporal edge. The arterioles of the retina diverge from and the veins converge toward the disc; in 80% of normal patients, venous pulsations may be seen, an indication that the intracranial pressure is <200 mm Hg.

The ophthalmoscopic examination may help to define the underlying mechanism through direct visualization of parenchymal and vascular retinal changes. Ophthalmoscopy allows detection of diabetic, ischemic, or hypertensive retinopathy; retinal hemorrhage; and various types of emboli. The arteriolar and venous caliber and appearance should be examined. Disappearance of spontaneous venous pulsations may be the earliest sign of venous congestion, which may be associated with increased intracranial pressure. The retina should be inspected for microaneurysms, papilledema, papillitis, optic atrophy or disc pallor, areas of exudates, abnormal pigmentation, and subhyaloid hemorrhages.

Retinal emboli may be associated with central retinal artery or branch occlusion. The three most common types of retinal emboli are cholesterol, fibrin-platelet, and calcium emboli. **Cholesterol emboli** are composed of cholesterol crystals that generally originate from an ulcerated atheromatous intimal lesion of the ipsilateral internal carotid artery and appear as shiny orange-yellow lesions, and they are often situated at the bifurcation of retinal arterioles. **Fibrin-platelet emboli** are grayish white lesions that usually are indicative of an underlying atheromatous lesion of the ipsilateral carotid system, and they tend to cause arteriolar occlusions much more commonly than do cholesterol emboli. **Calcium emboli** are less common and consist of white particles of calcium that generally originate from calcific aortic stenosis. Septic, talc, polytef (Teflon), cornstarch, and some other emboli may also be seen in the retina but are very uncommon.

Atherosclerosis may manifest ophthalmoscopically in the retinal arterial walls. **Hypertension** may be associated with various changes, including retinal arteriolar narrowing, sclerosis, or even occlusion. Hypertensive retinopathy usually involves retinal edema, cotton-wool patches, hemorrhages, and papilledema. In addition to hypertension, retinal hemorrhages and exudates maybe caused by other systemic disorders, such as diabetes mellitus, systemic lupus erythematosus, and blood dyscrasias. Retinal changes associated with **diabetes mellitus** may be similar to the changes associated with hypertension, but microaneurysms, dilated veins, and neurovascularization are often present.

Other ophthalmoscopic findings ipsilateral to carotid occlusive lesions include venous stasis (low-flow) retinopathy and asymmetric (lesser) hypertensive arteriolar changes. Venous stasis (low-flow) retinopathy resembles diabetic retinopathy but tends to be located more peripherally (microaneurysm formation, venous engorgement, retinal hemorrhages, neovascularization) and may be associated with secondary glaucoma.

In **papillitis** caused by passive congestion, the disc becomes abnormally vascular (hyperemic) and slightly elevated (edema), and small hemorrhages may be seen (cecocentral scotoma may be present). In **retrobulbar** neuritis, however, because of the location of the inflammatory lesion in the posterior portion of the optic nerve, the disc is not swollen. Papillitis is typically unilateral, and the disc seems similar to that seen in papilledema. Visual acuity is usually severely affected early, in comparison with papilledema, which may be associated with more chronic changes in visual acuity.

Papilledema is indicative of increased intracranial pressure and in its early stage is characterized by hyperemia of the rim of the disc. Later, the vessels on the surface of the disc are engorged, and disc swelling, hemorrhages, and nerve fiber infarctions (cotton-wool spots) may occur. In massive papilledema, large areas of the nerve fiber layer may become infarcted. Development of papilledema within 12 to 24 hours of a neurologic event frequently indicates increased intracranial pressure from intracranial mass lesions, such as brain trauma or hemorrhage; pronounced papilledema at the onset of symptoms usually indicates lesions of longer duration, such as brain tumor or abscess.

Subhyaloid hemorrhage is a preretinal hemorrhage that is commonly associated with intracranial hemorrhage, particularly aneurysmal subarachnoid hemorrhage, but may be seen with severe brain trauma or any condition that produces suddenly increased intracranial pressure.

In **anterior ischemic optic neuropathy**, altitudinal or segmental disc swelling, hyperemia, disc margin hemorrhages, and other signs of disc infarction are often noted after the sudden or subacute onset of an altitudinal or segmental visual field loss. Potential causes include diabetes mellitus, hypertension, inflammatory vasculitis, hypercoagulable state, and unknown cause (idiopathic). **Occlusion of the central retinal vein** often produces extensive hemorrhage in the region of the optic disc, disc swelling, dilated veins, and partial visual loss. **Central retinal artery occlusion** causes sudden visual field loss associated with a pale disc and retina. Weeks to months later, the disc whitens as a result of optic atrophy.

Special Ophthalmic Examinations

Special examinations include **perimetry** to assess the peripheral and central visual fields with manual or automated methods; **ophthalmodynamometry** to measure relative pressures in the central retinal arteries, used as an indirect means of assessing the pressure of the carotid arterial system (see Chapter 7, Ophthalmodynamometry); **Schiötz tonometry** to measure intraocular pressure, in which a pressure of 20 mm Hg or more is considered above average and most often reflects underlying glaucoma; and **fluorescein angiography** to detail the choroidal and retinal vasculature.

CRANIAL NERVES

Cranial nerve functions, symptoms of cranial nerve deficits, and some of the syndromes that affect the cranial nerves are reviewed in Tables 5-4 and 5-5.

Olfactory Nerve (I)

The olfactory nerve is seldom damaged in cerebrovascular disease but may be affected by large intracranial aneurysms. Each of the patient's nostrils should be tested individually with an

Table 5-4.   Location and general function of the cranial nerves and major signs and symptoms of impaired function

Cranial Nerve	Major Anatomic Structures and Relationships	General Function	Major Signs and Symptoms of Impaired Function
Olfactory (I)	Orbital surfaces of the frontal lobe (olfactory nerve, bulb, tract, lateral olfactory gyrus, amygdaloid nucleus, septal nuclei, hypothalamus)	Smell	Anosmia; parosmia, cacosmia
Optic (II)	Retina, optic nerve, optic chiasm, optic tract, lateral geniculate bodies, optic radiation, visual cortex of occipital lobe	Vision	Impaired visual acuity and visual fields (scotoma)
Oculomotor (III)	Midbrain (nucleus or fascicular portion), subarachnoid space, cavernous sinus, superior orbital fissure, orbit	Eye movement (levator palpebrae muscle), pupillary constriction	Downward and outward deviation of affected eye, horizontal and vertical diplopia, ptosis, pupil dilatation
Trochlear (IV)	Dorsal midbrain (nucleus and fascicles), undersurface of tentorial edge, cavernous sinus, superior orbital fissure, orbit	Eye movement (superior oblique muscle)	Vertical diplopia with tilt greatest on downward gaze to the side opposite the lesion. Corrects with tilting head toward the lesion
Trigeminal (V)	Pons (motor portion), semilunar ganglion in middle cranial fossa (sensory portion), brainstem nuclei, gasserian ganglion (ophthalmic, maxillary, mandibular divisions)	Facial sensation, jaw movement	Trigeminal neuralgia or ipsilateral dissociated (nucleus) or total (nerve roots or ganglion) hemianesthesia of face; weakness, atrophy of masticatory muscles; loss of corneal reflex

Nerve	Location	Function	Clinical findings
Abducens (VI)	Lower pons, sulcus between pons and medulla, prepontine cistern, cavernous sinus, superior orbital fissure, orbit	Eye movement (lateral rectus muscle)	Inward deviation of affected eye; ipsilateral gaze palsy with horizontal diplopia worse when looking toward paralyzed side
Facial (VII)	Caudal pons, cerebellopontine angle, internal auditory meatus, facial canal in petrous bone, tympanic and mastoid segments	Facial movement; taste on anterior two thirds of tongue	Peripheral type of facial nerve palsy (Bell's palsy) with or without ipsilateral loss of taste on anterior two thirds of tongue; impairment of lacrimation, salivation, and hyperacusis
Vestibulocochlear (VIII)	Pons, upper medulla, internal auditory meatus, vestibular and cochlear nerves, cochlea (organ of Corti), ampullae and semicircular canals, utricle, saccule	Hearing and balance	Sensorineural deafness or vertigo, nausea or vomiting, horizontal or rotatory nystagmus
Glossopharyngeal (IX)	Medulla, jugular foramen, cerebellopontine angle, space between internal carotid artery and internal jugular vein, pharynx, base of tongue	Palatal and pharyngeal movement, taste to posterior one third of tongue	Mild dysphagia, homolateral loss of taste over posterior one third of tongue, depressed pharyngeal or gag reflex
Vagus (X)	Medulla; jugular foramen; auricular, meningeal, pharyngeal, and cardiac rami; recurrent laryngeal nerve	Palatal, pharyngeal, and laryngeal movement; control of visceral organs	Ipsilateral palatal, pharyngeal, and laryngeal paresis (dysphagia and dysphonia) associated with unilateral laryngeal anesthesia and depressed gag reflex

(Continued)

Table 5-4. *Continued*

Cranial Nerve	Major Anatomic Structures and Relationships	General Function	Major Signs and Symptoms of Impaired Function
Spinal accessory (XI)	Medulla (cranial part), spinal cord (spinal part), foramen magnum, jugular foramen	Sternocleidomastoid, trapezius muscles	Paresis and atrophy of sternocleido-mastoid and trapezius muscles
Hypoglossal (XII)	Medulla (hypoglossal trigone of floor of fourth ventricle), medullary-pontine junction, hypoglossal canal	Tongue movement	Ipsilateral paresis and atrophy with or without fasciculations in one half of tongue: dysarthria

Table 5-5.   Syndromes involving cranial nerves

Eponym (Syndrome)	Structures Involved	Symptoms/Signs	Usual Cause
Foster Kennedy	Frontal lobe, olfactory (I) nerve	Ipsilateral anosmia, optic atrophy with contralateral papilledema	Tumors, saccular aneurysms of anterior portion of circle of Willis
Claude	Tegmentum of midbrain, oculomotor (III) nerve nucleus and red nucleus, brachium conjunctivum	Oculomotor palsy, horizontal diplopia with contralateral ataxia and cerebellar tremor	Infarction, hemorrhage, basilar aneurysm compression, tumor
Benedikt	Tegmentum of midbrain, subthalamic region, corticospinal tract, oculomotor (III) nerve nucleus, red nucleus, brachium conjunctivum	Oculomotor palsy with contralateral ataxia, cerebellar tremor, corticospinal signs	Infarction, hemorrhage, basilar aneurysm compression, tumor
Nothnagel	Tectum of midbrain (brachium conjunctivum below the decussation), oculomotor (III) nerve	Oculomotor palsy with ipsilateral cerebellar disturbance	infarction, hemorrhage, basilar aneurysm compression, tumor
Weber	Tectum of midbrain and cerebral peduncle, oculomotor (III) nerve	Oculomotor palsy with contralateral hemiparesis	Infarction, hemorrhage, basilar aneurysm compression, tumor
Parinaud	Dorsal midbrain (periaqueductal gray matter)	Paralysis of upward gaze and accommodation; light-near dissociation, retraction nystagmus	Tumor, hydrocephalus, infarction, hemorrhage
Millard-Gubler	Base of pons, abducens (VI) and facial (VII) nerves	Facial and abducens palsy with contralateral hemiplegia	Infarction, tumor

(Continued)

Table 5-5. *Continued*

Eponym (Syndrome)	Structures Involved	Symptoms/Signs	Usual Cause
Foville	Base of pons, nerve VII	Facial and conjugate gaze palsies, contralateral hemiplegia	Infarction, tumor
Gradenigo	Ophthalmic division of trigeminal (V) and abducens (VI) nerves	Retro-orbital pain, palsy of nerve VI, deafness, excessive lacrimation	Inflammation at level of petrous apex, infection; tumor, trauma, aneurysm
Raeder	Ophthalmic division of nerve V (sometimes IV, VI)	Miosis and ptosis (no facial anhidrosis), facial or retro-orbital pain	Tumor at level of petrous apex, infection, trauma, aneurysm
Tolosa-Hunt	Cranial nerves III, IV, V, VI	Retro-orbital pain with multiple ophthalmoplegia	Inflammation in cavernous sinus
Wallenberg	Lateral tegmentum of medulla, spinal nerves V, IX, X, XI	Dysphagia, dysarthria, gait and limb ataxia, ipsilateral dissociated hemianesthesia of face, contralateral hemisensory loss in limbs and trunk, Horner's syndrome	Occlusion of ipsilateral vertebral artery or posterior inferior cerebellar artery
Vernet	Glossopharyngeal (IX) and vagus (X) nerve roots	Dysphagia, dysphonia, depressed gag reflex, homolateral vocal cord paralysis, loss of taste or pain on posterior one third of tongue, soft palate with ipsilateral paresis of nerve XI	Tumors, aneurysms, abscess, basal skull fracture at jugular foramen

Collet-Sicard	Cranial nerves IX, X, XI, XII	Unilateral paralysis of trapezius, sternocleidomastoid muscles, vocal cord, half of tongue, loss of taste on posterior one third of tongue, hemianesthesia of palate, pharynx, and larynx	Tumors of parotid gland, carotid body, secondary and lymph node tumors, tuberculous adenitis
Villaret	Cranial nerves IX, X, XI, XII; sometimes sympathetic chain; sometimes cranial nerve VII	Same as for Collet-Sicard syndrome, ipsilateral Horner's syndrome, sometimes facial nerve palsy	Same as for Collet-Sicard syndrome at retroparotid or retropharyngeal space
Schmidt	Cranial nerves X, XI	Paralysis of vocal cord (cranial nerve X) and sternocleidomastoid muscle (cranial nerve XI)	Tumor, aneurysm, abscess (before nerve fibers leave skull)
Jackson	Cranial nerves X, XI, XII	Same as for Schmidt's syndrome, hemiparalysis of tongue (cranial nerve XII)	Same as for Schmidt's syndrome, perhaps intraparenchymal

aromatic material such as camphor or wintergreen. An impaired sense of smell is most commonly associated with rhinitis, head injury, heavy cigarette smoking, or nasal obstruction but sometimes may be caused by space-occupying lesions of the frontal lobe (tumors of the sphenoid or frontal bone, meningiomas, pituitary tumors, and saccular aneurysms of the anterior portion of the circle of Willis), producing the so-called **Foster Kennedy syndrome** characterized by ipsilateral anosmia and optic atrophy with contralateral papilledema (Table 5-5).

Optic Nerve (II)

The optic nerve is tested by measuring visual acuity, color vision, and peripheral vision (visual fields) and by inspecting the retina and the optic disc with an ophthalmoscope.

Oculomotor (III), Trochlear (IV), and Abducens (VI) Nerves

The oculomotor, trochlear, and abducens nerves subserve ocular movements (III, IV, and VI), lid elevation (III), and pupillary constriction (III). To evaluate the function of these nerves, the physician should assess each of the patient's eyes separately for the completeness of ocular movements, lid retraction, the presence of ptosis, pupillary abnormalities, abnormal spontaneous eye movements, and abnormal convergence.

An **oculomotor nerve (III) palsy** (Fig. 5-3) results in lateral deviation (divergent strabismus) of the affected eye in association with absence or limitation of convergence, horizontal and vertical diplopia, ipsilateral ptosis, and pupillary dilation caused by lesions in the midbrain, interpeduncular cistern, cavernous sinus, or orbit.

Lesions in the **midbrain,** which may result from infarction, hemorrhage, basilar aneurysm, demyelination, or tumor, may produce the syndromes outlined in Table 5-5.

Lesions in the **interpeduncular cistern** include aneurysmal compression of the posterior communicating or basilar arteries (oculomotor paresis may be incomplete) and basal meningitis. More distally, the third cranial nerve rests on the tentorial edge and may be compressed by uncal herniation. The dilated and fixed pupil may be affected before the extraocular muscle function in this type of compressive syndrome because the pupillomotor fibers travel predominantly in the outer portions of the nerve. Nerve trunk infarction may occur anywhere along its course as a result of hypertension, diabetes mellitus, or inflammatory arteriopathy; the pupil typically is spared.

In the **cavernous sinus,** lesions that affect the third cranial nerve may also affect the fourth, fifth, and sixth cranial nerves, the optic nerve, and oculosympathetic fibers as a result of intracavernous aneurysm, cavernous sinus thrombosis, pituitary adenoma, meningioma, metastasis, and nasopharyngeal carcinoma. The combination of third cranial nerve paresis and small, poorly reactive pupils is highly suggestive of a cavernous sinus lesion. Lesions in the **orbit or orbital fissure** include tumor, periostitis, or sphenocavernous lesion associated with fourth, fifth, and sixth cranial nerve dysfunction.

Trochlear (IV) and abducens (VI) nerve palsies result in mild convergent strabismus associated with limited movement of the affected eye to the paralyzed side, vertical diplopia when

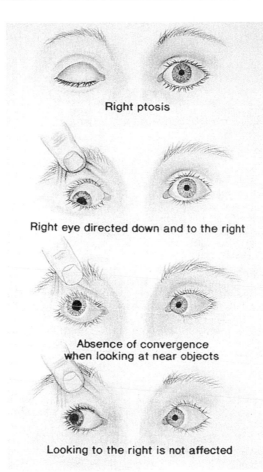

Right ptosis

Right eye directed down and to the right

Absence of convergence
when looking at near objects

Looking to the right is not affected

Figure 5-3.   **Right oculomotor (III) nerve dysfunction.**

the person looks downward (**fourth nerve palsy**) (Fig. 5-4), and horizontal diplopia when the person looks toward the side of the lesion (**sixth nerve palsy**) (Fig. 5-5). The palsies may be caused by the same lesions that cause palsy of the third cranial nerve. However, lesions of the fourth cranial nerve in the midbrain are usually associated with other midbrain syndromes, such as hemiparesis and hemisensory loss, predominantly involving the leg. Nuclear or intramedullary lesions of the sixth cranial nerve are usually associated with ipsilateral gaze palsy to the same side, contralateral hemiparesis, hemisensory loss, and ipsilateral lower motor neuron facial weakness; upper and lower face weakness is caused by palsy of the seventh cranial nerve. Pontine lesions, typically of vascular origin, may produce various syndromes, as outlined in Table 5-5.

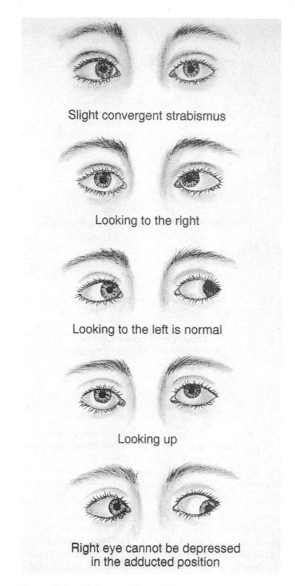

Slight convergent strabismus

Looking to the right

Looking to the left is normal

Looking up

Right eye cannot be depressed
in the adducted position

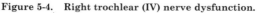

Figure 5-4.   Right trochlear (IV) nerve dysfunction.

Trigeminal Nerve (V)

The trigeminal nerve may be damaged by many conditions, including cerebrovascular disorders (supranuclear or nuclear infarct or hemorrhage, basilar aneurysm), tumor, infection, and trauma. The sensory portion of the trigeminal nerve is evaluated

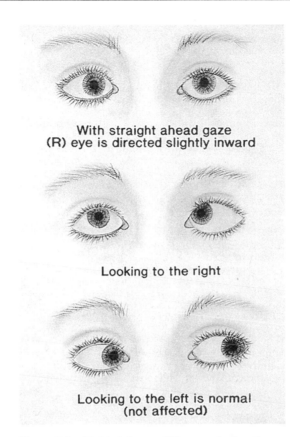

With straight ahead gaze (R) eye is directed slightly inward

Looking to the right

Looking to the left is normal (not affected)

Figure 5-5.   Right abducens (VI) nerve dysfunction.

by testing pain, temperature, and light touch sensation (including corneal reflex) over the whole face. The motor portion of the fifth cranial nerve is tested by having the patient clench the jaw and move the jaw from side to side against resistance and by checking the jaw jerk.

Unilateral **supranuclear lesions** (such as a thalamic lesion) may result in anesthesia of the contralateral face; bilateral supranuclear lesions produce an exaggerated jaw reflex. **Nuclear lesions that affect the dorsal mid pons** may produce ipsilateral trigeminal paresis; atrophy; and fasciculations of the muscles of mastication with associated contralateral hemiplegia, ipsilateral dissociated (loss of pain or temperature sensation, touch retained) hemianesthesia of the face, contralateral hemisensory loss of the limbs and trunk, and ipsilateral tremor.

Lesions that affect the spinal tract of the fifth cranial nerve include brainstem infarction, syringobulbia, demyelination, and tumor. The best known vascular syndrome that affects this tract is the **lateral medullary (Wallenberg) syndrome**, caused by a posterior-inferior cerebellar artery infarct and most often a result of occlusion of the ipsilateral vertebral artery; symptoms include dysphagia, dysarthria, gait unsteadiness, ipsilateral limb ataxia, vertigo, and hoarseness. Examination shows ipsilateral Horner's syndrome, ipsilateral dissociated hemianesthesia of the face, contralateral hemianesthesia in the limbs and trunk, gait ataxia, and ipsilateral limb ataxia.

Trigeminal nerve lesions may result from various pathologic processes, such as tumor, acute infection, chronic meningitis, trauma, or aneurysm located in the **preganglionic cisternal course** of the nerve, at the cerebellopontine angle, and in the petrous apex, orbital fissure, and cavernous sinus. Some syndromes that affect the trigeminal nerve are reviewed in Table 5-5.

Facial Nerve (VII)

Evaluation of facial nerve function begins with watching the patient talk and smile. The physician should be alert for asymmetric eye closure, elevation of one corner of the mouth, and flattening of the nasolabial fold. The patient is instructed to wrinkle the forehead, close the eyes while the physician attempts to open them, purse the lips while the physician presses the cheeks, and show the teeth (Fig. 5-6). Corneal reflexes should be tested and any asymmetries noted. Facial nerve palsies may be caused by vascular, neoplastic, demyelinating, or infectious processes at different anatomic levels. Vascular damage to the seventh cranial nerve usually occurs at supranuclear, pontine (infarction, hemorrhage), and, rarely, cerebellopontine angle (aneurysm) levels (Fig. 5-6, Table 5-5).

Vestibulocochlear Nerve (VIII)

Hearing function is tested in several ways, such as tone audiometry, speech threshold testing, and impedance measures. **Pure tone audiometry** measures hearing sensitivity as a function of frequency and can be tested either by air conduction through earphones or by bone conduction through a tuning fork on the skull. Bone conduction tests include the **Weber test**, in which a vibrating tuning fork is placed over the midline of the skull; normally, hearing is equal in both ears without lateralization. In the **Rinne test**, the vibration of the tuning fork is applied to the mastoid bone until vibration disappears; the tuning fork then is placed next to the ear, 1 inch from the external auditory meatus. The test is normal when the vibrations are still perceived in the ear. In **conductive deafness**, bone conduction is better than air conduction; thus, the Weber test lateralizes to the affected ear, and the Rinne test is abnormal. In **nerve deafness**, both bone and air conduction are impaired, but air conduction remains greater than bone conduction; thus, the Weber test lateralizes to the normal ear, and the Rinne test is normal. Beyond these neurologic examination techniques, other special studies, such as speech discrimination tests and impedance measures made with a tympanogram and acoustic reflex, may be performed.

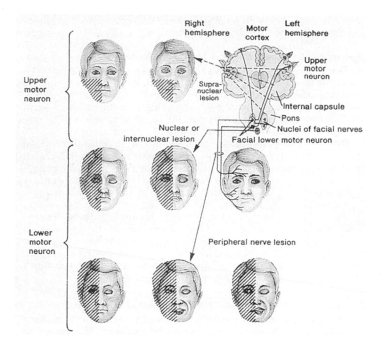

Figure 5-6. Facial paralysis—upper and lower motor neuron.

The **vestibular component** of eighth cranial nerve function may be evaluated with the **Romberg test.** The patient, standing with eyes closed and feet together, will fall or veer to the side that has vestibular dysfunction.

Vascular causes of central vestibular dysfunction include vertebrobasilar ischemia or infarction with symptoms of vertigo or dizziness, typically associated with other brainstem signs such as diplopia, dysarthria, ataxia, unilateral or bilateral homonymous hemianopia, alternating unilateral or bilateral sensory or motor deficits, **labyrinthine ischemic stroke** (caused by occlusion of the internal auditory artery and resulting in vertigo, tinnitus or deafness, and nausea or vomiting), and **Wallenberg's syndrome.** Other causes are **cerebellar infarction or hemorrhage** with associated nystagmus; truncal and limb ataxia; and intention tremor and **basilar migraine**, which frequently affects young women and is characterized by occipital throbbing headache, bilateral visual symptoms, unsteadiness, dysarthria, vertigo, and limb paresthesia, with or without loss of consciousness. **Subclavian steal syndrome** is caused by stenosis of the proximal subclavian artery and results in retrograde flow down the vertebral artery with arm exercise and a clinical picture of vertebrobasilar insufficiency, such as vertigo or nystagmus, facial or extremity numbness, double vision, unsteadiness, weakness, and diminution of pulse and blood pressure in the affected arm.

Glossopharyngeal (IX) and Vagus (X) Nerves

The glossopharyngeal and vagus nerves should be examined together because their functions (speaking, swallowing, palatal movements, and gag reflex) are seldom individually impaired. When the palate is examined, the middle of the palate should rise in the midline when the patient is asked to say "ah." If one side is weak, the midline deviates to the intact side.

Bilateral supranuclear lesions, often of vascular origin because of bilateral infarction, result in pseudobulbar palsy with severe dysphagia, dysarthria, spastic tongue, depressed or exaggerated gag reflex, and emotional lability. **Nuclear or intramedullary lesions** that are caused by vascular disease, syringobulbia, demyelinating disease, or tumor commonly involve other brainstem structures. **Extramedullary lesions that affect these nerves** include tumor, aneurysm, and abscess and may cause a **cerebellopontine angle syndrome** of dysphagia, dysphonia, depressed gag reflex, tinnitus, deafness, vertigo, and facial sensory loss. Other syndromes that affect the ninth and 10th cranial nerves are reviewed in Table 5-5.

Spinal Accessory (XI) and Hypoglossal (XII) Nerves

The spinal accessory nerve innervates the sternocleidomastoid and trapezius muscles, which are tested by asking the patient to rotate the head against resistance and to shrug the shoulders against resistance. To examine the hypoglossal nerve, the physician asks the patient to open the mouth and protrude the tongue. When the hypoglossal nerve or nucleus is involved, the protruded tongue deviates toward the side of the lesion. The side of involvement also may show atrophy and fasciculations.

Supranuclear lesions (such as cerebral infarction at the level of the internal capsule) usually do not cause weakness of the tongue. However, upper motor neuron lesions that affect corticobulbar fibers that go to the hypoglossal nucleus typically lead to slowing of tongue movements and may cause contralateral weakness of half of the tongue, resulting in tongue deviation toward the side of the hemiplegia. **Nuclear lesions** (syringomyelia, intraparenchymal tumor, demyelinating disease, vascular insult) of the spinal accessory nerve are unusual but may result in paresis of the trapezius and sternocleidomastoid muscles with atrophy and fasciculations. Nuclear or intramedullary lesions of the hypoglossal nerve may result in **Dejerine's anterior bulbar syndrome** (ipsilateral paresis, atrophy, and fibrillations of the tongue associated with contralateral hemiplegia with facial sparing, contralateral loss of position, tactile and vibratory sensations on the trunk and limbs, and sparing of pain and temperature sensation).

Peripheral lesions of the 11th and 12th cranial nerves may be caused by trauma, carotid aneurysms, local infections, or neck surgery (complications may result in **floppy head syndrome** [isolated palsy of the 11th cranial nerve, weakness of neck extension against gravity]), or they may be associated with one of the syndromes reviewed in Table 5-5.

MOTOR SYSTEM

Muscle bulk, muscle tone, muscle power, and reflexes should be examined in each limb. **Muscle wasting** may indicate lower motor neuron disease, **hypertrophy** may suggest some form of myopathy, and prominent **fasciculations or fibrillations** may indicate anterior horn cell disease or nerve root damage. A **decrease in muscle tone** may indicate lower motor neuron disease, and **hypertonicity or spasticity** manifested by the "clasp-knife" phenomenon (initial resistance to passive movement is precipitously overcome) may indicate an upper motor neuron lesion. "Cogwheel" or "lead-pipe" ratchet-like **rigidity** involves a steady increase in resistance throughout the movement and may indicate an extrapyramidal lesion.

Severe weakness or plegia of the limbs is usually easily recognized. Individual muscle testing typically is necessary to detect mild weakness. Examination of alternating motion rates in the patient's fingers, hands, and feet also may clarify more subtle degrees of weakness. The presence of pronator drift also may indicate a subtle pyramidal tract lesion. To examine for drift, the physician may ask the patient to close the eyes and hold the arms outstretched with the hands supinated for as long as 1 minute—subtle drift starts with finger flexion, and the weak arm gradually pronates and drifts downward. In addition, the physician may observe a patient's voluntary movements (for instance, in dressing or walking); the weak limb will be used less than the strong limb.

In addition to examination of muscle power, **deep tendon reflexes** (biceps, brachioradialis, triceps, patellar, and Achilles), plantar reflex, and, in some circumstances, snout, grasp, palmomental, glabellar, and abdominal reflexes should be examined, with attention given to asymmetries between the two sides.

If limb weakness results from damage to the motor system at the upper motor neuron level (corticospinal pyramidal tract), deep tendon reflexes will be exaggerated in the affected limbs compared with the unaffected limbs, and extensor plantar responses and other pathologic reflexes in the affected limbs may be noted. Superficial reflexes will be depressed or absent on the affected side.

In contrast, if limb weakness results from motor system damage at the lower motor neuron level (anterior horn cell level and lower), deep tendon and superficial reflexes will be depressed (all or selectively, depending on the extent of damage and the level of damage) in the affected limbs. Examination of power, tone, and reflexes of individual muscles or muscle groups is essential to localize the lesion at the level of the spinal root or nerve. The clinical features that differentiate upper motor lesions from lower motor lesions are summarized in Table 5-6.

POSTURE, GAIT, AND COORDINATION

The cerebellar syndromes can be divided into four groups by location. The **rostral vermis syndrome**, involving the anterior lobe, leads to a wide-based stance and gait, ataxia of gait with proportionally little ataxia on the heel-to-shin maneuver with the patient lying down; normal or slightly impaired arm coordination;

Table 5-6. Clinical features that differentiate upper motor lesions from lower motor lesions

Upper Motor Neuron Lesions		Lower Motor Neuron Lesions	
(General clinical features: hemiplegia or hemiparesis [predominantly distal weakness]; spasticity; hyperactive deep tendon reflexes; clonus; absent abdominal reflexes; Babinski's sign, suck/snout and Hoffmann's reflexes)		(General clinical features: weakness with atrophy, hypotonia, decreased deep tendon and superficial reflexes, fasciculations in affected muscles of face, trunk, or extremities; vasomotor disturbances; absent Babinski's sign)	
Weaker Muscles	Stronger Muscles	Structure Involved	Clinical Features
Face (lower face)	Face (forehead)	Nucleus of cranial nerve III	Horizontal diplopia, downward and outward deviation of affected eye, bilateral incomplete ptosis, pupillary dilation
Upper extremities External rotator Deltoid Triceps Digit extensors Hypothenar Interossei	Upper extremities Pectoralis major Biceps Wrist flexors Digit flexors Thenar	Cranial nerve IV Cranial nerve VI	Vertical diplopia with tilt component Horizontal diplopia, worsens toward the paretic side, often as Foville's syndrome
		Cranial nerve VII	Unilateral weakness of ipsilateral upper and lower facial muscles (often as Millard-Gubler or Foville's syndrome)
Lower extremities Iliopsoas	Lower extremities Adductor thigh	Cranial nerves IX, X, XI, XII	Bulbar syndrome, Wallenberg, Vernet, Schmidt, Jackson, Collet-Sicard syndrome

Thigh abductors Hamstrings Peronei Toe flexors	Gluteus maximus Quadriceps Tibialis anterior Toe extensors Tibialis posterior	Anterior horn cells	Weakness, prominent atrophy, fasciculations in affected muscles of trunk and extremities
	Gastrocnemius Soleus	Root and radicular	Radicular pain, weakness, atrophy in myotomal distribution of the affected root, sensory loss, paresthesias
		Plexus	Weakness and distal atrophy in affected muscles with or without sensory disturbance
		Peripheral nerve	Weakness and atrophy of specific muscle group(s) involved with or without sensory, vasomotor, and trophic disturbances in distribution of specific nerve(s)

and infrequent presence of hypotonia, nystagmus, and dysarthria. The **caudal vermis syndrome** is caused by a flocculonodular and posterior lobe lesion; associated findings include axial dysequilibrium and staggering gait, little or no limb ataxia, and occasional spontaneous nystagmus and rotated postures of the head. A **hemispheric syndrome** with posterior lobe and variable anterior lobe involvement leads to incoordination of ipsilateral appendicular movements, particularly when they require fine-motor coordination. The **pan cerebellar syndrome** affects the cerebellum globally and leads to bilateral signs of cerebellar dysfunction that affects the trunk, limbs, and cranial musculature.

To examine posture and coordination, the physician should ask the patient to stand with heels and toes together, first with eyes open and then with eyes closed (**Romberg test**). The presence of loss of balance with the eyes open or closed may indicate a cerebellar or cerebellar-spinal pathway deficit. This ataxia is usually associated with other cerebellar symptoms such as **asynergia** (lack of synergy of the various muscles performing complex movements), **dysmetria** (abnormal in movement), **dysdiadochokinesia** (difficulty with rapid alternating movements), **intention tremor**, **rebound phenomena** (the outstretched arm[s] overcorrects when displaced), **decreased muscle tone**, or **nystagmus** (the fast component of the nystagmus is usually to the side of the cerebellar damage). Deep tendon reflexes may be normal or decreased.

Gait disorders are detected on examination by instructing the patient to walk normally "as though you are walking down the street," on the toes, on the heels, and in tandem, "one foot in front of the other, heel touching toe." Gait ataxia with uncoordinated steps, falling, or near falling may indicate a cerebellar deficit or spinocerebellar tract impairment. Most people who are older than 60 years have some degree of tandem gait ataxia. Gait ataxia alone usually indicates anterior cerebellar lobe dysfunction and is most commonly caused by aging or alcohol intake, although mass lesions (including tumors, AVMs, and abscesses) and cerebellar hemorrhage and infarction are occasional causes.

Appendicular ataxia, or incoordination of the arms or legs, is usually ipsilateral to a cerebellar hemispheric lesion or lesion of the cerebellopontine angle (including infarction; hemorrhage; or other mass lesion such as hemangioma, metastasis, and astrocytoma). Such incoordination is manifested by intention tremor and clumsiness independent of weakness on finger-to-nose and heel-to-shin testing.

Truncal ataxia, usually involving both gait ataxia and ataxia when the patient is sitting, may be apparent only when the patient attempts to correct sitting posture after it is slightly displaced. Lesions that produce such disturbances are usually located in or near the cerebellar vermis or its brainstem connections. The differential diagnosis of such lesions includes sensory ataxias and cerebellar ataxias. Sensory ataxias, which worsen when the patient has eyes closed, are often the result of separate vestibular or proprioceptive disturbances. Cerebellar ataxias are generally about the same whether the patient has eyes open or closed.

SENSATION

The sensory examination is usually conducted with the patient's eyes closed while the physician tests each half of the body (face, trunk, and limbs) separately. Each neurologic examination should include at least one type of testing of the spinothalamic tract system (such as pain or temperature) and function of the dorsal column (such as proprioception or vibration). Lateral spinothalamic system modalities may also reflect thalamic function (as does vibration); the modalities of joint position (proprioception), stereognosis, two-point discriminations, and graphesthesias involve higher cortical functions.

Clinically, **lesions of the parietal cortex** usually produce a contralateral discriminatory type of hemisensory loss (impaired two-point discrimination, astereognosis, sensory ataxia) or, if partial, selective sensory deficit in the face, arm, trunk, or leg.

Lesions of the thalamus or the internal capsule usually result in contralateral hemisensory loss (including the face) of all modalities. In addition, thalamic lesions may produce other sensory disturbances, such as **thalamic pain**, an unpleasant or severe burning, dysesthetic pain on the contralateral side of the body, or **anesthesia dolorosa** (reduction of pinprick sensation in the painful area).

Brainstem lesions may produce ipsilateral loss of pain and temperature or loss of sensation and numbness over the ipsilateral side of the face and contralateral loss of all modalities in the limbs, depending on the size and the location of the lesion.

Spinal cord lesions involving only the spinothalamic tract on one side cause loss of pain, temperature, and light-touch sensations below and contralateral to the lesion, but in lesions that involve half of the spinal cord (**Brown-Séquard syndrome**), the spinothalamic tract signs plus ipsilateral loss of proprioception and discriminatory touch sensation occur as far as the level of the lesion. Complete cord lesions result in bilateral loss of all modalities, and central cord lesions usually lead to bilateral loss of pain and temperature sensation with sparing of proprioception and discriminatory sensation and sacral sparing of pain and temperature.

To determine whether the patient has central or peripheral nervous system damage and at which level, the physician first must evaluate systematically two or more of the above-mentioned sensory modalities in the spared half of the body (face, arm, trunk, or leg) and then evaluate the affected side, comparing the normal side with the corresponding area on the opposite side and with contiguous dermatomes. Familiarity with sensory distributions over the various parts of the body is important (Fig. 5-7).

COGNITIVE FUNCTION

An adequate assessment of cognitive function is possible only when the patient is alert and oriented to time, place, and person and when the patient is not aphasic. Evaluation of the patient's intellectual or mental ability includes assessment of language, memory (short-term, recent, and long-term), calculation, abstract reasoning, judgment, perceptual and constructional functions, right–left orientation, and finger gnosis.

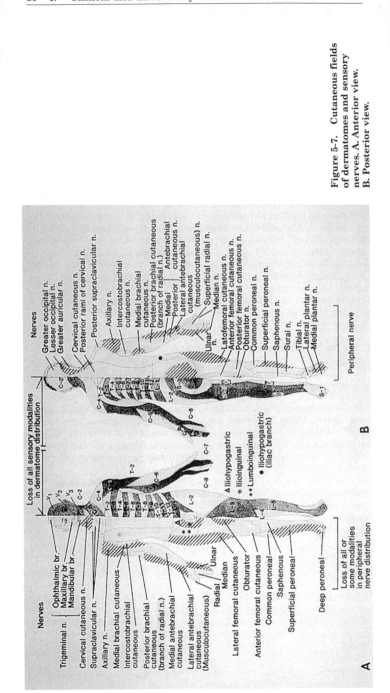

Figure 5-7. Cutaneous fields of dermatomes and sensory nerves. A. Anterior view. B. Posterior view.

Language

Language can be defined as the understanding and the production of individual words and grouping of words for the communication of ideas and feelings. Language should be evaluated early in any examination of mental status, because the presence of language deficits can influence performance on several parts of the mental status examination. Specific attention must be paid to **spontaneous speech**, including the characteristics such as the nature of speech output, presence of a dysarthria, and specific aphasic errors. Paraphasia is an important aphasic error, with substitution of an incorrect word or sound for the correct one and loss of fluency of speech. **Comprehension** is tested by asking a patient to follow one-, two-, and three-step commands, presented both orally and on paper. A patient is asked to repeat a word or a sentence, of increasing difficulty, after the examiner to reveal repetition abnormalities, including possible paraphasias, grammatical errors, omissions, additions, and failures to approximate the examples given.

Naming and word finding are tested by asking the patient to describe a picture or to name various objects. Both reading comprehension and reading aloud should be tested to demonstrate possible alexia (reading deficit). **Writing** is tested by asking the patient to write letters, numbers, names of common objects, and a short sentence from dictation to detect possible agraphia. Aphasic patients are nearly always agraphic and frequently alexic. More than 99% of right-handed people have a left hemisphere dominance for language, and approximately 60% to 80% of left-handed people have a left hemisphere dominance or mixed dominance for language.

The common aphasia syndromes may be classified according to four major examination findings: speech fluency, repetition, comprehension, and naming (Table 5-7). All aphasias are associated with naming difficulties. Transcortical aphasias do not involve lesions in perisylvian locations; thus, they manifest relative sparing of repetition.

Pure alexia without agraphia, in which the patient understands words that are spelled aloud and can write but is unable to read, may result from lesions of the posterior portion of the corpus callosum and the occipital lobe in the dominant hemisphere. **Alexia with agraphia** indicates inability to read or write and may be caused by lesions in the dominant inferior parietal lobule, in the angular gyrus. **Pure agraphia** occurs rarely and generally with the left hand because of lesions of the anterior corpus callosum; agraphia associated with dyscalculia, right–left confusion, and finger agnosia (**Gerstmann syndrome**) is more common in patients with lesions in the dominant parietal lobe.

Nonorganic speech and language disorders may occur in some patients who have functional disturbances and convert anxiety into a halting, telegraphic speech. Comprehension, repetition, naming, reading, and writing are normal; appropriate psychotherapy alters the abnormal speech patterns. An acute aphonia with total inability to adduct the vocal cord and make audible sounds but normal breathing and no evidence of stridor also responds well to speech therapy. In elective mutism, patients may demonstrate willful reluctance or an outright refusal to speak, but

Table 5-7.   Classification of aphasias

Subtype	Location	Examination Findings			
		Fluent	Repetition	Comprehension	Naming
Broca's	Frontal operculum	No	−	+	−[a]
Wernicke's	Superior temporal	Yes	−	−	−
Conduction	Supramarginal gyrus, arcuate fasciculus	Yes	——	+	−
Anomic	Angular gyrus, toxic or metabolic encephalopathy; poorly localized	Yes	+	+	−
Global	Middle cerebral artery distribution	No	−	−	−
Transcortical					
Motor	Anterior arterial border zone	No	+	+	−
Sensory	Posterior arterial border zone	Yes	+	−	−
Mixed	Entire border zone	No	+	−	−

+ = normal or relatively unaffected; − = abnormal; —— = markedly abnormal.
[a]May be good, relative to paucity of spontaneous speech.

they have no demonstrable language deficit. These patients usually respond to behavior modification.

Memory

To assess short-term (immediate) **memory**, the physician should ask the patient either to recall a sequence of random numbers or to recall the names of items after 5 minutes. To assess recent memory, the physician may ask the patient to recall events of the past few days or to describe the duration of the hospital stay. Long-term (remote) memory may be assessed by asking the patient about his or her date of birth, home address, the years of World War II, or details of other events that have occurred more than 5 years previously.

Memory impairment involves bilateral lesions, and results of the mental status examination may help in differential and topical diagnoses. For instance, **impaired recent memory** is often caused by lesions of the limbic system, whereas **remote memory impairment** is often associated with diffuse cortical lesions. Also, patients with acute cerebrovascular disorders, epilepsy, or recent brain injury may have loss of memory for events that led to the current illness (**retrograde amnesia**); permanent loss of memory of events for a period after a current illness is highly characteristic of brain trauma (**posttraumatic or anterograde amnesia**).

Short Mental Status Examination

A detailed mental status examination can be very time-consuming. For practical use by physicians and neurologists who do not have special neuropsychological training, the short mental status examination that has been used at the Mayo Clinic provides an efficient and reproducible way of evaluating general cognitive function (Table 5-8). **Orientation** is tested by asking the patient to give his or her (1) full name; (2) address; (3) current location (building); (4) city; (5) state; and (6) the current date, either the day of the week or the day of the month, (7) month, and (8) year. Each correct response is worth 1 point (maximum score is 8). To assess **attention**, the physician tells the patient, "I will give you a series of numbers. Please pay close attention to them, wait until I am finished, and then repeat the numbers to me in the same order as I have given them." Usually, a span of five to seven digits is given to the patient. The number of digits that are repeated correctly is the patient's score; the maximum score is 7, and the minimum score is 0.

To assess **learning** functions, the patient is told, "I shall now give you four words. I would like you to learn them, keep them in mind, and repeat them to me from time to time when I ask you to do so." The four words are "apple," "Mr. Johnson," "charity," and "tunnel." The patient is asked to repeat the words. If he or she learns the words on the first trial, then a score of 4 points is given. If the patient is unable to learn all four words, then a point is earned for each word learned. The number of trials (a maximum of four) that are required to learn the words is recorded separately, but for scoring, the number of trials greater than one is subtracted from the points earned for each word learned.

Table 5-8.   Short mental status examination

Subtest	Maximum Possible Score
Orientation	8
Attention	7
Learning	
Number of words learned (maximum of 4)	4
Number of trials (maximum of 4) for acquisition	
Arithmetic calculation	4
Abstraction	3
Information	4
Construction	4
Recall	4
Total score	38

Source: From Kokmen E, Naessens JM, Offord KP. A short test of mental status: description and preliminary results. *Mayo Clinic Proc.* 1987;62: 281–288, with permission of Mayo Foundation.

Arithmetic calculation ability is tested by asking the patient to multiply 5 by 13, to subtract 7 from 65, to divide 58 by 2, and to add 11 and 29. Each correct answer earns 1 point, and the maximum score is 4. Interpretation of similarities by use of word pairs is used as a test of **abstraction**. The word pairs are "orange/banana," "horse/dog," and "table/bookcase." One point for each word pair is given only for definitely abstract interpretations (for example, horse/dog = animal). Concrete interpretations or inability to note a similarity earns 0 points for that word pair. The maximum score is 3. For assessment of **information**, the patient is asked to name the current president and the first president of the United States, to state the number of weeks per year, and to define an island. Each correct answer earns 1 point, and the maximum score is 4. **Construction** ability is tested by asking the patient to draw the face of a clock showing 11:15 and to copy a three-dimensional cube (impaired constructional functions may result from lesions in the nondominant parietal lobe). The patient is able to view the diagram of the cube while drawing his or her own version. For each construction, an adequate conceptual drawing is scored as 2, a less-than-complete drawing as 1, and inability to perform the task as 0 (the maximum score for the construction task is 4).

At the end of the short mental status examination, **recall** ability is tested. The patient is asked to recall the four words from the learning subtest: "apple," "Mr. Johnson," "charity," and "tunnel." No cues or reminders are given. The patient earns 1 point for each word recalled, and the maximum score is 4. The total score for each patient is the sum of the scores on the eight subtests. The highest possible score on the test is 38. Any patient who scores <29 should have a more detailed evaluation for dementia and related disorders. A single test such as this one **should not be the sole basis** of a diagnosis of dementia or any other cognitive disturbance.

Other Intellectual Function Tests

Construction may be tested by having the patient draw a clock, including the numbers, and arrange the hands to indicate a specific time (lesions in the nondominant parietal lobe may result in constructional apraxia). **Right–left orientation** is tested by asking the patient to identify right from left for his or her own body parts (this function maybe impaired because of lesions in the dominant angular gyrus). For assessment of **finger gnosia**, the patient may be asked to name his or her own fingers and to point to and name the appropriate finger of the examiner (impaired finger gnosia may result from focal dominant parietal lesions or, occasionally, from more diffuse lesions).

The differential diagnosis of dementia and other forms of cognitive dysfunction is discussed in Chapter 2.

Approach to the Comatose Patient

Coma is a state of unarousable unresponsiveness (impairment of consciousness) in which the patient is unable to sense or respond noticeably to the environment. When managing a comatose patient, the physician should initiate therapeutic actions that are aimed at maintaining vital functions to help to avoid permanent brain damage from potentially reversible conditions while performing diagnostic procedures to define the cause of the comatose state. Management of specific coma-producing processes (for example, stroke, trauma, infections, tumor) requires careful evaluation of the patient because this state may derive from various systemic and intracranial causes. The following is a general outline for the clinical approach to the comatose patient, including a discussion of how to distinguish among various cerebrovascular and noncerebrovascular causes of coma. Further aspects regarding the management of comatose patients with stroke are discussed in Chapter 11.

MAJOR TYPES OF COMA

Wakefulness is maintained by a diffuse system of upper brainstem and thalamic neurons and the reticular activating system (RAS) and its connections to the cerebral hemispheres. Therefore, depression of either the RAS or generalized hemispheric activity may produce impaired consciousness. Three major types of coma result from various pathophysiologic mechanisms by which consciousness may be impaired (Fig. 6-1): (1) **focal cerebral lesion with mass effect** on deep diencephalic structures caused by intracerebral hematoma, subdural or epidural hematoma, tumor, abscess, large supratentorial infarct (although large hemispheric infarct may not produce coma caused by increasing edema for 1 to 4 days after stroke); (2) **intrinsic brainstem lesions that** affect the RAS, including infarct, hemorrhage, tumor, abscess, and cerebellar masses that cause direct brainstem compression; and (3) **processes that cause diffuse bilateral cortical and brainstem dysfunction**, occurring most commonly in cases of **metabolic encephalopathy, hypoxic encephalopathies,** and **infectious or inflammatory central nervous system (CNS) disease.** The differential diagnosis of coma is reviewed in Table 6-1.

NEUROLOGIC EXAMINATION

Because coma has many causes, a systematic approach is required for the examiner to quickly establish the location and the probable nature of the lesion, define appropriate laboratory tests, and outline appropriate intervention. Before the neurologic examination is performed, one must be certain that the patient's airway, breathing, and circulation are evaluated. Emergency treatment of airway compromise or insufficient ventilation may require suction, supplemental oxygen, or intubation. Hemodynamic instability also should be treated appropriately

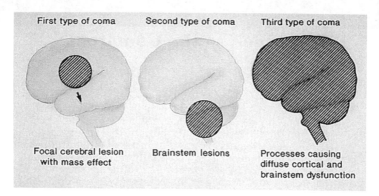

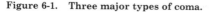

Figure 6-1.   Three major types of coma.

before more comprehensive neurologic evaluation. **Neurologic examination should include evaluation of the following five major neurologic functions:**

1. Level of consciousness
2. Respiratory pattern
3. Pupillary size and response to light
4. Ocular position at rest and after vestibular stimulation
5. Motor and reflex activity

Level of Consciousness

Level of consciousness can be determined by applying verbal, tactile, visual, and painful stimuli. Initially, the patient should be observed for the presence of spontaneous movement or postures. Spontaneous purposeful movement suggests intact brainstem pathways. The degree of stimulus that is necessary to evoke a response should be recorded. One initially attempts verbal stimuli, followed by tactile stimuli, then painful stimuli, which include sternal rub or fingernail or toenail pressure. The type of movements evoked with these maneuvers also should be noted. Patient movements may include appropriate withdrawal, which indicates intact spinal cord, brainstem, and cortical pathways. One should consider corticospinal tract dysfunction if movement is asymmetric. Decerebrate or decorticate posturing is also of localizing significance (see Motor and Reflex Activity, p. 93).

The **Glasgow coma scale** is an objective scale that may prove useful for measuring the depth of coma or the level of consciousness in patients who have had stroke. This scale (Appendix B) has a score range from 3 (minimum score, deepest coma) to 15 (maximum score, normal consciousness). Assessment of the level of coma alone does not establish the cause, but documentation of progression or regression of the level of coma is vitally important.

Respiration

Generally, normal respiration is characterized by rhythmic breathing with a frequency of approximately 10 to 15 breaths/minute (a normal breath is approximately 500 ml of

Table 6-1.   Major types of coma

Type	Examples
Focal cerebral lesion with mass effect	Intracerebral hematoma, subdural or epidural hematoma, tumor, abscess, large supratentorial infarct
Brainstem lesions	Brainstem infarct, hemorrhage, tumor, abscess, basilar migraine Cerebellar masses with brainstem compression, including tumor, hemorrhage, abscess, infarction

Processes that cause diffuse cortical and brainstem dysfunction	Metabolic
	  Endogenous
	    Hypoglycemic, hyperosmolar coma; diabetic acidosis
	    Renal or hepatic failure
	    Thyroid, pituitary, adrenal dysfunction
	    Hyponatremia or hypernatremia, hypokalemia or hyperkalemia, acidosis or alkalosis, hypocalcemia or hypercalcemia
	    Wernicke's encephalopathy
	  Exogenous
	    Alcohol, sedatives, narcotics, antidepressants, anticonvulsants, anesthetic agents, carbon monoxide
	  Other
	    Severe hypothermia, hyperthermia
	Hypoxia or anoxia
	  Cardiac disorders: cardiac arrest, severe congestive heart failure
	  Chronic obstructive pulmonary disease
	Infectious disorders
	  Meningitis
	  Encephalitis
	  Systemic infections
	Other diffuse disorders
	  Subarachnoid hemorrhage
	  Postictal state
	  Concussion
	  Hypertensive encephalopathy
	  Hydrocephalus
	  Degenerative neurologic disorders

inspired air). Some respiratory patterns can have a localizing significance and help in the diagnosis of coma (Fig. 6-2).

Cheyne-Stokes respiration is a periodic pattern in which episodes of hyperpnea alternate with apnea and suggests bilateral, deep hemispheric lesions or diffuse cortical and brainstem dysfunction. This respiration pattern may be the first sign of

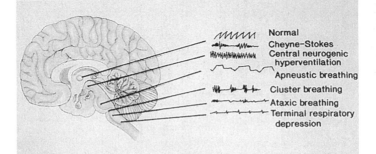

Figure 6-2.   Respiratory patterns characteristic of lesions at
different levels of the brain. Adapted from The localization of lesions
causing coma. In: Brazis PW, Masdeu JC, Biller J. *Localization in
clinical neurology*. 3rd ed. Boston: Little, Brown; 1996: 565–595.

transtentorial herniation in patients with a unilateral supratentorial lesion. The pattern may also be seen in normal individuals and in those with metabolic disorders and other causes of diffuse cortical and brainstem dysfunction. **Central neurogenic
hyperventilation**, a regular, rapid, deep, machinery-like breathing, usually indicates a lesion of the brainstem tegmentum
between the low midbrain and the middle third of the pons or
diffuse cortical or brainstem dysfunction. A systemic, acid-base
imbalance also must be considered if hyperventilation is noted.
Central neurogenic hyperventilation that results in metabolic
acidosis may be caused by pneumonia (often accompanied by an
expiratory grunt, cyanosis, and fever), neurogenic pulmonary
edema, or diabetic or uremic acidosis and may occur in hepatic
coma and salicylate poisoning. **Apneustic breathing** consists of
a prolonged inspiratory cramp followed by an expiratory pause
and usually denotes a lesion (especially infarction or primary
hemorrhage) in the pons. **Ataxic breathing**, which is irregular
and variable, and **cluster breathing**, with irregular pauses
between breaths, are often terminal patterns that signify a high
medullary dysfunction. With further depression of the medulla,
respiration becomes more erratic and may eventually decrease
(**suppression**) and then stop (**apnea**).

Pupils

Pupillary size, symmetry, and reactivity to light (Fig. 6-3) all
are important in the evaluation of the comatose patient. The
response of the pupils to light in a comatose patient should be
tested with a bright light to be certain of the response. Pupillary
light response is relatively resistant to metabolic abnormalities,
and the preservation of light response in association with other
signs of midbrain dysfunction indicates a probable metabolic
cause. Although the presence of the light reflex is the single most
important physical sign that differentiates diffuse (cortical and
brainstem dysfunction) from structural brain disease, metabolic
disorders can mimic structural brain disease. Glutethimide,

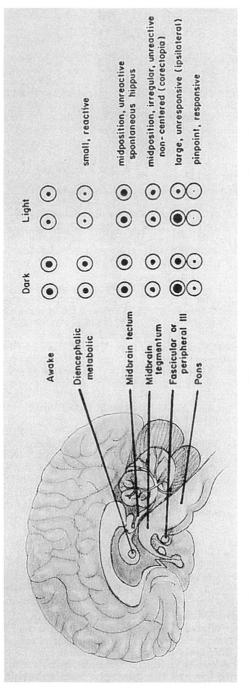

Figure 6-3. Pupillary responses characteristic of lesions at different levels of the brain. Adapted from The localization of lesions causing coma. In: Brazis PW, Masdeu JC, Biller J. *Localization in clinical neurology*. 3rd ed. Boston: Little, Brown; 1996: 565–595.

scopolamine, and atropine may cause fixed and dilated pupils; opiates may cause constricted pupils.

Bilateral dilated (6 to 7 mm) and fixed pupils usually signify brain death but may also occur with barbiturate intoxication or severe hypothermia. Midposition (4 to 5 mm), equal, and reactive pupils usually occur in patients with diffuse cortical and brainstem dysfunction; midposition pupils that are fixed to light indicate a midbrain lesion. Unilateral pupillary dilation may indicate uncal herniation through the tentorial notch or a third cranial nerve compressive lesion. Bilateral very small (pinpoint) and reactive pupils suggest pontine hemorrhage, infarction, or narcotic use.

Ocular Position and Movements

Careful assessment of eye position and movements in comatose patients is often very helpful for localizing the offending lesion(s) (Fig. 6-4). Spontaneous, roving, conjugate eye movements indicate intact brainstem pathways. Dysconjugate ocular movements typically indicate abnormal brainstem function. Lateral gaze deviation is also localizing, as noted below.

Unilateral or bilateral paralysis of abduction may be caused by increased intracranial pressure that results from a massive hemispheric lesion. Conjugate lateral gaze deviation may be caused by frontal or pontine lesions. In frontal hemispheric destructive lesions, the **eyes deviate toward the damaged hemisphere** and away from the affected limbs; in pontine lesions, the **eyes deviate away from the damaged brainstem** and toward the affected limbs (forced lateral gaze). In irritative lesions, such as a seizure, the eyes deviate away from the frontal seizure and are directed toward the hemiparetic limb. **Absence of eye movements** with reactive pupils suggests a process that causes diffuse cortical and brainstem dysfunction. Deviation of one eye laterally and down, complete ptosis, and pupil dilation are characteristic of damage to the ipsilateral third cranial nerve (Fig. 6-4).

In a patient with a hemispheric lesion, the eyes are fully deviated but can be brought beyond the midline toward the other side by either cold water caloric stimulation (oculovestibular caloric reflex) or passive head turning (doll's eye maneuver). **Cold water caloric stimulation** (10 to 20 ml of ice-cold water introduced into the ear canal, with the head inclined at 30 degrees) helps to evaluate brainstem function between the upper medulla and the midbrain: In a patient with a functioning brainstem, the eyes will deviate slowly toward the stimulated side. In a patient with a pontine lesion, ipsilateral caloric stimulation may bring the eyes only to the midline. In a comatose patient with intact brainstem function, rotation or flexion of the head produces eye movements in a direction opposite the direction of head movement **(oculocephalic [doll's eye] reflex);** in patients with brainstem dysfunction, this maneuver produces no eye movement, or ocular movement may not be conjugate.

Nystagmus (rapid, jerking eye movements) in a comatose patient may be caused by brainstem or cerebellar dysfunction as a result of vascular disease, demyelination, infection, neoplasm, alcohol intoxication, or toxicity from phenytoin (in cases of localized cerebellar damage, the direction of the fast phase of

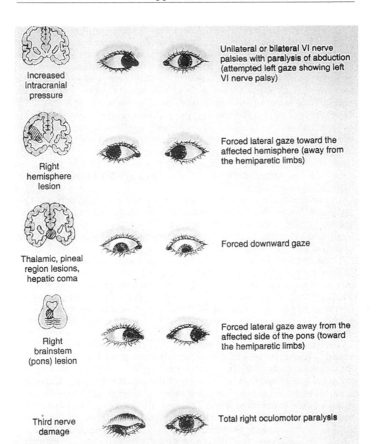

Increased intracranial pressure — Unilateral or bilateral VI nerve palsies with paralysis of abduction (attempted left gaze showing left VI nerve palsy)

Right hemisphere lesion — Forced lateral gaze toward the affected hemisphere (away from the hemiparetic limbs)

Thalamic, pineal region lesions, hepatic coma — Forced downward gaze

Right brainstem (pons) lesion — Forced lateral gaze away from the affected side of the pons (toward the hemiparetic limbs)

Third nerve damage — Total right oculomotor paralysis

Figure 6-4. Examination of eye position and movements in comatose patients.

nystagmus tends to occur to the affected side of the cerebellar lesion). In conscious patients with functional coma, nystagmus develops when caloric testing is performed.

Forced downgaze usually occurs with thalamic hemorrhage, a mass lesion in the pineal region, or diffuse cortical and brainstem dysfunction; rapid downgaze followed by slow upgaze is more characteristic of a caudal pontine lesion. Unilateral loss of the **corneal reflex** signifies a pontine lesion (bilateral loss or diminution of the corneal reflexes may be observed in the deep stages of coma, indicating depression of brainstem function).

Motor and Reflex Activity

An important component of the neurologic examination of the comatose patient is to determine whether hemiplegia or other focal neurologic signs are present. Because the comatose patient is unable to respond, the face and the limbs should be observed to detect subtle asymmetries of neurologic function. When one cheek puffs out with each expiration, one eyelid does not close completely after passive lifting and release (compared with the other side of the face), or there is homolateral absence of the corneal reflex, the affected side of the face is usually paretic or plegic. Absence of **movements** on one side of the body or asymmetry of movements is suggestive of hemiparesis. Symmetric limb responses, especially when associated with reactive pupils and full eye movements, suggest diffuse cortical and brainstem dysfunction. Focal **seizures** may point to a localized cerebral lesion. Multifocal seizures, myoclonic jerks, or asterixis are suggestive of diffuse cortical and brainstem dysfunction.

In addition to general observation of the position of the patient's body and limbs, paralysis of the limbs can be determined through the examination of muscle tone. By lifting each limb and allowing it to fall (the paralyzed limb falls rapidly and heavily, and the spared one falls more gradually) or by flexing the patient's knees so that the heels approach the buttocks (with the patient supine, the paralyzed leg falls farther to the side and more rapidly when the knees are released), paralysis may become apparent. Bilateral paratonic rigidity or gegenhalten (plastic-like increase in muscle resistance to passive movements of the extremities) is suggestive of diffuse cortical and brainstem dysfunction.

The predominant posture of the limbs and the body should be noted. **Decorticate rigidity** (arm[s] flexed and adducted, and leg[s] extended) usually results from deep hemispheric lesions above the red nucleus (cerebral white matter, internal capsule, or thalamus) (Fig. 6-5). Lesions below the level of the vestibular nuclei usually produce flaccidity and absence of all postures and movements. **Decerebrate rigidity** (opisthotonos, jaw clenching, stiff limb extension, internal rotation of the arms, and plantar flexion of the feet) typically suggests a lesion in the upper brainstem between the red nucleus in the midbrain and the upper medulla, but a similar-appearing posture also may be noted in bilateral diencephalic and cortical dysfunction (Fig. 6-5). **Deep tendon reflexes** usually add little to the testing of motor activity and are seldom needed to localize the abnormality that is causing coma. Deep tendon reflexes may be normal or slightly reduced on the hemiplegic side, and the plantar reflexes may be absent or extensor. Asymmetries of deep tendon reflexes and limb movements, facial grimace in response to painful stimulation, and the presence of **pathologic reflexes** (Babinski's sign) or clonus of the affected limbs all indicate the probable presence of a structural lesion. Occasionally, all deep tendon reflexes may be lost or very depressed in comatose patients immediately after a stroke, but, more common, the reflexes are hyperactive on the side opposite the cerebral lesion. Bilateral Babinski's signs may occur in a patient with a massive unilateral lesion if cerebral edema has caused midbrain compression. However, Babinski's signs and clonus also can be present in some metabolic comas.

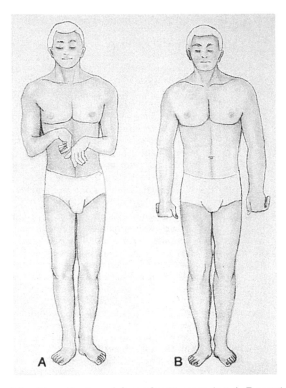

Figure 6-5. Decorticate and decerebrate posturing. A. Decorticate posture may occur with severe unilateral hemispheric lesion with central herniation, a deep hemispheric lesion, or a high brainstem lesion at or above the level of the red nucleus (midbrain) level. B. Decerebrate posture usually indicates a lesion in the brainstem between the red nucleus in the midbrain and the upper medulla.

Summary

Key findings in the three main types of coma described are summarized in Table 6-2. After brief neurologic examination, one should be able to localize the neurologic abnormality and define a differential diagnosis for the coma (Table 6-1).

ADDITIONAL EVALUATION: HISTORY AND GENERAL EXAMINATION

Although the neurologic examination aids in localizing a lesion, the cause of the coma still may not be clear. Additional historical and general examination findings are useful for narrowing the differential diagnosis and outlining appropriate treatment.

History

Having determined which type of coma is present, the physician must define the underlying cause of the comatose state. A properly taken **history** is essential in the differential diagnosis.

Table 6-2.   Clinical features of major types of coma[a]

Type	Clinical Features
I: Focal cerebral lesion with mass effect[b]	Cheyne-Stokes respiration, bilateral paralysis of abduction, eye deviation toward damaged hemisphere and away from affected limbs, eye deviation overcome by cold caloric or oculovestibular testing, forced downgaze, decorticate posture, hemiplegia with unilateral Babinski's sign and reduced tendon reflexes on hemiplegic side, focal seizures ± unilateral third nerve palsy with early pupil dilation in cases of early herniation
II: Brainstem lesions	Apneustic breathing; ataxic breathing; central neurogenic hyperventilation; midposition pupils fixed to light; pinpoint, reactive pupils; eye deviation away from damaged brainstem and toward affected limbs; eye deviation not overcome by cold caloric or oculovestibular testing; rapid downgaze and slow upgaze; nystagmus; skew deviation of eyes; decerebrate posture; hemiplegia (with unilateral Babinski's sign); unilateral loss of corneal reflex
III: Processes that cause diffuse cortical and brainstem dysfunction[c]	Cheyne-Stokes respiration, central neurogenic hyperventilation or slow or shallow regular breathing, equal and reactive pupils, intact or impaired corneal reflex, brisk ocular response to passive head turning, divergent strabismus, no focal neurologic signs, decerebrate rigidity, asterixis, tremor, multifocal seizures, myoclonic jerks

[a]All forms of coma may produce any of the levels of consciousness.
[b]Other brainstem findings may appear with increasing brainstem compression from mass effect.
[c]The features of this type of coma can be remembered easily with the phrase "nothing works but everything works," referring to the initial appearance of unresponsiveness ("nothing works") but the intact or relatively intact function of respiration, pupils, ocular position and involvement, and motor and reflex activity ("but everything works").

Questioning of friends, relatives, and ambulance personnel should focus on the exact **circumstances** and **mode of onset** of the condition (acute onset of symptoms is typical for intracerebral hemorrhage, subarachnoid hemorrhage, or embolic vertebrobasilar infarction; gradual development of symptoms is more characteristic of an expanding mass lesion or various metabolic or infective causes of coma). Questions should elicit information about **previous illnesses** such as transient ischemic attack or stroke, diabetes mellitus (may cause hypoglycemia or, less likely, hyperglycemia), epilepsy (may cause postictal state), drug abuse, previous head injury (may cause diffuse white matter injury, acute intracranial hematoma, chronic subdural hematoma), or psychiatric disorders (may be associated with drug overdose or functional coma); **previous bacterial or viral infection** (may cause meningitis or encephalitis); **malignancy** (may produce intracranial metastasis); and **previous medications or alcohol intake** (may help to define primary illness, drug overdose, or alcohol abuse).

In patients with **type I coma** (focal cerebral lesion with mass effect), historical features may clarify the cause of the coma. The differential diagnosis includes intracerebral hematoma (history of hypertension, acute onset of deficit with early change in level of consciousness), subdural or epidural hematoma (history of head injury, with a lucid interval in epidural hematoma), large supratentorial infarct (recent onset of a focal neurologic deficit that fits a single arterial territory), tumor (history of malignancy, preceding headache, seizures, mental disturbances, papilledema), and abscess (preceding subacute progression of focal neurologic signs, headache, depressed mental status, evidence of a contiguous or systemic source of infection). In most patients with the first type of coma, a specific diagnosis is established by characteristic findings on computed tomography (CT) of the head.

Brainstem ischemia, hemorrhage, tumor, abscess, or compression should be considered in patients with **type II coma**. Historical features mimic those described for entities that cause type I coma.

In patients with **type III coma** caused by diffuse cortical and brainstem dysfunction, the differential diagnosis should include metabolic or hypoxic encephalopathies and infectious or inflammatory CNS disorders. Historical features of a previous medical disorder associated with one of the causes reviewed in Table 6-1; history of drug or alcohol use; recent cardiac or respiratory disease; report of previous infection or fever; or other history of seizure, hypertension, or head injury may suggest the diagnosis.

General Physical Examination

The differential diagnosis of comatose patients should also be based on the general physical examination, with special attention given to the patient's head, blood pressure (BP), pulse, heart, breathing, skin, chest, abdomen, extremities, temperature, and signs of meningeal irritation.

On examination of the **head**, lacerations, bruising, "raccoon eyes," Battle's sign, localized tenderness, crepitus, and cerebrospinal fluid (CSF) leakage from the ears or nostrils suggest head injury. Periorbital ecchymosis associated with CSF leakage from an ear or the nose is an indication of cranial fracture. An enlarged head or tense anterior fontanelle in an infant indicates increased intracranial pressure. Internal auditory meatus pus or an infected sinus may be indicative of cerebral abscess or meningitis.

Hypotension and cardiac arrhythmias may occur in coma as a result of alcohol or barbiturate intoxication, myocardial

infarction (decreased cardiac output), internal hemorrhage, septicemia, and addisonian crisis. Hypotension may also occur in
diabetic or metabolic coma, dissecting aortic aneurysm, and
Gram-negative bacillary septicemia. A cardiac murmur may indicate underlying valvular disease with endocarditis. A **slow pulse
rate** in combination with hypertension and hyperventilation or
periodic breathing may be indicative of an increase in intracranial pressure. An **exceptionally slow pulse rate** suggests primary heart block but may also be caused by medication overdose.
Marked hypertension usually occurs in patients with hypertensive encephalopathy or intracranial hemorrhage and in those
with other causes of greatly increased intracranial pressure.

Respiratory patterns were previously discussed (see
Respiration). In addition, the patient's breath may reveal the
smell of liquor in cases of alcohol intoxication, fetor hepaticus in
cases of liver failure, the spoiled-fruit smell of ketoacidosis in
cases of diabetic coma, the uriniferous smell of uremia, or the
burnt-almond odor of cyanide poisoning.

Tongue biting suggests epilepsy or a postictal state. **Needle
marks** on limbs may indicate drug abuse, and "snout" rash indicates solvent abuse. **Emaciation, hepatomegaly,** or **lymphadenopathy** may be indicative of an underlying malignancy
and intracranial metastases. **Generalized cutaneous petechiae**
suggest thrombotic thrombocytopenic purpura, a bleeding
diathesis that causes intracerebral hemorrhage, or systemic
infection with meningococcus. Signs of trauma (multiple bruises,
especially on the scalp), stigmata of liver disease, skin infection,
or embolic phenomena also have diagnostic importance.
Cyanosis of the lips and nail beds suggests inadequate oxygenation caused by pulmonary or circulatory insufficiency or
methemoglobinemia. **Cherry red coloration** is typical of carbon
monoxide poisoning, and **yellow coloration** may indicate underlying liver or kidney disease. **Telangiectases and hyperemia of
the face** and conjunctival area are characteristic of alcoholism;
marked pallor is associated with internal hemorrhage; and a
macular hemorrhagic rash may be caused by meningococcal
infection, staphylococcal endocarditis, typhus, or Rocky Mountain
spotted fever. **Excessive sweating** suggests hypoglycemia or
shock, but **excessively dry skin** points to diabetic acidosis or
uremia. Dehydration results in reduction of **skin turgor**. **Needle
marks** indicate possible narcotic intoxication.

Pyrexia suggests systemic infection; cerebral abscess; meningitis; or subarachnoid, intracerebral, or pontine hemorrhage. If it is
associated with dry skin, it should raise the suspicion of heat
stroke. **Hypothermia** may be a complication of exposure during
the winter months or may be caused by alcoholic or barbiturate
intoxication, peripheral circulatory failure, or myxedema.

The chest and cardiac examinations may reveal evidence for
infective lung or valvular disease predisposing to cerebral
abscess or meningitis. The presence of abdominal muscle rigidity
suggests possible abdominal hemorrhage or infection.

Resistance and pain on neck flexion (the patient's head cannot
be completely flexed forward onto the chest, or flexion causes
pain), **Kernig's sign** (extending the knee with the thigh flexed at
the hip causes resistance and pain), and **Brudzinski's sign**

(flexion of the knees in response to head flexion) all can be indicative of meningeal irritation caused by subarachnoid bleeding, meningitis, meningoencephalitis, or meningeal carcinomatosis. However, in some patients with subarachnoid hemorrhage, the signs of meningeal irritation may not develop until 12 to 24 hours after the ictus. Resistance to movement of the neck may also be caused by generalized muscle rigidity (as in phenothiazine intoxication) or by disease of the cervical spine. If any signs of meningeal irritation are present, emergency CT should be performed. In the absence of an intracranial mass or other identifiable lesion causative for symptoms, a lumbar puncture should also be undertaken.

Laboratory Studies

Investigations in the acute stage of coma include **routine tests** such as complete blood cell count and determination of electrolyte, creatinine, serum glucose, calcium, aspartate aminotransferase, and bilirubin values. Urinalysis, chest radiography, electrocardiography, and arterial blood gas studies also should be done. **Toxin screening**, when clinically indicated (such as patients with type III coma), should be done on blood and urine to screen for opiates, barbiturates, sedatives, antidepressants, cocaine, and alcohol. If routine screening blood tests, arterial blood gas studies, urine and serum toxin screening, and head CT do not reveal an abnormality, additional metabolic screening may be necessary. This screening may include determination of **ammonia, serum magnesium, B_{12}, serum amylase, folic acid, and serum cortisol values; thyroid function tests**; and evaluation of **porphyrins**.

In virtually all cases of coma, especially with signs of trauma, focal neurologic signs, or raised intracranial pressure, head **CT or magnetic resonance imaging** is indicated. In patients with types I and II coma and evidence or suspicion of increased intracranial pressure, CT of the head without contrast should be performed as a primary procedure; in other instances, it should be done immediately after the initial laboratory procedures. In patients with type III coma, CT may still be necessary if the cause of the diffuse process is not readily apparent from the laboratory studies. Electroencephalography may provide evidence of subclinical epilepsy (seizure discharge), herpes simplex encephalitis (nonspecific but suggestive findings, including spike and slow wave activity over the temporal lobes, delta waves, or periodic lateralized epileptiform discharges), or metabolic encephalopathy (diffuse abnormalities, which may include triphasic waves).

Lumbar puncture should be performed in patients with a possible diagnosis of meningitis or encephalitis, clinical suspicion of subarachnoid hemorrhage associated with negative findings on CT, and cases with normal findings on CT in which the origin of coma is obscure. **Lumbar puncture is generally contraindicated** if CT reveals an intracranial mass lesion; if there are other signs of increased intracranial pressure, such as papilledema; if clinical findings suggest a focal, probable mass lesion and CT is unavailable; or if the patient has a bleeding disorder.

Initial Management

As described earlier, initial management should include stabilization of a patient's airway, breathing, and circulation. Subsequent neurologic and general examinations quickly narrow the differential diagnosis. If the cause of the coma does not become clear after the first few minutes of the evaluation, therapeutic intervention on an empiric basis may be initiated. These initial treatments include 25 ml of 50% dextrose, given immediately after serum glucose determination. One should be certain to give thiamine, 100 mg intravenously, because a patient with heavy alcohol intake or other factors that lead to poor nutrition may be thiamine deficient, and glucose intake may precipitate Wernicke's syndrome. Naloxone hydrochloride (Narcan) may be given (0.4 mg intravenously every 5 minutes) if acute narcotic overdose is possible. Flumazenil (0.2 mg per minute intravenously, up to a total dose of 1 mg) may be administered if there is any concern regarding benzodiazepine overdose. There is a risk for rapid arousal; a risk for aspiration pneumonia; and, particularly among those with seizure disorder or concurrent tricyclic antidepressant overdose, a risk for seizure with use of flumazenil.

The initiation of other interventions should be based on the results of the clinical examination, laboratory studies, and cranial imaging. Other measures that may need to be considered for urgent use include antibacterial, antiviral, or antiparasitic agents for possible meningitis or encephalitis; anticonvulsants for seizures; hyperventilation or osmotic agents for increased intracranial pressure; or neurosurgical consultation for a focal cerebral mass lesion (see Chapter 11).

COMA-LIKE SYNDROMES

Several syndromes may mimic comatose states because they produce apparent unresponsiveness. "Waxy flexibility" in a patient without voluntary or responsive movements and with eyes open may suggest a psychiatric state such as **catatonia**. On recovery, patients fully recall events that occurred during their catatonic stupor. Patients with **psychogenic unresponsiveness** voluntarily try to appear comatose and may resist eyelid elevation, blink to threat when the lids are held open, and move the eyes concomitantly with head rotation. Pupils are normal and reactive, and cold caloric testing provokes nystagmus rather than gaze deviation.

Akinetic mutism refers to the appearance of a partially or fully awake patient who is immobile and silent as a result of lesions of both frontal lobes, masses in the region of the third ventricle, or hydrocephalus. In the **locked-in syndrome**, patients are able to communicate by means of blinks or vertical eye movements but otherwise are completely paralyzed. This syndrome results from lesions involving the ventral pons, such as infarction, hemorrhage, or central pontine myelinolysis. A similar state may occur in severe cases of acute polyneuritis or myasthenia gravis, but unlike basilar artery stroke, vertical eye movements are not selectively spared in these conditions.

Nonconvulsive status epilepticus is usually characterized by rhythmic blinking of the eyelids or conjugate jerking of the eyes associated with continuous seizure activity on electroencephalography. If this diagnosis is suspected, then intravenous administration of benzodiazepine (e.g., lorazepam, 1 to 4 mg) should result in improvement.

PERSISTENT VEGETATIVE STATE AND BRAIN DEATH

Comatose patients who are chronically unresponsive with preserved brainstem function are said to be in a **persistent vegetative state** (spontaneous pulse, respiration, and BP but no apparent awareness of their environment, no ability to communicate, and only reflex or random motor activity responses to stimuli). This state may follow cardiac arrest, trauma, or drug overdose or be an end stage of a chronic degenerative disease and should be diagnosed only when there are no concomitant medical or toxic conditions. The patient who is in a persistent vegetative state must be observed for a sufficient time (at least 1 month, even longer in children) to establish the permanence of the syndrome and to look for any signs of neurologic improvement.

Brain death, or irreversible coma, results from total cessation of cerebral function and blood flow at a time when cardiopulmonary functions may remain preserved but depend on ventilatory assistance (no respiratory movements are observed when the ventilator is disconnected). The patient is **fully unresponsive** to external stimuli. **Movements** and **brainstem reflexes**, including spontaneous respiration, **are absent**; pupils are midposition to fully dilated with no pupil reaction to light, no orbicularis oculi contraction in response to corneal stimulation, and no vestibuloocular and oculocephalic reflexes, and no gag reflex is present. An appropriate apnea test should reveal no respiratory movements. Spinal cord reflexes, including deep tendon reflexes, may persist, but decorticate or full decerebrate posturing precludes the diagnosis of brain death. The **electroencephalogram is flat or isoelectric**, and the patient is unresponsive to pain or other stimuli. Transcranial Doppler ultrasonography may also be used to confirm brain death on the basis of a pattern of small systolic peaks in early systole without diastolic flow or reverberating flow. Conventional arteriography reveals no filling at the level of the carotid bifurcation or circle of Willis. **Exogenous and endogenous toxins and hypothermia must be excluded**. Brain death should be diagnosed only when it persists for some period of observation (usually 12 to 24 hours, but often longer if there is any doubt about the preconditions).

PROGNOSIS OF COMA

A definitive prognosis cannot be given for each comatose patient, but the physician can provide some guidance on the basis of existing natural history data. In this respect, examination of the level of consciousness and determination of the duration of coma, pupillary responses, eye movements, age, underlying disease, and general medical condition provide valuable prognostic information. The signs of brain death predict an extremely poor outcome. Unfavorable signs during the first hours after admission of a patient with nontraumatic coma are the absence of any two of the following: pupillary responses, corneal reflexes, or oculovestibular responses.

The survival rate for patients whose pupillary responses or reflex eye movements are absent 24 hours after the onset of coma is approximately 10%. Nontraumatic coma that lasts more than 1 week; poor motor responses at 3 days despite awakening on day 1; absence of visual, auditory, and somatosensory evoked responses; and persistent coma or vegetative state at 1 week are also unfavorable prognostic signs. In comatose patients, the survival rate decreases with prolonged coma, concurrent medical illness, complications, or advanced age. However, children, young adults, and patients with head trauma, toxic overdose, or metabolic coma are more likely to recover even when ominous signs are present. Patients who have motor responses or spontaneous eye movements with visual fixation at 3 days after onset or obey commands at 7 days after onset have a survival rate of approximately 75%.

Laboratory Evaluation

Laboratory and radiologic investigations allow anatomic localization of the cerebrovascular event and assist in the determination of its pathogenesis. Techniques that are available to aid the physician in the diagnosis and management of potential cerebrovascular disease include computed tomography (CT), magnetic resonance imaging (MRI), cerebral arteriography, noninvasive neurovascular studies, and other ancillary studies. The proper use of these techniques requires an understanding of the underlying disease process, the principles of the test involved, and the advantages and limitations of each procedure. Specific attention should be focused on how each investigation influences the management of a patient.

COMPUTED TOMOGRAPHY

Soon after its introduction in 1973, CT became the preferred method for imaging tissue damage from stroke, and its use was extended to the body and the spine. In CT of the head, multiple rotating beams of x-rays pass through the patient's head, and diametrically opposed detectors measure the extent of absorption values for multiple, small blocks of tissue (voxels). Computerized reconstruction of these areas on a two-dimensional, gray-scaled display (pixels) provides the characteristic CT scan appearance. Modern CT scanners have spatial resolution from 1 to 2 mm (for routine scanning, slices are usually 5 to 10 mm thick). White and gray matter usually is differentiated easily (Fig. 7-1), and the major arteries may be visualized after the infusion of contrast material.

CT Findings in Patients with Ischemic Lesions

The ability of CT to reveal an ischemic lesion depends on the resolution of the scanner, the size and the location of the lesion, and time after onset of symptoms (Table 7-1). After a person has had a transient ischemic attack (TIA), the CT scan may be normal, or it may show an area of decreased density compatible with a small infarction (or, rarely, an area of increased density compatible with a small hematoma) in the distribution of the TIA. Therefore, TIA is considered a clinical diagnosis. The main role of CT in patients with TIA is to rule out an unexpected pathologic lesion, such as intracranial hemorrhage, vascular tumor, or arteriovenous malformation (AVM), which may change the investigative approach and management.

On admission, the CT is negative in approximately one third of patients in whom ischemic stroke has been diagnosed clinically. However, a negative result does not exclude the diagnosis of ischemic stroke. A CT scan may not detect relatively small infarctions in the vertebrobasilar system, infarcts near the skull base (because of bone-related artifact), infarcts that are <5 mm in diameter, or infarcts with little edema. Furthermore, within the first 24 hours after cerebral infarction, the CT scan may be negative in approximately 50% of cases. For patients in whom the

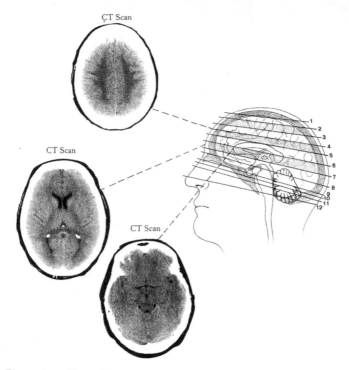

Figure 7-1.   Normal CT head scans.

presence of the ischemic stroke is not defined clearly by an area of decreased attenuation, one must scrutinize the scan carefully for the following suggestive findings: (1) flattening of the sulci (sulcal effacement), (2) loss of gray–white delineation (in the middle cerebral artery [MCA] distribution, this may manifest as loss of the insular ribbon), (3) loss of the outline of the lentiform nucleus, and (4) subtle area of subcortical hypointensity. A hyperdense middle cerebral artery may suggest clot within the artery. Clinicians should remember that the location of the lesion is important for making the diagnosis of cerebral infarction and helping to identify the underlying pathophysiologic mechanism that produced it. For example, infarcted tissue within a vascular territory of one or more major arteries may suggest large vessel disease or a cardiac source for emboli. In contrast, a tiny lesion in the basal ganglia area may suggest small vessel disease (for example, a lacunar infarct) or a lesion in a border zone between different vascular territories (watershed infarction) may suggest proximal occlusive disease with hemodynamic infarction.

Characteristic CT findings in patients with ischemic stroke include an area of decreased density, which often appears 12 to 48 hours after the stroke. The hypodensity initially is mild and poorly defined, but on the third or fourth day after the

Table 7-1. Common CT findings in patients with cerebral infarction and intracranial hemorrhage, by time from event to evaluation

Lesion Type	Interval between Stroke Onset and CT Evaluation	CT Finding
Infarction[a]	<24 hr	Mass effect with subtle gyral flattening or poorly demarcated zone of slightly reduced density
	24–48 hr	Mild and poorly defined area of decreased density
	3–5 d	Well-defined margins of decreased density; signs of cytotoxic edema (hypodensity involving both gray and white matter in the area affected by ischemia) and mass effect may be noted
	6–13 d	More homogeneous appearance of hypodense lesion, with sharp margination and abnormal contrast enhancement
	14–21 d	Fogging effect (infarcted area may become isodense with normal surrounding brain but may be detected with contrast enhancement as hypodense zone)
	>21 d	Smaller and better defined area of hypodensity with sharply demarcated margins of infarct (cystic space); ipsilateral ventricular enlargement may occur later
Hemorrhage	First 7–10 d[b]	Well-defined, homogeneous, hyperdense rounded, oval, or more irregular mass lesion, often with surrounding edema appearing as a narrow hypodense margin
	11 d–2 mo	Becomes a hypodense area with peripheral ring enhancement (hemosiderin deposition), an enlarged homolateral ventricle (in small

Table 7-1.   *Continued*

Lesion Type	Interval between Stroke Onset and CT Evaluation	CT Finding
		hematomas, hypodense area may become isodense)
	>2 mo	Isodense area (large hematomas can leave a hypodense defect with attenuation values similar to those of CSF) with decreased intensity of enhancement

CSF = cerebrospinal fluid.
[a]Changes of large infarctions may be detected earlier.
[b]In cases of large hematoma, the first 3 to 4 weeks.

stroke, the density decreases (in this period, edema is maximal and manifests as decreased density involving both gray and white matter in the area affected by ischemia), the margins of the lesion become better defined, and the lesion is better visualized (Fig. 7-2). Later, the edema and mass effect gradually subside, and the hypodensity becomes less evident. This change sometimes leads to radiologic disappearance of the infarcted area, which may become indistinguishable from the normal surrounding brain. The fogging effect occurs usually during the second or third week after the stroke and corresponds to the period of invasion by macrophages and proliferation of capillaries.

Thus, the peak period for detection of brain infarction by standard CT techniques is between the third and tenth days after stroke. However, small infarcts, particularly lacunes and brainstem infarcts, may not be visible on CT scans even after an appropriate delay. After the third week, phagocytosis of affected tissue ensues, the infarcted area gradually becomes replaced by cystic spaces filled with fluid, and the CT scan again shows a smaller and better defined area of hypodensity with sharply demarcated margins of the infarct. In this phase, the density of the affected area is closely matched to the density of cerebrospinal fluid (CSF).

The combination of a hyperdense zone and a hypodense adjacent white matter is characteristic of a **hemorrhagic infarction**, which more commonly occurs in embolic vascular occlusions and usually involves the cerebral cortex with sparing of the subcortical white matter. The hyperdense hemorrhagic portion usually appears smaller than a hypodense component representing infarct, and this hemorrhage is usually absorbed within 3 weeks. CT findings in patients with **hypertensive encephalopathy** usually include signs of generalized cerebral edema and mass effect, including compression of lateral ventricles, basal cisterns, and cortical sulcal spaces.

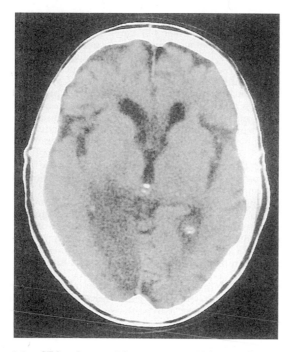

Figure 7-2.   CT head scan without contrast, 72 hours after onset of symptoms: area of decreased density in distribution of right posterior cerebral artery, consistent with cerebral infarction.

Under normal circumstances, **contrast agents** do not enter the brain, but if the blood–brain barrier is disrupted by a stroke, tumor, abscess, or other process, then contrast material leaks into that area and produces better visualization (enhancement). Therefore, the use of a contrast agent (usually iodinated, water-soluble contrast medium administered intravenously) allows visualization of a small percentage of otherwise isodense and undetectable infarcts, particularly in the second to fourth weeks after stroke, when the fogging effect is present. After 1 month, the area of infarction typically will not enhance with adminis-tration of contrast medium. Other indications for contrast administration are suspected AVM, intracranial tumor, and intracerebral abscess. Contrast agents (particularly in high doses) may also have neurotoxic effects and cause clinical dete-rioration. MRI has lessened the need for CT scanning with con-trast, but the technique may still be of use in patients who can-not undergo MRI.

In patients with **venous infarction** caused by venous sinus or cortical venous thrombosis, CT of the head usually reveals extensive areas of edema with patchy contrast enhancement and multiple small hemorrhages. In the case of sagittal sinus throm-bosis, changes tend to occur in a bilateral parasagittal pattern.

CT Findings in Patients with Hemorrhagic Lesions

Immediately after a person has had a hemorrhagic stroke, CT detects freshly extravasated blood (areas of increased density) in virtually all cases of intracerebral hemorrhage and in 80% to 90% of patients with subarachnoid hemorrhage (small amounts of subarachnoid blood may not be detected). **Characteristic CT findings in patients with acute intracerebral hematoma** (the first few days after ictus) include a well-defined, homogeneous, hyperdense mass lesion of a rounded, oval, or more irregular shape. The initial hyperdensity of the hematoma then begins to decline. The average lesion decreases in density by 1.4 Hounsfield units per day as a result of hemoglobin breakdown, progressing through an isodense (subacute) phase to a hypodense (chronic) phase. Therefore, the differentiation between infarction and intracerebral hematoma is readily made by CT at any time within the first 7 to 10 days after stroke (or as long as 3 to 4 weeks with large hematomas, in which disappearance of the hyperdensity is slower). In the chronic phase, a hematoma is often reduced to a slit-like cavity (with attenuation values similar to those of CSF) or may even disappear. **Subarachnoid hemorrhage** is even more transient, and CSF examination should be considered within 1 day to as long as 6 weeks after the ictus when the clinical history suggests this diagnosis and the CT scan is negative. In patients with **intraventricular hemorrhage**, CT demonstrates a hyperdense cast outlining the ventricular system.

Administration of an intravenous contrast agent is usually unnecessary in the early stages of intracerebral hemorrhage, and no significant changes show on CT in the first 7 to 10 days. However, a contrast CT (or MRI study) is required when the plain CT scan shows white matter abnormalities around the acute hematoma or abnormal densities adjacent to or surrounding the hematoma, because these findings may indicate possible underlying AVM, aneurysm, tumor, or abscess. Often, contrast CT or MRI is delayed a few weeks to provide a better chance for visualizing possible underlying lesions.

Epidural hematomas appear on CT as biconvex to lenticular, hyperdense, homogeneous extracerebral zones adjacent to the inner table of the skull with sharp margins. In cases of subacute epidural hematoma, CT usually shows a biconvex mixed-density lesion (the detached dura can often be seen on plain CT or on contrast CT as a thin, hyperdense stripe between the hematoma and the brain). In patients with **acute subdural hematoma**, the CT scan shows hyperdense, homogeneous, crescent-shaped lesions located between the calvarium and the underlying cortex, often accompanied by marked ipsilateral edema and mass effect. **Chronic subdural hematoma** usually appears as a hypodense, crescent-shaped, extracerebral lesion that is characteristically surrounded by a well-defined capsule.

Computed Tomography Angiography

Noninvasive real-time modalities such as **CT angiography** (**CTA**; including four-dimensional and three-dimensional CTA) using spiral CT scanners are increasingly replacing conventional cerebral arteriography in the evaluation of craniocervical arterial lesions such as carotid artery stenosis and intracranial aneurysms. Compared with magnetic resonance angiography (MRA), which is discussed in the next section, CTA may be less costly, may require less physician supervision, provides faster patient throughput, and is better tolerated by claustrophobic patients. However, CTA does utilize some ionizing radiation and requires contrast doses associated with slightly higher complication rates.

MAGNETIC RESONANCE IMAGING

For **MRI**, the patient is placed within a uniform, powerful magnetic field. The procedure is based on the resultant interaction within body tissues between pulsed magnetic waves and nuclei of interest. Hydrogen nuclei (such as those in water) absorb energy and are deflected from their alignment. As the nuclei return from a stage of excitation to their rest state, a signal is induced in a receiver, which converts it into a diagnostic image. During the process of energy release en route to tissue relaxation, two tissue-specific relaxation constants (T1, longitudinal or spin-lattice relaxation time, and T2, transverse or spin-spin relaxation time) can be used to reconstruct **T1-weighted images**, in which CSF has decreased signal intensity relative to the brain and fat has increased signal (ventricles appear dark, and gray matter is darker than white matter), and **T2-weighted images**, in which CSF has increased signal relative to the brain (ventricles appear white, and gray matter is lighter than white matter) (Fig. 7-3).

Disease processes such as edema, ischemia, hemorrhage, tumor, abscess, and demyelination typically cause an increase in free water concentration and hence an increase in the observed T1 and T2 relaxation times. An MRI scan can be obtained to accentuate either the T1 or the T2 characteristics of the tissue. The T1 and T2 signal characteristics of cerebral infarction and cerebral hemorrhage are outlined in Table 7-2, and a cerebral infarction is shown in Figure 7-4.

MRI produces images that generally are more detailed than those of CT and that provide more information about tissue characteristics. In many cases of stroke, this technique is not superior to CT, but MRI does have some **advantages over CT**: (1) any plane can be selected (coronal, sagittal, oblique); (2) there is no ionizing radiation; (3) it is more sensitive to tissue changes (small infarcts may be detected earlier, within the first few hours, and more precisely); (4) cavernous malformations or small AVMs may be more easily visible; (5) there are no bone-related artifacts to obscure small infarctions in the vertebrobasilar system and infarcts near the skull base; (6) iodinated contrast agents are not required (paramagnetic contrast agents such as gadolinium allow differentiation of new strokes from old ones on the basis of their enhancement); (7) cerebral infarction may be differentiated from cerebral hemorrhage even after several weeks have passed; and (8) T2-weighted gradient echo MRI sequences are very sensitive to the presence of hemorrhage, including previous small intracerebral hemorrhages.

The **major disadvantages of MRI** compared with CT are that (1) slice thickness is limited (3 mm wide), (2) bone imaging is limited to the display of marrow, (3) scanning time is relatively

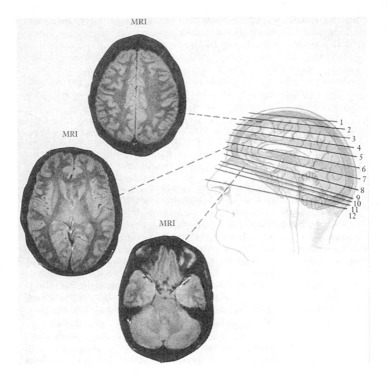

Figure 7-3.   Normal MRI head scans.

long, (4) claustrophobia occurs in approximately 10% of patients, (5) some patients do not fit into the machine, and (6) MRI cannot be done if a pacemaker or other ferromagnetic materials such as shrapnel or certain surgical clips are in the body.

Since the initial investigations into the use of MRI techniques to demonstrate vascular structures in the mid-1980s, **magnetic resonance angiography (MRA)** has become available on a widespread basis. MRA is a subtype of MRI that can noninvasively visualize extracranial and intracranial arterial and venous circulations. Major advantages over standard x-ray arteriography include imaging without administration of potentially toxic contrast media and without the risks associated with arterial puncture and catheterization. The technique is especially useful for the noninvasive identification of intracranial aneurysms (a three-dimensional image that can be rotated through 360 degrees may be obtained, a feature that is helpful for differentiating arterial loops from aneurysms). MRA also enables identification of increased intracranial vascularity that may occur with AVMs. However, MRA does not clearly distinguish high-grade, cervical vessel stenosis from occlusion; may tend to overestimate the degree of carotid arterial stenosis; cannot clearly detect intimal irregularities; does not provide

Table 7-2. Major MRI signal characteristics of cerebral infarction and cerebral hemorrhage

Type of Lesion I Hemorrhage Composition	MRI Signal Characteristics	
	T1-Weighted Image	T2-Weighted Image
Cerebral infarction	Dark	White
Cerebral hemorrhage, time (days) from stroke to MRI		
1–3 (acute) deoxyhemoglobin formation	Isodense	Dark
3–7 (early subacute) intracellular methemoglobin	White	Isodense
7–14 (late subacute) cell breakdown, free methemoglobin	White	White
>21 (chronic) hemosiderin formation	Isodense, may have dark rim	Very dark rim

MRI = magnetic resonance imaging.

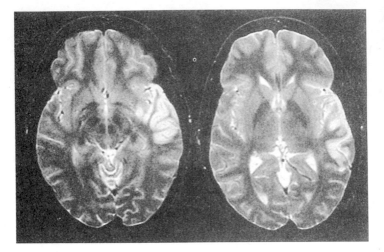

Figure 7-4.   MRI head scan 72 hours after onset of symptoms: area
of increased T2 signal in anterior temporal region consistent with
cerebral infarction.

sequential information on the filling of the cerebral circulation;
and generally has limited use in evaluation of the distal
intracranial vessels. Overall, for evaluating extracranial carotid
arteries, the ability of MRA to detect carotid arterial stenosis is
similar to that of color duplex ultrasonography. The sensitivity
and the specificity of MRA for detection of hemodynamically significant stenoses in the vertebrobasilar system is also excellent.

Significant advantages are offered by newer rapid magnetic
resonance techniques, particularly **diffusion-weighted MRI**,
which is more sensitive than CT in detecting acute ischemia and
can visualize major ischemia more easily than plain CT scan.
Diffusion-weighted imaging (DWI) follows the random motion of
water molecules throughout the brain, and, unlike standard T2
MR technique, which may detect an ischemic lesion as early as
3 hours after the ictus, DWI can detect the lesion within minutes. The increase in signal on DWI can persist for approximately 14 days after the onset of ischemia.

Perfusion-weighted MRI involves following the temporal
passage of a rapidly injected intravenous contrast agent through
contiguous slices of brain tissue as seen by rapid MRI techniques. Patients with acute ischemic stroke, low tissue perfusion
(suggesting low blood flow), and relatively normal DWI (suggesting little or no cytotoxic edema associated with early infarction) have been considered to have **diffusion–perfusion mis-
matches**, which may reflect a greater likelihood of reversibility
of the ischemic deficit after thrombolytic therapy.

Magnetic resonance spectroscopy provides information
about the biochemical state of the ischemic brain. Its diagnostic
and prognostic importance have not yet been delineated clearly.
In addition, its clinical use for patients in the acute phase of

stroke is limited by long acquisition times and wider slice thickness, precluding sufficient detail to be useful in some stroke syndromes.

CEREBRAL ARTERIOGRAPHY

Cerebral arteriography remains the only method for complete study of both the extracranial and the intracranial vasculature. It allows visualization of all phases of the cerebral circulation, including the distal intracranial arteries and venous drainage.

Arteriography is the most reliable method for demonstrating occlusion, recanalization, ulceration, and intraluminal thrombus in large arteries as well as stenosis and irregularity of distal intracranial segments of large and small arteries. It is also used for detailed study of aneurysms and AVMs. However, arteriography does not reliably image vessels that are <0.5 mm in diameter and is usually not helpful for determining the cause of deep lacunar infarctions.

Even in the most skilled hands, neurologic complications occur either during or soon after cerebral arteriography in 2% to 4% of patients with cerebrovascular disease, including transient neurologic deficit in 1.8% to 2.9%, permanent neurologic deficit in 0.1% to 0.6%, and death in 0.1% to 0.5%. These complications may result from embolization of arteriosclerotic plaque or thrombus dislodged by the catheter tip, from the toxic effect of the contrast medium, or from vasospasm after injection of the contrast agent. The risk for complications increases with advanced age or impaired renal function and may be reduced with use of nonionic contrast material (such as iohexol, iopamidol).

Important indications for cerebral arteriography are (1) stroke syndromes in which arteritis or luminal thrombus is a diagnostic consideration; (2) subarachnoid hemorrhage to determine the presence of an underlying aneurysm or vascular malformation; (3) intracerebral hemorrhage not clearly caused by hypertension or amyloid angiopathy, with negative noninvasive imaging with MRI and MRA; and (4) better delineation of the characteristics of an arterial aneurysm or AVM.

Digital subtraction angiography (DSA) uses a computerized technique to subtract or de-emphasize unwanted images to accentuate intracranial and extracranial vascular structures. It may be performed with intravenous (IV) administration of contrast material or intra-arterial injection of contrast material. The major advantages of DSA over standard arteriography are that (1) it is faster, (2) it requires less contrast material for intraarterial injection and therefore has less risk for complications, and (3) IV DSA causes less discomfort and still allows some visualization of extracranial vessels and very good visualization of intracranial veins. DSA also has some disadvantages compared with standard arteriography: (1) IV DSA results in superimposition of vessels, which may mask an abnormality; (2) IV DSA has limited spatial resolution, which may prevent visualization of small intracranial vessels; (3) even a small movement, such as swallowing by the patient during DSA, can produce artifacts that result in image blurring; and (4) the quantity of contrast medium used for intravenous injection is much more than that needed for standard arteriography and is more likely to cause renal damage (especially in older patients and those with diabetes mellitus and/or impaired renal function) and allergic reactions.

ELECTROCARDIOGRAPHY AND ECHOCARDIOGRAPHY

The heart should be assessed in all patients with cerebrovascular disease. **Electrocardiography** may rapidly reveal evidence of myocardial ischemia or infarction, dysrhythmias (especially atrial fibrillation), or left ventricular hypertrophy as potential causes of ischemic stroke or TIA. Continuous **electrocardiographic** (Holter) **monitoring** for detecting chronic or intermittent cardiac arrhythmia may be used in patients who have possible embolic events and in whom another source of the event is not defined. Transthoracic (TTE) and transesophageal **echocardiography** (TEE) are relatively safe methods of evaluating cardiac anatomy and allow detection of potential cardiogenic sources of cerebral embolism, such as left atrial thrombi, left atrial appendage thrombi, atrial septal aneurysm, and patent foramen ovale with right-to-left shunt; left ventricular thrombus; ventricular aneurysm; valvular or cardiac mass lesions; and cardiomyopathy (Table 7-3). Other findings, which are less likely to be associated with a high frequency of TIA and stroke, include spontaneous echocardiographic contrast, mitral valve prolapse, hypokinetic left ventricular segments, and valvular strands. Aortic arch atheromatous debris seems to be a marker for systemic atherosclerosis rather than a common primary source of emboli, but this is still under evaluation. More recently, indicators of diastolic dysfunction, such as increased

Table 7-3.   TEE and TTE for detecting cardiac sources of embolism

Detected Better by TEE	Detected Better or Equally Well by TTE
Atrial septal aneurysm	Left ventricular thrombus
Atrial septal defect	Myxomatous mitral valvulopathy with prolapse
Patent foramen ovale	Mitral annular calcification
Atrial myxoma	Mitral stenosis
Atrial thrombus	Aortic stenosis
Atrial appendage thrombus	Aortic valve vegetations
Aortic arch atheroma/thrombi	
Mitral valve vegetations	
Infective endocarditis	
Nonbacterial thrombotic endocarditis	

TEE = transesophageal echocardiography; TTE = transthoracic echocardiography.
Source: From Sherman DG, Dyken ML Jr, Fisher M, et al. Antithrombotic therapy for cerebrovascular disorders. *Chest.* 1992;102[Suppl]: 5295–537S.

left atrial volume (more accurately depicted on TTE than TEE) have been associated with an increased risk for developing certain ischemic stroke risk factors, including atrial fibrillation and congestive heart failure.

TEE should be reserved for patients with one or more cerebral ischemic events of unknown or uncertain cause, in whom the detection of a cardiac source would lead to a change in therapy.

NONINVASIVE NEUROVASCULAR STUDIES

The various noninvasive neurovascular studies can be divided into two major groups: indirect studies, such as ophthalmodynamometry, ocular pneumoplethysmography, and periorbital directional Doppler ultrasonography; and direct studies, such as real-time B-scan ultrasonic arteriography, duplex scanning, and transcranial Doppler ultrasonography (see previous discussions of CTA, under Computed Tomography, and MRA, under Magnetic Resonance Imaging).

Indirect techniques use the ophthalmic and external carotid arterial systems for indirect assessment of the more proximal carotid system hemodynamics. All indirect techniques are designed to detect the presence or the absence of lesions that compromise 75% or more of the luminal area (equivalent to 50% or more reduction in diameter in all planes) somewhere within the internal carotid system proximal to and including the ophthalmic artery. None of the techniques can localize the lesion within the internal carotid system, detect mild stenosis or ulceration within lesions, or reliably differentiate high-grade stenosis from occlusion.

Direct techniques provide physiologic or morphologic data about the external and internal carotid arteries in the neck and some proximal intracranial arteries. The B-mode and duplex scanning techniques are particularly sensitive for detecting mild degrees of stenosis at or near the carotid bifurcation, but the results of these studies may be adversely affected by calcified plaques that prevent transmission of the Doppler signal and produce acoustic shadowing. Technical difficulties also often occur in patients who have large, short necks or a very high carotid bifurcation. The differentiation of fresh thrombus from moving blood with B-scanning is also problematic, but difficulties can be overcome with the Doppler flow velocity analysis instrumentation incorporated into the duplex scanner.

The clinical application of noninvasive cerebrovascular studies varies widely. Although arteriography remains the most informative study regarding the cerebral circulation, noninvasive studies provide useful information without the risks associated with arteriography and, in recent years, have increasingly replaced conventional arteriography. Noninvasive studies are often used to select which patients may be the most likely to benefit from carotid arteriography and endarterectomy procedures. The studies also may be used repeatedly to follow the condition of the carotid circulation in patients who receive various forms of medical or surgical treatment. As the quality of MRA and CTA studies has increased, these tests have been used increasingly to screen for and assess patients with intracranial aneurysms. The results of all of the above tests must be interpreted in light of the clinical situation, because patients with symptoms may have test results that are negative.

Although the direct tests now are used much more frequently than the indirect tests, the indirect tests may be more cost-effective in certain situations, such as screening for high-grade asymptomatic carotid stenosis. In addition, the indirect and direct tests complement each other and may be useful in combination because they provide different types of information. Major principles underlying each of the various noninvasive techniques are outlined in Table 7-4.

Ophthalmodynamometry

Ophthalmodynamometry provides a measure of the central retinal artery pressure and yields information about pressure-significant (75% or more stenosis of the area) ipsilateral lesions of the internal carotid system proximal to and including the central retinal artery. The examiner applies pressure to the side of the globe of the eye with a calibrated, handheld ophthalmodynamometer while observing the patient's central retinal artery with an ophthalmoscope. As the intraocular pressure is increased, the point at which pulsations appear is the diastolic pressure and the point at which pulsations are eliminated is the systolic pressure. Criteria for abnormality include a 15% or more decrease in the systolic pressure of the retinal artery or a 50% or more decrease in the diastolic pressure of the retinal artery in one eye compared with that in the other. Absolute systolic retinal artery pressures <40 mm Hg are also considered abnormal in the absence of systolic hypertension. The procedure requires great technical expertise, and results may be subject to wide variation.

Ocular Pneumoplethysmography

Ocular pneumoplethysmography provides a simultaneous measure of the systolic pressures of the ophthalmic arteries by an air-filled system. Suction is applied to the anesthetized sclera by eye cups that serve as pressure transducers, and the resulting scleral displacement creates an increase in intraocular pressure that can be measured precisely. Recordings are made during continuous release of the applied vacuum (300 to 500 mm Hg). The point at which the ophthalmic artery pressure overcomes intraocular pressure and produces ocular pulsations represents the systolic pressure of the ophthalmic artery. Asymmetry in ophthalmic artery systolic pressure of 5 mm Hg or more indicates a pressure-significant stenosis of the internal cerebral artery on the side with lower pressure proximal to the central retinal artery.

The systolic pressures of the ophthalmic arteries also are expressed routinely as fractions of the systolic pressures of the brachial arteries. When these ratios decrease below calculated critical values, pressure-significant stenoses can be identified with or without asymmetries in the systolic pressure of the ophthalmic arteries. This technique also may be used for measuring collateral pressure around either carotid system by common carotid artery compression maneuvers performed during ocular pneumoplethysmographic testing. The technique

Table 7-4. Major principles underlying indirect and direct noninvasive techniques

Technique	Factor Measured	Lesions Detected by Luminal Area Stenosis (%)	Accuracy (Agreement with Arteriogram; %)	Limitations[a]
Indirect				
Ophthalmodynamometry	Retinal arterial pulse pressure	75–100	60–76	Do not detect ulceration, do not differentiate high-grade stenosis from occlusion, do not evaluate posterior circulation, do not detect lesions with <75% area of stenosis, do not localize pressure-significant lesions
Ocular pneumoplethysmography	Systolic ophthalmic arterial pressure	75–100	90–95	
Periorbital Doppler ultrasonography	Flow (collateral flow)	75–100	50–90	
Direct				
Real-time B-scan ultrasonic arteriography	Morphology of the arterial wall	<10–100	75–85	Do not detect lesions outside carotid bifurcation area, do not evaluate posterior circulation, affected by calcium in arterial wall
Duplex scanning	Blood velocities and arterial wall morphology	<10–100	90–95	

(Continued)

Table 7-4. *Continued*

Technique	Factor Measured	Lesions Detected by Luminal Area Stenosis (%)	Accuracy (Agreement with Arteriogram; %)	Limitations[a]
Transcranial Doppler ultrasonography	Blood velocities	<10–100	75–85	Inadequate bony windows resulting in nondiagnostic transcranial Doppler studies in 4% to 10% of patients

[a]Limitations of the techniques can be minimized to some extent by using tests in combination, especially direct and indirect tests.

is highly reproducible when performed by trained technicians and is not subject to as much operator-dependent variation as other noninvasive neurovascular studies.

Periorbital Directional Doppler Ultrasonography

Periorbital directional Doppler ultrasonography assesses the direction and the quality of blood flow in the periorbital arteries and the response of these variables to arterial compression maneuvers about the face and neck. Because the periorbital arteries are terminal branches of the ophthalmic artery, blood flow is normally directed out of the orbit and may be augmented by external compression of carotid artery branches.

After locating one or more periorbital vessels near the orbital rim, the examiner positions the Doppler probe over the vessel to be studied. Reversed flow indicates extracranial collateral flow, usually resulting from a pressure-significant stenosis of the ipsilateral internal carotid system. The source of collateral flow is often better defined by sequentially compressing the superficial temporal, infraorbital, and facial arteries on each side of the head. A diminution or obliteration of periorbital flow indicates that the compressed vessel supplies collateral flow via the external carotid system. Compression of the common carotid artery may detect pressure-significant stenosis of the internal carotid system when intracranial collateral circulation from the circle of Willis maintains periorbital blood flow in the normal direction. In such instances, periorbital blood flow is unchanged or augmented by ipsilateral compression of the common carotid artery.

Real-Time B-Scan Ultrasonic Arteriography

A two-dimensional image of the vessel wall is created by sound waves that are generated and recorded from an **ultrasonic B-mode probe**. Because the sound waves are reflected differently from interfaces of different acoustic impedance, the common and proximal internal and external carotid arteries in the neck can be identified. The blood column is generally sonolucent, but the vessel wall and atherosclerotic deposits are comparatively dense. Both transverse and longitudinal scans are obtained, and the percentage of stenosis in any given area is estimated.

Duplex Scanning

The **duplex scanner** combines real-time B-scan ultrasound with Doppler flow velocity analysis in the same instrument. The B-scan component allows imaging of the walls of the common carotid, internal carotid, and external carotid arteries, and a pulsed Doppler cursor is placed within the lumen of any of the arteries to record flow velocity signals that subsequently can be analyzed by audiofrequency or color-coding methods. The ability of continuous-wave Doppler sonography to identify reliably both obstructive cervical carotid artery disease and subclavian artery obstructions makes it particularly useful in screening patients who are being considered for surgical revascularization.

Color-coded duplex sonography allows characterization of fresh thrombotic material adjacent to the vessel wall and facilitates detection of ulceration within carotid artery lesions. The sensitivity of color-coded duplex sonography compared with that of conventional arteriography for detecting carotid occlusive disease is >90%; thus, this technique is useful for rapid identification of patients who are at high risk for stroke from high-grade stenosis of the carotid bifurcation area and for studies of the development of atherogenesis and carotid plaques.

Transcranial Doppler Ultrasonography

Transcranial Doppler ultrasonography was introduced in 1982 as a noninvasive procedure for assessment of the intracranial cerebral circulation. The principle of transcranial Doppler is that a range-gated, low-frequency, pulsed-Doppler ultrasonic beam of 2 MHz crosses the intact skull at points known as windows and allows noninvasive study of the hemodynamic characteristics (blood flow velocity, direction of flow, collateral patterns, and state of cerebral vasoreactivity) of the basal cerebral blood vessels (Fig. 7-5). Such criteria as window used, depth of sampling, direction of flow, and velocity measurements allow specific identification of the intracranial arteries. As with other noninvasive techniques, the physician must be familiar with the capabilities and the limitations of transcranial Doppler technology to make clinical decisions that are based on test results. Clinicians will find transcranial Doppler studies most helpful if they have specific questions about the status of the intracranial circulation.

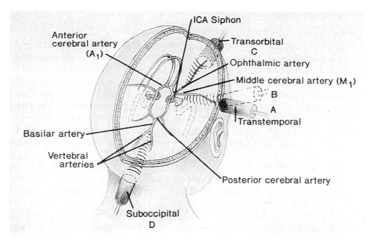

Figure 7-5.   Transcranial Doppler ultrasound windows.
Transtemporal approach (A and B) is used to insonate middle cerebral artery stem (M_1); A_1 segment of anterior cerebral artery (A_1); distalmost segment of internal carotid artery siphon (ICA Siphon); and P_1 and P_2 segments of posterior cerebral artery. Transorbital window (C) is used for insonation of ophthalmic artery and immediately supraclinoid and infraclinoid segments of internal carotid artery siphon. Suboccipital transcranial window (D) is used for insonation of distal intracranial segments of both vertebral arteries and basilar artery.

The procedure is safe and can be relatively fast (taking 20 to 60 minutes), but it requires patience to detect the signal and then to find the best angle for insonation at a given depth, because even minor anatomic variations can cause misleading changes in signal strength. Intracranial stenosis is identified by increased blood flow velocities to levels >2 standard deviations from normal, and spectrum analysis of the signals allows estimation of the degree of the stenosis. A challenge test of contralateral compression of the carotid artery can be done to determine whether the effects of unilateral extracranial stenosis are compensated or lack anatomic collaterals.

Established clinical indications and potential applications for transcranial Doppler testing are outlined in Table 7-5. Transcranial Doppler ultrasonography is currently used for detection of stenoses of the major intracranial arteries, monitoring and early diagnosis of vasospasm in patients with aneurysmal subarachnoid hemorrhage, assessing intracranial collateral flow in patients with extracranial arterial occlusive disease, detecting intracranial arterial stenosis, identifying the feeding

Table 7-5. Established clinical indications and potential applications for transcranial Doppler testing

Established Clinical Indications	Potential Applications
1. Assessment of pattern and extent of intracranial collateral circulation in patients with known regions of severe stenosis or occlusion in the internal carotid arteries, vertebral arteries, or subclavian arteries	1. Preoperative, intraoperative, and postoperative monitoring of neurosurgical patients (such as monitoring of patients during carotid endarterectomy and other revascularization procedures; intraoperative and postoperative study of the hemodynamic behavior of AVMs)
2. Detection of hemodynamically significant stenosis in the major intracranial arteries at the base of the brain	2. Monitoring intracranial pressure in patients with head injury, intracranial hemorrhage, brain tumor, or hypoxia
3. Assessment and follow-up of patients with vasoconstriction of any cause, especially vasospasm that occurs after subarachnoid hemorrhage	3. Research applications (e.g., investigation of cerebral hemodynamic changes in response to physiologic and pharmacologic stimuli investigation of pathophysiologic mechanisms involved in stroke in patients with sickle cell disease, migraine, cerebral vasculitis, and other conditions)
4. Detection of AVMs and study of their feeding arteries and the hemodynamic effects of treatment	
5. Confirmation of clinical diagnosis of brain death	

AVM = arteriovenous malformation.
Source: Adapted from Petty GW, Wiebers DO, Meissner I. Transcranial Doppler ultrasonography: clinical applications in cerebrovascular disease. *Mayo Clin Proc.* 1990;65:1350–1364.

arteries of AVMs and monitoring the hemodynamic effects of their treatment, confirming the clinical diagnosis of brain death, monitoring of brain-injured patients in intensive care units, and intraoperative and postoperative emboli monitoring of patients who have had neurosurgical procedures (including interventional neuroradiology). In addition to the obvious advantage of being noninvasive, transcranial Doppler ultrasonography is performed with lightweight, portable equipment; therefore, bedside assessment of critically ill hospitalized patients and also outpatients is possible. However, approximately 10% of all patients have inadequate bony windows to allow the pulsed-Doppler ultrasonic beam to insonate the intracranial vessels, which precludes completion of the study.

HEMATOLOGIC STUDIES

The **clinical and biochemical analysis** of peripheral blood is important in the evaluation of all patients with cerebrovascular diseases, because specific hematologic disorders may be the primary cause of cerebral ischemia or hemorrhage, and other hematologic abnormalities may predispose to cerebrovascular occlusive disorders.

Specific **hematologic disorders** that are associated with cerebrovascular events are hereditary deficiency of coagulation inhibitors or hereditary abnormalities of fibrinolysis, elevated concentration of coagulation factors, autoantibody syndromes, polycythemia vera, leukemia other hematologic malignancies, sickle cell disease, platelet disorders, and secondary polycythemias.

Several **tests** are available to aid the physician in the diagnosis and management of these hematologic conditions: determination of platelet count, hemoglobin and hematocrit values, leukocyte count, prothrombin time, partial thromboplastin time, bleeding time, fibrinogen level, lupus anticoagulant, and anticardiolipin antibody and homocysteine levels; hemoglobin electrophoresis; protein C and protein S assay; antithrombin III assay; evaluation for resistance to activated protein C; evaluation for the prothrombin gene mutation; and assessment for factor V Leiden deficiency. Some of the hematologic findings are greater risk factors for venous thrombosis rather than arterial thrombosis, so any positive findings must be put into the clinical context.

Other blood tests may be needed in patients with cerebrovascular disease. Blood urea nitrogen and serum creatinine analyses help to exclude renal disease, which might be a cause of chronic hypertension. Elevated total cholesterol and low-density lipoprotein cholesterol levels and a low level of high-density lipoprotein cholesterol and lipoprotein (a) often are associated with atheromatous plaques in the cerebral arteries and an increased risk for stroke. Although fasting blood glucose and glycosylated hemoglobin levels are generally good indicators of diabetes mellitus and diabetes control, transient hyperglycemia and glycosuria may also follow hemorrhagic or ischemic stroke.

Marked elevation of the erythrocyte sedimentation rate occurs in temporal arteritis but also occurs in other conditions, such as systemic infection and malignancy. The leukocyte count in the peripheral blood is usually normal in patients with ischemic stroke, but it may be increased after intracerebral hemorrhage or ischemic stroke caused by septic embolus (usually indicating an infection when associated with a polymorphonucleocytosis). Increased platelet aggregability may be associated with TIA or cerebral infarction, particularly in young patients. The treponemal antibody absorption test helps to exclude syphilis. The C-reactive protein (CRP) is an acute-phase protein; the level may be useful in defining the presence of inflammation in the arterial wall. CRP elevation may predict an increased risk for myocardial infarction and sudden cardiac death, but its use as a predictor of future cerebral infarction is less certain.

LUMBAR PUNCTURE

Lumbar puncture (LP) is not performed routinely in cases of stroke but is reserved for circumstances in which CT and MRI are nondiagnostic or unavailable or for specific diagnostic problems, especially in cases of possible subarachnoid hemorrhage, meningitis, encephalitis, or inflammatory disorders. In cases of possible subarachnoid hemorrhage, when the patient's clinical history is suggestive but the CT (or MRI) scan is negative, LP is usually indicated (often postponed 6 to 12 hours after the ictus). LP that is done at least 12 hours after the subarachnoid hemorrhage can detect reliably xanthochromia, but xanthochromia usually disappears by 21 days after the ictus. Relative contraindications to LP include (1) increased intracranial pressure, especially in cases of an intracranial mass lesion (for example, hematoma or tumor), particularly in the posterior fossa, and (2) hypocoagulable states.

When LP is performed, strict aseptic technique is required, and correct positioning of the patient is essential (Fig. 7-6). The patient's back should be perpendicular to the bed, knees drawn up to the chest, the neck flexed, and the head level with the LP needle. The L3-L4 interspace lies directly between the two superior iliac crests and is most easily identified for LP. Local anesthetic should be injected intradermally in the center of the selected interspace and into deeper tissues along the anticipated tract of the spinal puncture needle (but not into the subarachnoid space).

After waiting several minutes, the physician should insert the LP needle with the stylet in place through the patient's skin at a slight angle toward the patient's head, parallel to the spinous processes. As the needle penetrates the ligamentum flavum, there is often a sudden decrease in resistance, after which the stylet is removed and CSF is collected (if no fluid emerges, then the needle may be rotated and withdrawn a few millimeters). After the LP is completed, the patient should be encouraged to remain lying down for the next 6 to 8 hours (preferably supine) and to drink extra fluid. These measures help to avoid spinal headache, which occurs in approximately 10% of patients as a result of persistent leakage of CSF from the subarachnoid space. Spinal headache is usually positional in nature, exacerbated with standing or sitting, and relieved by lying down. The headache can usually be treated with bed rest, analgesics, and hydration. The post-LP headache treatments of proven efficacy include oral or IV caffeine, epidural saline, and epidural patches with autologous blood, whereas neither the duration of recumbency after a

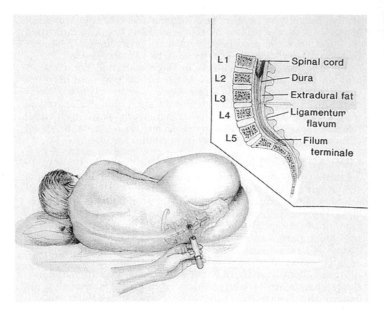

Figure 7-6.   Technique of LP.

diagnostic LP nor the use of increased fluids seems to influence or prevent the occurrence of post-LP headache.

To differentiate whether blood found in CSF is the result of subarachnoid hemorrhage or a traumatic tap (puncture of a blood vessel by the spinal needle), the CSF should be collected in three tubes. A traumatic tap usually results in a diminishing number of erythrocytes in each successive tube. If this change is noted, it is advisable to discard the initial few milliliters and collect only the clear fluid, which should be centrifuged promptly. Clear supernatant fluid characterizes the traumatic puncture, whereas a xanthochromic supernatant indicates that the blood has been in contact with the CSF for at least several hours and, therefore, antedates the LP. However, the supernatant fluid can be clear if a spontaneous subarachnoid hemorrhage has occurred within 1 to 2 hours of collection of the fluid, and xanthochromia may occur in traumatic LP, with erythrocyte counts exceeding 200,000 per µl. Differentiation of subarachnoid hemorrhage from traumatic LP may also be possible with the D-dimer assay, although this is still being evaluated.

The opening pressure should be recorded during the procedure, and the CSF should be examined for appearance, cell count, and glucose and protein levels. Some characteristics of normal and abnormal CSF are presented in Table 7-6.

The CSF is bloody in almost all patients with subarachnoid hemorrhage, in 85% of those with intraparenchymal hemorrhage, and in only 10% of those with cerebral infarction. The leukocyte count of the CSF is usually normal in patients with

Table 7-6. Some characteristics of normal and abnormal CSF

CSF Characteristics	Normal CSF	CSF Abnormalities and Their Possible Causes
Appearance	Clear and colorless	**Bloody CSF:** traumatic tap, subarachnoid hemorrhage, intraparenchymal hemorrhage, intraventricular hemorrhage **Yellowish color in the CSF (xanthochromia):** recent subarachnoid bleeding, subdural hematoma, intracerebral hematoma, purulent meningitis, Guillain-Barre syndrome, acoustic neuroma, spinal block, hyperbilirubinemia **Turbid to cloudy:** acute purulent meningitis, acute tuberculous or syphilitic meningitis
Opening pressure	60–140 mm Hg	**High pressure:** meningitis, mass lesion (e.g., tumor, abscess, hematoma, large infarction), benign intracranial hypertension **Low pressure:** spinal block, intracranial hypotension
Cells	<5 lymphocytes or mononuclear cells	**Lymphocytosis** Infections: bacterial (resolving or partially treated), viral, fungal, mycobacterial, syphilis, Lyme, HIV, parasitic, parameningeal (e.g., sinusitis, mastoiditis, subdural empyema, epidural abscess) Vascular: cerebral infarct, cerebral angiitis, cerebral hemorrhage, sinus thrombosis Inflammatory: multiple sclerosis, systemic vasculitides affecting CNS, Guillain-Barre syndrome, sarcoidosis Neoplastic: meningeal carcinomatosis and lymphomatosis, some primary CNS tumors Other: chemical meningitis, drug-related, Mollaret's meningitis, Behçet's disease

(Continued)

Table 7-6. *Continued*

CSF Characteristics	Normal CSF	CSF Abnormalities and Their Possible Causes
		Polymorphonuclear leukocytes: bacterial infections, early in viral, fungal, and mycobacterial infection, brain abscess, subdural empyema, spinal epidural abscess, sphenoid sinusitis/abscess, septic cerebral emboli (infective endocarditis), chemical meningitis, Mollaret's meningitis
		Erythrocytes: traumatic tap, subarachnoid hemorrhage, intraventricular hemorrhage
Malignant cells	No	Meningeal carcinomatosis
Total protein	15–45 mg/dl	**Protein concentration** may be increased in association with various types of infection (see above for lymphocytosis and polymorphonuclear leukocytes), cerebral infarction, intracranial hemorrhage, spinal block, cerebral tumor (benign or malignant), meningeal carcinomatosis or lymphomatosis, inflammatory disorders (e.g., cerebral angiitis, chemical meningitis, Mollaret's meningitis, Behçet's disease, sarcoidosis)
IgG index	<8.4 mg/dl	**Gamma globulin, IgG, or IgM value** usually is increased in demyelinating disease of any kind; with neurosyphilis and subacute sclerosing panencephalitis; with other inflammatory diseases of the CNS; and with cirrhosis, sarcoidosis, myxedema, multiple myeloma
Newborn's IgM	37–374 ng/ml	
Gamma globulin	6%–13% of total protein	
Oligoclonal bands	0–1 band	**Raised** in patients with demyelinating diseases, neurosyphilis, subacute sclerosing panencephalitis, fungal meningitis, progressive rubellar panencephalitis

Myelin basic protein	0–4 ng/ml	
Glucose	45–80 mg/dl or 60%–80% plasma glucose	**Reduced** in various infections, including parameningeal infections (e.g., purulent, tuberculous, fungal, syphilis, granulomatous, mumps, herpetic meningoencephalitis), subarachnoid hemorrhage (most often in the first week), carcinomatous meningitis, Mollaret's meningitis, Behçet's disease, chemical meningitis, blood hypoglycemia

CNS = central nervous system; CSF = cerebrospinal fluid; HIV = human immunodeficiency virus; IgG = immunoglobulin G; IgM = immunoglobulin M.

cerebral infarction (a pleocytosis as high as 50 cells per μl is occasionally found). In cases of septic cerebral embolism and in rare cases of intracerebral hematoma, a moderate or severe pleocytosis as high as 4000 cells per μl may be found even in the absence of infection, as a result of an aseptic meningeal reaction. The aseptic nature of the reaction can be verified by a normal CSF glucose level and the absence of micro-organisms in the fluid. The CSF protein content increases in direct proportion to the amount of blood present in the fluid (1000 erythrocytes per 1 mg of CSF protein). However, hemolyzed erythrocytes (such as those found in subarachnoid bleeding) may increase the CSF protein to many times this ratio.

In cases of suspected acute infection of the central nervous system, with or without potential cerebrovascular symptoms, an examination of CSF should be performed. Urgent Gram stain, antigen detection, and cultures for bacteria are indicated; and fungal, viral, and mycobacterial cultures are required in selected cases. In patients with positive serum serologic results for syphilis or other reason to suspect neurosyphilis, a Venereal Disease Research Laboratory study of CSF is needed. Herpes zoster, herpes simplex, and Lyme disease studies may also be performed in certain situations.

ANCILLARY STUDIES

Electroencephalography

The **electroencephalogram** (**EEG**) records cortical electrical activity. In cases of stroke, the EEG is better for localizing the lesion than it is for identifying which type of stroke is present. For instance, in the case of an intracerebral hemorrhage, focal polymorphic delta activity (with or without bilateral projected dysrhythmia) may be seen on the side of the lesion, but these abnormalities are often similar to those caused by brain tumor or acute cerebral infarction. However, EEG abnormalities that are caused by acute stroke, in contrast to those that are caused by a tumor, tend to diminish progressively during the resolution of a cerebrovascular lesion. A subdural hematoma usually produces slowing or reduction in background cerebral voltage over the site of the hematoma, which seldom occurs with cerebral infarction or hemorrhage.

Within a few hours or days after an acute cortical infarction, the EEG sometimes contains periodic lateralized epileptiform discharges (PLEDS), which are frequently associated with clinical focal (partial) seizures, but these discharges are not pathognomonic for cerebral infarction, because they may result from many other types of nonvascular lesions. A small, deep cerebrovascular lesion (for instance, in the internal capsule) may produce little or no EEG abnormality, and TIAs almost never produce persistent EEG abnormalities.

The EEG may be helpful diagnostically in comatose patients who have cerebrovascular lesions involving the brainstem (typically showing prominent alpha activity and lacking normal reactivity) and as a supplementary investigation for confirming brain death in stroke patients with irreversible coma (flat or isoelectric EEG).

Plain Radiography

Because of the development of advanced radiologic and ultrasound techniques, routine skull radiography has less diagnostic value in the evaluation of patients with cerebrovascular disease, but it still has some potential applications. Skull fractures (which characteristically accompany epidural hematomas), developmental anomalies (platybasia, basilar impression, occipitalization of the atlas), bony erosion, and hyperostosis may be detected. Cervical spondylosis can cause compression of the vertebral artery in the neck when the head is turned, with resultant obstruction to blood flow and the production of symptoms of vertebrobasilar insufficiency.

Chest radiography provides an estimation of heart size and may reveal the presence of unsuspected pulmonary tumors or other disorders. It is a routine investigation in the evaluation of patients with cerebrovascular disease.

TESTS OF UNDETERMINED APPLICATION

Positron emission tomography (PET) and single photon emission CT (SPECT) are methods for imaging various aspects of brain metabolism (functional neuroimaging). However, the clinical usefulness of these methods in the evaluation of patients with cerebrovascular disorders remains uncertain; currently, neither PET nor SPECT is available on a widespread basis.

In the **SPECT** technique, a gamma camera counts (from multiple sites around the head) the density of signals that are emitted from an injected agent minutes after it is given intravenously. Scanning provides a two-dimensional image that depicts the radioactivity emitted from each pixel and detects relative regional ischemia in occlusive cerebrovascular disease. The technique is of limited usefulness in the acute stroke setting and has other limitations, including expense, tracer preparation issues, and availability.

PET uses short-lived, positron-emitting isotopes (radionuclides) in a technique similar to that of CT, but because an onsite or nearby cyclotron is needed to supply the isotopes, this study is available in only a few centers. Regional brain biochemical activity is reflected in the emitted metabolic end products of such important substrates as oxygen and glucose. Therefore, PET scanning is of particular value for investigating the relationship between cerebral blood flow and oxygen utilization in focal areas of ischemia. Although PET remains impractical in the acute stroke setting, its clinical usefulness in other settings, such as identifying patients who have carotid occlusion and may benefit from external carotid–internal carotid bypass, is currently being investigated.

SUGGESTED READING FOR PART I

Alexandrov A, ed. *Cerebrovascular Ultrasound in Stroke Prevention and Treatment*. New York: Blackwell Publishing, Inc.; 2004.

Anticardiolipin antibodies and the risk of recurrent thrombo-occlusive events and death. The Antiphospholipid Antibodies and Stroke Study Group (APASS). *Neurology*. 1997;48:91–94.

Babikian VL, Feldmann E, Wechsler LR, et al. Transcranial Doppler ultrasonography: year 2000 update. *J Neuroimaging*. 2000;10:101–115.

Boonyakarnkul S, Dennis M, Sandercock P, et al.: Primary intracerebral hemorrhage in the Oxfordshire Community Stroke Project: 1. Incidence, clinical features and causes. *Cerebrovasc Dis*. 1993;3:343–349.

Caplan L, DeWitt L, Breen J. Neuroimaging in patients with cerebrovascular disease. In: Greenberg JO, ed. *Neuroimaging*. New York: McGraw-Hill; 1999:493–520.

Cheitlin MD, Alpert JS, Armstrong WF, et al. ACC/AHA Guidelines for the Clinical Application of Echocardiography. A report of the American College of Cardiology/American Heart Association Task Force on Practice Guidelines (Committee on Clinical Application of Echocardiography). Developed in collaboration with the American Society of Echocardiography. *Circulation*. 1997;95:1686–1744.

Cheung RT, Zou LY. Use of the original, modified, or new intracerebral hemorrhage score to predict mortality and morbidity after intracerebral hemorrhage. *Stroke*. 2003;34:1717–1722.

Comess KA, DeRook FA, Beach KW, et al. Transesophageal echocardiography and carotid ultrasound in patients with cerebral ischemia: prevalence of findings and recurrent stroke risk. *J Am Coll Cardiol*. 1994;23:1598–1603.

Culebras A, Kase CS, Masdeu JC, et al. Practice guidelines for the use of imaging in transient ischemic attacks and acute stroke. A report of the Stroke Council. American Heart Association. *Stroke*. 1997;28:1480–1497.

DeRook FA, Comess KA, Albers GW, et al. Transesophageal echocardiography in the evaluation of stroke. *Ann Intern Med*. 1992;117:922–932.

Donnan GA. Investigation of patients with stroke and transient ischaemic attacks. *Lancet*. 1992;339:473–477.

Evans RW, Armon C, Frohman E, et al. Assessment: prevention of post-lumbar puncture headaches. Report of the Therapeutics and Technology Assessment Subcommittee of the American Academy of Neurology. *Neurology*. 2000;55:909–914.

Fishman RA. *Cerebrospinal Fluid in Diseases of the Nervous System*. 2nd ed. Philadelphia: WB Saunders; 1992.

Gibbs RG, Newson R, Lawrenson R, et al. Diagnosis and initial management of stroke and transient ischemic attack across UK health regions from 1992 to 1996: experience of a national primary care database. *Stroke*. 2001;32:1085–1090.

Goldstein LB, Matchar DB. Clinical assessment of stroke. *JAMA*. 1994;271:1114–1120.

Gomes AS. Aortic arch studies and selective arteriography. In: Moore WS, ed. *Surgery for cerebrovascular disease*. New York: Churchill Livingstone; 1987:399–416.

Hanson SK, Grotta JC, Rhoades H, et al. Value of single-photon emission-computed tomography in acute stroke therapeutic trials. *Stroke.* 1993;24:1322–1329.

Hardemark HG, Wesslen N, Persson L. Influence of clinical factors, CT findings and early management on outcome in supratentorial intracerebral hemorrhage. *Cerebrovasc Dis.* 1999;9:10–21.

Harjai KJ. Potential new cardiovascular risk factors: left ventricular hypertrophy, homocysteine, lipoprotein(a), triglycerides, oxidative stress, and fibrinogen. *Ann Intern Med.* 1999;131:376–386.

Job FP, Ringelstein EB, Grafen Y, et al. Comparison of transcranial contrast Doppler sonography and transesophageal contrast echocardiography for the detection of patent foramen ovale in young stroke patients. *Am J Cardiol.* 1994;74:381–384.

Johnston DC, Goldstein LB. Clinical carotid endarterectomy decision making: noninvasive vascular imaging versus angiography. *Neurology.* 2001;56:1009–1015.

Jones EF, Donnan GA, Calafiore P, et al. Transoesophageal echocardiography in the investigation of stroke: experience in 135 patients with cerebral ischaemic events. *Aust N Z J Med.* 1993;23:477–483.

Kimura K, Minematsu K, Wada K, et al. Lesions visualized by contrast-enhanced magnetic resonance imaging in transient ischemic attacks. *J Neurol Sci.* 2000;173:103–108.

Kittner SJ, Sharkness CM, Sloan MA, et al. Infarcts with a cardiac source of embolism in the NINDS Stroke Data Bank: neurologic examination. *Neurology.* 1992;42:299–302.

Kucharczyk J, Moseley M, Barkovich AJ, eds. *Magnetic Resonance Neuroimaging.* Boca Raton: CRC Press; 1994.

Lang DT, Berberian LB, Lee S, et al. Rapid differentiation of subarachnoid hemorrhage from traumatic lumbar puncture using the D-dimer assay. *Am J Clin Pathol.* 1990;93:403–405.

Nederkoorn PJ, van der Graaf Y, Hunink MG: Duplex ultrasound and magnetic resonance angiography compared with digital subtraction angiography in carotid artery stenosis: a systematic review. *Stroke.* 2003;34:1324–1332.

Newell DW, Aaslid R, eds. *Transcranial Doppler.* New York: Raven Press; 1992.

Niedermeyer E. Cerebrovascular disorders and EEG. In: Niedermeyer E, Lopes da Silva F, eds. *Electroencephalography: basic principles, clinical applications, and related fields.* Baltimore: Williams & Wilkins; 1993:305–327.

Nuwer MR, Arnadottir G, Martin NA, et al. A comparison of quantitative electroencephalography, computed tomography, and behavioral evaluations to localize impairment in patients with stroke and transient ischemic attacks. *J Neuroimaging.* 1994;4:82–84.

Peter JB. *Use and Interpretation of Laboratory Tests in Neurology.* 2nd ed. Santa Monica: Specialty Laboratories; 1993–1994.

Petty GW, Wiebers DO, Meissner I. Transcranial Doppler ultrasonography: clinical applications in cerebrovascular disease. *Mayo Clin Proc.* 1990;65:1350–1364.

Quast MJ, Huang NC, Hillman GR, et al. The evolution of acute stroke recorded by multimodal magnetic resonance imaging. *Magn Reson Imaging*. 1993;11:465–471.

Riles TS, Eidelman EM, Litt AW, et al. Comparison of magnetic resonance angiography, conventional angiography, and duplex scanning. *Stroke*. 1992;23:341–346.

Scarabino T, Carriero A, Giannatempo GM, et al. Contrast-enhanced MR angiography (CE MRA) in the study of the carotid stenosis: comparison with digital subtraction angiography (DSA). *J Neuroradiol*. 1999;26:87–91.

Shrier DA, Tanaka H, Numaguchi Y, et al. CT angiography in the evaluation of acute stroke. *AJNR Am J Neuroradiol*. 1997;18:1011–1020.

Shuaib A, Lee D, Pelz D, et al. The impact of magnetic resonance imaging on the management of acute ischemic stroke. *Neurology*. 1992;42:816–818.

Stroke—1989. Recommendations on stroke prevention, diagnosis, and therapy. WHO Task Force on Stroke and Other Cerebrovascular Disorders. *Stroke*. 1989;20:1407–1431.

Viroslav AB, Hoffman JC Jr. The use of computed tomography in the diagnosis of stroke. *Heart Dis Stroke*. 1993;2:299–307.

Wiebers DO, Dale AJD, Kokmen E, et al., eds. *Mayo Clinic Examinations in Neurology*. 7th ed. St. Louis: Mosby; 1998.

Differential Diagnosis and Clinical Features of Cerebrovascular Disease

Differential Diagnosis Made Easy

General Approach

Differential diagnosis in cerebrovascular disease can be divided into ischemic and hemorrhagic disorders. After establishing that a condition is cerebrovascular and determining whether it is ischemic or hemorrhagic (see pages 3 to 4), the clinician must try to identify the underlying pathophysiologic mechanism for the condition. This step constitutes the bulk of the differential diagnosis in cerebrovascular disease and facilitates optimal treatment. Although the underlying mechanism cannot be identified with certainty in many cases (as much as 40%), the number of such cases can be minimized by following a systematic approach to classification and differential diagnosis.

ISCHEMIC CEREBROVASCULAR DISORDERS

Ischemic cerebrovascular disorders are often classified according to temporal profile, including transient ischemic attack (resolution of symptoms within the first 24 hours), ischemic stroke (symptoms that last longer than 24 hours), reversible ischemic neurologic deficit (term occasionally used for ischemic stroke with resolution of symptoms after 24 hours but within 3 weeks), and progressive ischemic stroke (progressive deficit, often for as long as 24 to 72 hours). However, such classification does not help to define pathophysiologic mechanisms, because each of the temporal profiles may be associated with any of the various underlying mechanisms for cerebral ischemic events.

An easy method for categorizing all ischemic conditions, which relates to the underlying pathophysiology, is to classify the mechanisms into four main groups, proceeding from proximal to distal in the arterial system: (1) cardiac disease, (2) large vessel disease (craniocervical occlusive disease), (3) small vessel disease (intracranial occlusive disease), and (4) hematologic disease (Table 8-1).

Traditional clinical and radiologic features that are considered to differentiate cardioembolic events from cerebral ischemic events of other causes have lower predictive value than previously reported. These features may be suggestive of cardioembolic cause, but the clinician must acknowledge that overlap exists. Abrupt onset of maximal neurologic deficit and hemorrhagic transformation, particularly at a subcortical site, may indicate a proximal embolic source. Suggestive clinical syndromes include cortical events, isolated Wernicke's aphasia, posterior cerebral artery ischemia with homonymous hemianopia, and top of the basilar syndrome. The findings of seizures and headache are not useful in differentiating mechanism.

Lacunar infarctions are small infarcts in noncortical cerebral sites and the brainstem and result from penetrating arteriole

Table 8-1. Four major groups of diseases associated with ischemic cerebrovascular disorders

Cardiac disorders	**Valve-related emboli:** rheumatic heart disease, calcific aortic stenosis, cardiac surgery, prosthetic heart valve, infective endocarditis, nonbacterial thrombotic endocarditis
	Intracardiac thrombus or tumor: left atrial thrombus, left ventricular thrombus, recent myocardial infarction, congestive heart failure, cardiomyopathy, atrial myxoma, cardiac fibroelastoma
	Rhythm disturbances: atrial fibrillation, atrial flutter, sick sinus syndrome, other major rhythm disturbances
	Systemic venous thrombi with right-to-left cardiac shunt: interatrial or interventricular septal defect, pulmonary vein thrombosis, pulmonary arteriovenous malformation
Large vessel diseases (craniocervical occlusive diseases)	**Atherosclerosis:** cervical arteries, aortic arch, and major intracranial arteries
	Fibromuscular dysplasia: the internal carotid arteries above the carotid bifurcation
	Carotid artery dissection: traumatic, spontaneous, or caused by fibromuscular dysplasia, aortic dissection
	Takayasu's disease (see also noninfectious arteritis, below)
	Other: vasospasm (migraine), moyamoya disease, homocystinuria, Fabry's disease, pseudoxanthoma elasticum
Small vessel diseases (intracranial occlusive diseases)	**Hypertension**
	Infectious arteritis caused by bacterial; fungal; tuberculous meningitides; or other infective processes of central nervous system, such as tertiary syphilis, malaria, Lyme disease, rickettsial diseases, mucormycosis, aspergillosis, trichinosis or schistosomiasis, herpes zoster, basal meningitis (*Cryptococcus, Histoplasma, Coccidioides*)
	Noninfectious arteritis: systemic lupus erythematosus; polyarteritis nodosa; granulomatous angiitis; temporal arteritis; drug use and abuse, including cocaine, heroin, amphetamine,

Table 8-1. *Continued*

	phencyclidine, and LSD; irradiation arteritis; Wegener's granulomatosis; sarcoidosis; Behçet's disease
Hematologic diseases	Polycythemia, thrombocythemia, thrombotic thrombocytopenic purpura, sickle cell disease, dysproteinemia, leukemia, disseminated intravascular coagulation, antiphospholipid antibody syndromes (lupus anticoagulant, anti-cardiolipin antibodies), protein C and protein S deficiency, resistance to activated protein C, antithrombin III deficiency, prothrombin gene mutation, factor V Leiden deficiency, elevated homocysteine level

LSD = lysergic acid diethylamide.

occlusion. Characteristic symptoms allow clinical characterization as a lacunar syndrome but do not suggest a clear localization, although a narrowed differential diagnosis is possible. These infarcts do not typically cause aphasia, hemianopia, significantly altered level of consciousness, seizures, or sensory or motor deficit in a single limb. Common clinical syndromes include pure motor hemiparesis with weakness in the face, arm, and leg and pure sensory stroke with numbness in the face, arm, and leg. Ataxic hemiparesis with dysmetria and weakness in the involved limbs characterizes another lacunar syndrome; dysarthria and nystagmus may also be noted. The dysarthria–clumsy hand syndrome leads to dysarthria, facial weakness, and slight weakness in the hand (see Chapter 16).

HEMORRHAGIC CEREBROVASCULAR DISORDERS

Hemorrhagic cerebrovascular diseases can be categorized into five main categories according to location from outside to inside: epidural hematoma, subdural hematoma, subarachnoid hemorrhage, intracerebral (cerebral, intraparenchymal) hemorrhage, and intraventricular hemorrhage (Table 8-2). The clinical features of hemorrhagic cerebrovascular disease vary, depending on the site and the size of the hemorrhage, but in many cases, the location helps to define its cause (see Chapter 17).

Table 8-2.   Location and associated causes of hemorrhagic cerebrovascular disorders (intracranial hemorrhage)

Location of Hemorrhage	Cause
Epidural hematoma	Head trauma; less commonly, anticoagulants, primary and metastatic neoplasm, bleeding diatheses
Subdural hematoma	Head trauma; less commonly, anticoagulants, primary and secondary neoplasm, AVM, bleeding diatheses
Subarachnoid hemorrhage	Intracranial aneurysm, AVM, head trauma, extension from intracerebral hemorrhage, bleeding diatheses, anticoagulant use, cerebral vasculitis, venous thrombosis, arterial dissection, primary and metastatic neoplasm, spinal lesions, drugs including alcohol abuse and cocaine use
Intracerebral (cerebral, intraparenchymal) hemorrhage	Hypertension, intracranial aneurysm, AVM, cerebral amyloid angiopathy, bleeding diatheses, anticoagulants, thrombolytic drugs, moyamoya disease, arterial dissection, infection, abscess, primary and metastatic brain neoplasm, venous thrombosis, drugs including cocaine, phenylpropanolamine, alcohol, and heroin use
Intraventricular hemorrhage	Hypertension, intracranial aneurysm, AVM, neoplasm of the choroid plexus, primary and metastatic brain neoplasms (see causes of intracerebral hemorrhage, above)

AVM = arteriovenous malformation.

Temporal Profile of Ischemic Cerebrovascular Diseases

The general description of focal cerebral ischemic events is based on the patient's temporal profile. The clinician should attempt to go beyond the profile, identify the underlying cause, and design a mechanism-based treatment approach. When the cause cannot be identified, treatment is less specific, again based on the temporal profile, results of available studies, probable cause given the patient's age and history, and physical examination findings.

TRANSIENT ISCHEMIC ATTACKS

Transient ischemic attacks (TIAs) are focal episodes of neurologic dysfunction caused by ischemia. They are typically rapid in onset, lasting 10 seconds to 15 minutes but occasionally as long as 24 hours. The longer the episode, the greater the likelihood of finding a cerebral infarction on computed tomography (CT) or magnetic resonance imaging (MRI). Overall, cerebral infarction in a distribution that is appropriate for the clinical symptoms is detected by radiologic imaging in approximately 30% to 50% of patients with TIA. TIAs can usually be localized to a portion of the brain that is supplied by a single vascular system. The symptoms usually reach maximum intensity within 2 minutes, often within a few seconds. Fleeting episodes that last only 1 or 2 seconds and symptoms such as unconsciousness without other symptoms of vertebrobasilar ischemia and a prolonged "marching" of symptoms are not likely to be TIAs. Positive symptoms such as tingling, repetitive rhythmic shaking of a limb, and scintillating scotomata are also uncommonly ischemic in nature. The frequency of episodes varies: Some patients experience a single attack, but others experience multiple attacks at different intervals or at increasing frequency (crescendo TIAs).

Amaurosis fugax (transient monocular blindness) is included as part of the definition of carotid system TIA, but certain **isolated symptoms**, such as vertigo, light-headedness, syncope, dysarthria, dysphagia, diplopia, dizziness (or wooziness), bowel or bladder incontinence, loss of vision associated with alteration of level of consciousness, focal symptoms associated with migraine, amnesia, and confusion are not, by definition, considered TIA.

The duration, stereotyped nature, and frequency of repetitive spells may suggest a pathophysiologic mechanism. For example, repetitive (as many as 5 to 10 per day), short-lived (<15 minutes), stereotyped spells suggest a hemodynamic mechanism with proximal arterial narrowing or occlusion associated with reduced cerebral perfusion (low flow) and inadequate collateral circulation or thrombosis at the low-flow arterial narrowing. Stereotyped focal spells may also result from seizures, migraine, positional vertigo, or other causes. The other end of the spectrum is the patient who presents with symptoms suggesting TIAs in multiple distributions occurring over a short period of time. This suggests a proximal source of embolus, a hypercoagulable state, or some disorder that can affect multiple arteries simultaneously, such as an inflammatory disorder.

TIAs should be differentiated from other conditions that result in transient focal neurologic deficit. **Migraine** is often characterized by visual auras (particularly scintillating scotoma) that march or expand across the vision of both eyes during 10 to 30 minutes. Other focal neurologic symptoms associated with migraine include marching paresthesias that characteristically start in one hand, motor disturbances (hemiplegic migraine), unilateral visual disturbances (retinal migraine), ocular movement abnormalities (ophthalmoplegic migraine), and aphasia. These symptoms sometimes occur without associated headache (migraine equivalent or migraine cine cephalgia), but they are usually followed by a unilateral throbbing headache that lasts hours to 1 or 2 days and are often associated with nausea or vomiting. Various combinations of posterior circulation symptoms that evolve over minutes, such as dysarthria, vertigo, alteration in level of consciousness, bilateral visual obscuration, and motor weakness (often occurring in young women and typically followed by a severe, often throbbing occipital headache), are referred to as **basilar migraine**.

Focal seizures commonly produce episodes of repetitive jerking, tingling, visual phenomena, or speech arrest, any of which may be followed by a generalized seizure. Typical electroencephalographic findings provide additional evidence of seizure. **Postseizure states** may also mimic or follow TIA or stroke (a focal ischemic neurologic deficit may trigger a seizure and postictal state that lasts as long as 24 hours), with the focal postictal transient deficit called a Todd's paralysis.

Multiple sclerosis occurs mainly in young patients and usually is characterized by recurrent fluctuating subacute onset (during hours or days) of symptoms with neurologic deficits that last 1 day or longer. Less commonly, the condition may be associated with gradually progressive neurologic deficit; rarely, symptoms may involve sudden-onset, short-lived spells of neurologic dysfunction called paroxysmal symptoms of multiple sclerosis, including isolated recurrent dysarthria, ataxia with hemiparesis, hemisensory symptoms, and episodic tonic spasm of the limbs. The condition typically progresses to involve various parts of the white matter of the brain and spinal cord. The diagnosis is clinical in nature, but it may be aided by ancillary studies such as MRI.

Attacks that are clinically indistinguishable from TIA can result from **small cerebral infarction or intracerebral hemorrhage.** These attacks usually last hours rather than seconds or minutes. The diagnosis is established by CT or MRI. **Arteriovenous malformations**, **brain tumors** (for instance, meningiomas, gliomas, metastases), or **subdural hematomas** may also be associated with TIA-like spells. Characteristic historical data and papilledema may or may not be present. The diagnosis is usually made with CT or MRI. Enlargement of a **saccular aneurysm** may present with transient symptoms and persistent, localized headache. Sometimes a clot that forms within the aneurysmal sac can embolize distally and cause TIAs; the diagnosis is based on arteriographic and CT or MRI findings.

Hypoglycemia with typical prodromal autonomic symptoms may mimic TIA. Prompt improvement after intravenous administration of 50% glucose helps to establish the diagnosis. **Familial paroxysmal ataxia** may also be associated with transient focal neurologic deficit and is difficult to diagnose without the characteristic family history. Many patients with episodic vertigo alone have **benign positional vertigo** unrelated to cerebral or brainstem ischemia. These patients tend to hold their head still or avoid certain head positions that exacerbate the vertigo, and the vertigo usually decreases with repeated actions that would typically precipitate the symptom (see Chapters 2 and 4). **Transient global amnesia (TGA)** is associated with the relatively sudden onset of anterograde amnesia often with some degree of retrograde amnesia (see Chapter 2). Whereas some of these episodes may be caused by a posterior circulation TIA, most are likely due to a benign, possibly migrainous cause. A key issue in differentiating this syndrome from a more definite TIA is that the patient with TGA should have no other neurologic deficit. Episodic isolated diplopia seldom relates to cerebrovascular disease. A common ocular cause is **divergence insufficiency**, which tends to develop with increasing age (see Chapters 2 and 4).

REVERSIBLE ISCHEMIC NEUROLOGIC DEFICIT

An ischemic stroke characterized by a focal neurologic deficit that persists for >24 hours but clears within 3 weeks is sometimes referred to as a **reversible ischemic neurologic deficit (RIND)**. Although the prognosis for subsequent stroke is slightly better than that of TIA, the management of TIA, RIND, and minor cerebral infarction is similar (see Appendix E-2).

ISCHEMIC STROKE

When the hemodynamic disturbance that results in stroke stabilizes, the stage of completed stroke occurs. Patients with completed ischemic stroke show no further deterioration or fluctuation of their focal neurologic deficit. Sometimes a seemingly stable ischemic stroke may change abruptly (stuttering) or may progress within hours or during a few days and result in progressive ischemic stroke that requires appropriate treatment and has a different prognosis.

PROGRESSIVE ISCHEMIC STROKE

Progressive ischemic stroke refers to a neurologic deficit that progresses or fluctuates and occurs in approximately 20% of patients with infarction in the distribution of the carotid system and in approximately 40% with infarction in the vertebrobasilar distribution. The progression may last as long as 24 to 48 hours with infarction of the carotid system and as long as 96 hours with infarction of the vertebrobasilar system. It is critical that the physician attempt to identify the underlying mechanism that is responsible for the progression. In doing so, one must consider not only the possible ischemic mechanisms that may be responsible but also other disorders that may mimic this clinical picture.

In the area of cerebral infarction, vessels in the marginally ischemic zone are maximally vasodilated, and blood flow in this region depends mainly on the patient's systemic blood pressure (BP). Some progression of the neurologic deficit as a result of widening of the marginally ischemic zone associated with a cerebral infarction may be attributed to a decrease in systemic BP. In some cases, the infarction becomes hemorrhagic and the patient has a concomitant worsening deficit. Secondary hemorrhage into infarction is more frequent in large embolic infarction, especially when the infarction is treated with anticoagulants. Gradual neurologic deterioration a few hours to 2 weeks after an arterial occlusion is a common clinical feature; the diagnosis is established by CT or MRI.

Other patients have deterioration because of cerebral edema associated with the area of cerebral infarction. Edema, which may continue to increase 3 to 5 days after the event, should be suspected in a patient who has a large hemispheric infarction with alteration of consciousness and progressive deterioration. Patients with progressing infarction have propagation of an intra-arterial thrombus or subsequent additional embolization from a proximal source with associated failure of collateral circulation and a decrease in the blood supply to the ischemic area. In contrast to patients with cerebral edema, many of these patients have sudden, stepwise increases in neurologic deficits.

Some patients who have a progressive neurologic course that may initially seem to be related to cerebral infarction have other types of intracranial pathologic processes causing their symptoms. Such processes include intracerebral hemorrhage, subdural hematoma, neoplasms (particularly malignant gliomas and metastatic tumors), infectious or inflammatory processes (e.g., encephalitis, brain abscess, demyelinating disease), and superimposed metabolic encephalopathies.

SUGGESTED READING FOR PART II

Albers GW, Caplan LR, Easton JD, et al. Transient ischemic attack—proposal for a new definition. *N Engl J Med.* 2002;347:1713–1716.

Albers GW, Hart RG, Lutsep HL, et al. AHA Scientific Statement. Supplement to the guidelines for the management of transient ischemic attacks: a statement from the Ad Hoc Committee on Guidelines for the Management of Transient Ischemic Attacks. Stroke Council, American Heart Association. *Stroke.* 1999;30:2502–2511.

Broderick JP, Adams HP, Barsan W, et al. Guidelines for the management of spontaneous intracerebral hemorrhage: a statement for healthcare professionals from a special writing group of the Stroke Council, American Heart Association. *Stroke.* 1999;30:905–915.

Brown RD Jr, Petty GW, O'Fallon WM, et al. Incidence of transient ischemic attack in Rochester, Minnesota, 1985–1989. *Stroke.* 1998;29:2109–2113.

Brown RD, Whisnant JP, Sicks JD, et al. Stroke incidence, prevalence, and survival: secular trends in Rochester, Minnesota, through 1989. *Stroke.* 1996;27:373–380.

Caplan LR, Pessin MS, Mohr JP. Vertebrobasilar occlusive disease. In: Barnett HJM, Mohr JP, Stein BM, et al., eds. *Stroke: pathophysiology, diagnosis, and management.* 2nd ed. New York: Churchill Livingstone; 1992:443–515.

Celani MG, Righetti E, Migliacci R, et al. Comparability and validity of two clinical scores in the early differential diagnosis of acute stroke. *BMJ.* 1994;308:1674–1676.

Falke P, Jerntorp P, Pessah-Rasmussen H. Differences in cardiac disease prevalence and in blood variables between major and minor stroke patients. *Int Angiol.* 1993;12:5–8.

Hart RG, Easton JD. Hemorrhagic infarcts. *Stroke.* 1986;17:586–589.

Johnston SC, Fayad PB, Gorelick PB, et al. Prevalence and knowledge of transient ischemic attack among US adults. *Neurology.* 2003;60:1429–1434.

Johnston SC, Smith WS. Practice variability in management of transient ischemic attacks. *Eur Neurol.* 1999;42:105–108.

Kimura K, Minematsu K, Yasaka M, et al. The duration of symptoms in transient ischemic attack. Neurology. 1999;52:976–980.

Koudstaal PJ, Algra A, Pop GA, et al. Risk of cardiac events in atypical transient ischaemic attack or minor stroke: the Dutch TIA Study Group. *Lancet.* 1992;340:630–633.

Koudstaal PJ, van Gijn J, Frenken CW, et al. TIA, RIND, minor stroke: a continuum, or different subgroups? Dutch TIA Study Group. *J Neurol Neurosurg Psychiatry.* 1992;55:95–97.

Libman RB, Wirkowski E, Alvir J, et al. Conditions that mimic stroke in the emergency department. Implications for acute stroke trials. *Arch Neurol.* 1995;52:1119–1122.

Lindsay KW, Bone I, Callander R. *Neurology and Neurosurgery Illustrated.* 2nd ed. Edinburgh: Churchill Livingstone; 1991.

Mazagri R, Shuaib A, Denath F, et al. Very brief transient ischemic attack. *South Med J.* 1994;87:87–88.

Melo TP, Bogousslavsky J. Specific neurologic manifestations of stroke. In: Ginsberg MD, Bogousslavsky J, eds. *Cerebrovascular disease: pathophysiology, diagnosis, and management.* Vol. 2. Massachusetts: Blackwell Science; 1998:961–985.

National Institute of Neurological Disorders and Stroke. Classification of cerebrovascular diseases III. *Stroke.* 1990;21:637–676.

Petty GW, Brown RD Jr, Whisnant JP, et al. Ischemic stroke subtypes: a population-based study of functional outcome, survival, and recurrence. *Stroke.* 2000;31:1062–1068.

van Swieten JC, Kappelle LJ, Algra A, et al. Hypodensity of the cerebral white matter in patients with transient ischemic attack or minor stroke: influence on the rate of subsequent stroke: Dutch TIA Trial Study Group. *Ann Neurol.* 1992;32:177–183.

Wain RA, Tuhrim S, D'Autrechy L, et al. The design and automated testing of an expert system for the differential diagnosis of acute stroke. *Proc Annu Symp Comput Appl Med Care.* 1991:94–98.

Whisnant JP, ed. *Stroke: Populations, Cohorts, and Clinical Trials.* Boston: Butterworth-Heinemann; 1993.

Wiebers DO, Dale AJD, Kokmen E, Swanson JW, eds. *Mayo Clinic Examinations in Neurology.* 7th ed. St. Louis: Mosby; 1998.

Williams LS, Bruno A, Rouch D, et al. Stroke patients' knowledge of stroke. Influence on time to presentation. *Stroke.* 1997;28:912–915.

Yasaka M, Yamaguchi T, Oita J, et al. Clinical features of recurrent embolization in acute cardioembolic stroke. *Stroke.* 1993;24:1681–1685.

Management Before Determination of the Mechanism of Cerebrovascular Disease

Telephone Interview and Triage

Although both the diagnostic evaluation and the initial care of many patients with acute cerebrovascular diseases are accomplished in the hospital, outpatient evaluation and treatment are provided for an increasing number of patients with cerebrovascular conditions. Outpatient management involves the efficient evaluation and treatment of underlying disease, the selection of appropriate therapy to lessen the risk for recurrence, and the treatment of physical or psychosocial complications of the disease. Many patients with transient ischemic attack (TIA), recent-onset mild to moderate symptoms from ischemic or hemorrhagic stroke, or even subarachnoid hemorrhage (SAH) may initially present in an ambulatory setting. A patient with a probable acute cerebrovascular event needs prompt and efficient evaluation to decide whether immediate hospitalization is indicated and, if not, to plan appropriate urgent outpatient evaluation and treatment.

ACUTE STROKE UNITS

Any patient with acute stroke should be admitted to a hospital stroke unit as soon as possible. There is robust evidence that stroke patients who receive organized inpatient care in a defined acute stroke unit (ASU) are more likely to be alive, independent, and living at home 1 year after the stroke. This is currently the single most effective management strategy that should be used routinely in all hospitals that admit patients with acute stroke. All patients with acute stroke, irrespective of age, stroke severity, or other considerations, should be admitted to the ASU for the initial evaluation and treatment. The following designated staffing in terms of full-time equivalents has been recommended for 10 dedicated beds in an ASU (approximately one bed per 40,000 residents serviced): a specialist physician (stroke physician, neurologist or another physician with training and experience in stroke medicine), 1 to 1.5; nurses, 7 to 12 (including one stroke educational nurse and one nurse in charge); physiotherapists 1 to 2; occupational therapist, 1 to 2; social worker, 0.4 to 0.7; and speech and language therapist, 0.2 to 0.6. It is also desirable to have a designated stroke unit director (usually a senior consultant physician), geriatrician, clinical pharmacologist, dietician, and neuropsychologist. There are three major types of stroke units: (1) ASU for acute care only (the average length of stay in such units is usually a few days), (2) comprehensive stroke unit that provides both acute care and rehabilitation (the average length of stay in such units is usually from several days to a few weeks), and (3) mobile stroke team. Current evidence shows superiority of the first two types of ASUs as opposed to a mobile stroke team. The key element of ASUs is a coordinated expert interdisciplinary team working in a geographically based setting with regular team meetings (at least weekly). The tasks of the team are to establish an accurate diagnosis, observe vital signs, maintain homeostasis, provide acute treatment, prevent complications, implement early rehabilitation and initiate secondary prevention strategies, and develop the most appropriate discharge and rehabilitation plan. On the basis of the existing evidence, the following are the six key indicators of the good quality of stroke care in a hospital: (1) >70% of patients with acute stroke should be discharged from a geographically defined ASU; (2) >90% of admitted patients with stroke should have a computed tomography/magnetic resonance imaging scan within 48 hours after the admission; (3) >80% of patients with acute stroke should be discharged by a consultant with a special interest in stroke; (4) >95% of patients who have stroke and are referred to the neurovascular outpatient clinic should be seen within 7 days; (5) appropriate patients should have carotid revascularization within 2 weeks of first assessment; and (6) all patients with ischemic stroke or TIA should be prescribed an appropriate antithrombotic drug.

INDICATIONS FOR OUTPATIENT MANAGEMENT

In general, outpatient evaluation may be considered for the following patients with cerebrovascular diseases: (1) patients with a TIA (or multiple TIAs) within 2 weeks of presentation, if the TIAs are unassociated with a probable cardioembolic source, if there is no evidence of a high-grade arterial stenosis as the probable cause, if there is no evidence of increasingly severe or frequent events, if the deficit associated with the event(s) was mild, and if the duration was not >60 minutes; (2) those who have had TIA or cerebral infarction >2 weeks before presentation; (3) those who have had recent ischemic cerebrovascular events that presented with transient monocular blindness alone and no evidence of carotid stenosis; (4) those who have had an intracerebral hemorrhage >30 days before presentation; (5) those who have chronic cerebrovascular disease, such as asymptomatic carotid or vertebral artery stenosis, asymptomatic and unruptured intracranial aneurysm, arteriovenous malformation, or cavernous malformation; and (6) those who refuse to be hospitalized. However, if symptoms of an acute cerebrovascular event recur during the period of outpatient diagnostic evaluation or treatment, immediate hospitalization is strongly recommended (the patient and the family are requested to report any new symptoms immediately to the physician).

TELEPHONE EVALUATION AND TRIAGE

Although interviewing the patient by telephone is less optimal diagnostically than an in-person interview and examination, several circumstances call for at least some kind of preliminary judgment by the physician about the patientís condition. A growing number of physicians are being called on to make a triage decision about patients with possible cerebrovascular disorders on the basis of telephone interviews. An algorithm for the evaluation of a patient by telephone is depicted in Appendix E-1.

Patients should be instructed to call the physician when any of the following warning signs of acute cerebrovascular disease develop, especially when they occur as well-defined, acute-onset spells involving one or more of the following: (1) loss of strength (or development of clumsiness) in some part of the body, especially on one side, including the face, arm, or leg; (2) numbness (sensory loss) or other unusual sensations in some part of the body, especially if on one side; (3) unexplained visual disturbances; (4) inability to speak properly or to understand language; (5) unsteadiness or falling; (6) any other kind of transient spells (vertigo, dizziness, swallowing difficulties, or memory disturbances); (7) headache that is unusually severe, abrupt in onset, or of unusual character; and (8) convulsions or other unexplained alteration in consciousness.

If the physician is to make the right decision about sending an ambulance or instructing the patient to come to the office or the hospital, then the patient must be interviewed in a step-by-step manner to facilitate answering **two fundamental questions**: (1) Is the problem vascular? (2) If so, is the situation an emergency?

The answer to the first question is based primarily on the **temporal profile of the onset of the presenting symptoms and their character.** The physician should elicit a detailed description of the presenting complaint, including the course of the illness and how it developed. Time and mode of onset, character and severity of the symptoms, and whether any progression or improvement has occurred require clarification.

The rapid onset and evolution of focal neurologic symptoms are characteristic of most types of acute cerebrovascular disorders, although some disorders such as SAH or mass effect from bilateral subdural hematoma may create generalized disturbances of neurologic function, regardless of the total duration or the severity of the symptoms. Because of the acute onset, most patients with cerebrovascular events can recall accurately the actual time of onset of their symptoms and what activity they were engaged in at the time.

However, one of the most dramatic acute cerebrovascular diseases, SAH, may present with headache alone, without focal neurologic dysfunction or other associated symptoms. In this situation, it is critically important to obtain a **detailed history of the headache** to distinguish **SAH** or from other causes such as **migraine** (usually starts in childhood or early adulthood, with unilateral throbbing headache, often with nausea, vomiting, and photophobia), **temporal arteritis** (commonly occurs in elderly patients and is associated with an enlarged, painful, tender temporal artery and pain in the jaw during chewing), **cluster headache**(usually unilateral, retro-orbital, searing pain, typically accompanied by unilateral lacrimation and nasal or conjunctival congestion), **muscle-contraction headache** (usually steady, deep, and generalized and associated with soreness of neck muscles), **brain tumor** (usually slowly progressive in frequency and severity, and headache tends to occur when the person awakens in the morning), **meningitis or encephalitis** (usually generalized and associated with fever and meningismus), **subdural hematoma** (history of recent head trauma), and **ocular disease** (see Chapter 2).

Sudden severe headache that commonly is described by the patient as "like being hit over the head by a hammer" or "the worst headache of my life" with no apparent cause is strongly suggestive of **SAH**. This type of headache is often accompanied by vomiting, stiff neck, or transient loss of consciousness. However, up to 30% of all SAHs may be atypical, and a small SAH, especially in older individuals, may not necessarily present with very severe headache or a catastrophic onset. In these cases, the element of abruptness in the new-onset headache suggests the diagnosis.

As outlined previously, it is important to distinguish TIA, defined as a temporary episode of focal ischemic neurologic deficit that completely resolves within 24 hours, from an episode of generalized cerebral ischemia (syncope) and from spells such as seizures and migraine, both of which may appear as episodes of transient focal neurologic dysfunction. The temporal profile of focal seizures generally involves progression and evolution within a few minutes (approximately 2 to 3 minutes), whereas the focal deficit that sometimes occurs with migraine usually builds or moves during 15 to 20 minutes before subsiding and often is associated with localized headache that normally occurs after the focal neurologic deficit. Another distinguishing characteristic of a TIA is that it tends to produce negative phenomena (i.e., weakness, difficulty in speaking or comprehending, or visual or sensory loss), but focal seizures tend to produce positive phenomena (tonic-clonic movements, tingling, visual hallucinations, or scintillating scotomata); migraine may produce either (more commonly, positive phenomena).

Other symptoms of particular importance for differentiating cerebrovascular disorders from other types of illness are reviewed in Chapter 2.

Any pertinent **medical history** (general health before the onset of the current illness, operations, or injuries) and **family history** should be ascertained as needed. A recent history of head injury, even if minor, should raise the possibility of subdural or epidural hematoma. Patients with acute cerebrovascular disease may have a history of stroke or TIA, carotid artery stenosis, heart disease, hypertension, hematologic disorder, tobacco use, high cholesterol level, or use of illicit drugs and a family history of stroke.

Having determined that the problem is vascular, the physician next must decide whether to send an ambulance, have the patient report to the emergency department or hospital admission desk, or instruct the patient to come to the office for medical consultation and outpatient management. Patients with sudden weakness or clumsiness; numbness of the face, arm, and leg on one side of the body; sudden decrease or loss of vision (particularly in one eye) or double vision with other symptoms of potential posterior circulation ischemia (not diplopia alone); loss of speech or difficulty talking or understanding written or spoken language; sudden, severe headache with no apparent cause; sudden unexplained dizziness (not unsteadiness alone) or vertigo in combination with other brainstem symptoms; or sudden ataxia (especially associated with any of the symptoms noted above) within the 2 weeks before presentation probably have acute cerebrovascular disease and should be referred to the hospital immediately for initial evaluation and consideration of hospitalization (see Appendix E-1). If the deficit that is associated with the event is marked, associated with a decrease in the level of consciousness, seizure, or respiratory or circulatory insufficiency, an ambulance should be sent. Sending an ambulance is also advised for cases that are associated with worsening or fluctuating neurologic deficits, traumatic cerebrovascular disorders (subdural or epidural hematoma), and other suspected urgent noncerebrovascular neurologic disorders such as meningitis or encephalitis. In other cases, the patient may be instructed to come to the office.

Management of Acute Stroke in Critically Ill Patients

While efforts are under way to determine the mechanism of acute cerebrovascular disease, the patient should be given supportive care to maintain general medical status. Particular attention should be directed to monitoring fluid intake and output and serum and urine electrolyte levels to ensure proper fluid balance. Constant observation in a neurologic intensive care unit (NICU) with monitoring of vital signs is advised for the first few days after large or progressive cerebral infarction and most intracerebral hemorrhages (ICHs) and subarachnoid hemorrhages (SAHs). In the absence of a NICU, admission to a medical ICU is recommended.

The initial physical examination should include general and neurologic (including neurovascular) examinations (see Chapters 4 to 6). Cardiac monitoring and observations every 4 hours with recording of vital signs (level of consciousness, blood pressure [BP], pulse, temperature, and respiration), pupillary size and reaction, and limb movements are recommended during at least the first few days after onset of an uncomplicated, acute, persistent cerebrovascular event, but half-hourly clinical observations and intermittent monitoring of blood gases and intracranial pressure (ICP) may be necessary for patients with severe stroke, especially those with impaired consciousness. Patients who have cerebral infarction and have received thrombolytic therapy or endovascular therapy should have frequent clinical assessment and monitoring of vital signs, including BP, particularly during the first 24 hours after treatment. In general, nursing staff should record neurologic observations and vital signs every 15 minutes for 2 hours after starting thrombolytic therapy, then every 30 minutes for 6 hours, and then hourly from the eighth hour until 24 hours after thrombolytics were started. Computed tomography should be performed as an emergency procedure for all critically ill patients with probable acute cerebrovascular disorders.

Immediate therapeutic measures for all comatose patients include establishing a good airway and insertion of a large-bore intravenous catheter to draw blood for studies and to maintain fluid and electrolyte balance. As noted in Chapter 6, for patients in whom the cause of coma is not readily known, naloxone, 0.4 mg intravenously, should be given with thiamine, 100 mg intravenously, followed by administration of 25 to 50 ml of 50% dextrose in water. If benzodiazepine overuse is suspected, then flumazenil may be administered. Fluid administration should be kept to a minimum (usually 1,000 ml normal saline/m^2 body surface area/day), unless the patient is hypotensive or clearly dehydrated (see below).

AIRWAY MANAGEMENT

Maintenance of a patent airway is the first priority in the care of an unconscious patient or any alert patient with respiratory problems such as shallow and irregular respirations or labored breathing. The most common causes of airway obstruction are posterior displacement of oropharyngeal soft tissue structures, nasopharyngeal vomitus, and secretions. The airway should be suctioned as necessary, with the patient placed in a lateral position to prevent airway obstruction (an oropharyngeal or nasal airway may also be useful). These measures are helpful for preventing atelectasis and bronchopneumonia. Supplemental oxygen (2 to 4 L per minute by nasal cannula) should be provided in the presence of decreased blood oxygen levels (arterial O_2 tension <90 mm Hg, O_2 saturation <95%).

Endotracheal intubation or assisted respiration is rarely indicated for patients with stroke but these procedures should be considered in circumstances of poor airway protection that are often caused by severe tongue and/or pharyngeal weakness with inability to clear secretions, insufficient oxygenation as a result of respiratory muscle fatigue, pneumonia or aspiration, or the need for markedly sedating medications because of a prolonged seizure. Endotracheal intubation and hyperventilation may also be considered for selected patients who exhibit increased ICP either alone or with other appropriate therapy for cerebral edema.

MANAGEMENT OF SYSTEMIC CARDIOVASCULAR DISORDERS

Treatment of general circulatory problems includes control of arrhythmias, restoration of cardiac output, and treatment of acute shock or hypovolemia. Hypotension is rarely a problem in stroke or transient ischemic attack, except when there is coincident myocardial infarction (MI), sepsis, or dehydration. To maintain normotension in these situations, plasma, low-molecular-weight dextran, or normal saline also may be administered. Volume expanders that contain an excessive amount of free water (such as D_5W) should be avoided, because this can worsen any evolving cerebral edema. In patients with low BP that is unresponsive to gentle volume expansion, sympathomimetic drugs (such as epinephrine) can be administered subcutaneously or intramuscularly to increase the systemic BP and increase cerebral perfusion. In cases of MI with vascular collapse, intravenously administered vasopressors are usually advised, with titration of the rate of infusion to maintain a stable, desired BP. If clinical heart failure is present, immediate treatment with inotropic agents (such as dobutamine) is indicated.

In patients with type I or type II coma (see Chapter 6), arterial BP usually is increased initially, but BP is commonly decreased in patients with type III coma or in those who are in the terminal stages of type I or type II coma. Medical treatment of transient hypertension that results from increased ICP associated with acute cerebrovascular disease (Cushing's reflex) usually is not required.

Persistent hypertension that results from increased ICP requires lowering of the ICP rather than antihypertensive medication. However, in patients who have acute ischemic stroke and whose diastolic BP is >140 mm Hg on two separate readings obtained 5 minutes or more apart, emergency antihypertensive therapy is usually started with a constant intravenous infusion of sodium nitroprusside (0.3 to 0.5 μg/kg/minute), which then can be titrated to the desired effect. The usual dose is 1 to 3 μg/kg/minute and should not exceed 10 μg/kg/minute. A gentle, carefully monitored reduction of BP is also recommended within 48 hours of onset of ischemic stroke for patients who have BP of 230 mm Hg or more systolic or 121 to 140 mm Hg diastolic on two separate readings obtained 30 minutes or more apart or associated with documented ICH, acute MI, left ventricular failure, renal failure as a result of accelerated hypertension, or dissection of the thoracic aorta. Reduction can be accomplished with intravenous agents such as labetalol, either in a constant infusion (2 mg per minute) or in an initial dosage of 10 to 20 mg intravenously during 1 to 2 minutes, repeated or doubled every 10 to 20 minutes until the desired BP is achieved or until a cumulative dose of 300 mg is reached. If a satisfactory response is not obtained, then sodium nitroprusside infusion should be considered.

Target BPs differ on the basis of the patient's history. In patients with no history of hypertension, the initial goal is usually from 160 to 170/95 to 100 mm Hg, whereas in those with a history of hypertension, an early goal of 170 to 180/100 to 110 mm Hg is more appropriate. Persistent (≥12 hours), milder levels (>180 to 230/105 to 120 mm Hg) of hypertension may be treated with intravenous labetalol (as outlined above) or oral agents, including labetalol and other beta-adrenergic blockers, angiotensin-converting enzyme inhibitors, or calcium channel blockers. Sublingual agents should be avoided, because the response is somewhat unpredictable and may lead to a precipitous decline in BP. If a patient receives thrombolytic therapy for cerebral infarction, then the BP goals should be <185/105 mm Hg, using the medications as outlined above.

MANAGEMENT OF INCREASED INTRACRANIAL PRESSURE

Increased ICP often complicates moderate- to large-sized ICHs and large cerebral infarcts. Although associated edema tends to develop more rapidly with hemorrhage, edema that is related to infarction may also be severe in the first 24 to 48 hours and often progresses during the first 3 to 7 days after infarction.

In general, the ICP should be kept at ≤20 mm Hg, and cerebral perfusion pressure should be kept at ≥70 mm Hg. The recommended treatments for increased ICP caused by ischemic or hemorrhagic stroke include hyperventilation, osmotherapy (most commonly with mannitol), renal-loop diuretics, hemicraniectomy and decompression, and ventricular drainage (Table 11-1). Glucocorticoids are another option, but there are very limited data supporting the efficacy of their use after cerebral infarction, ICH, or SAH. They are more effective in vasogenic edema rather than the type of edema that is predominant in patients with stroke, called cytotoxic edema. Simple measures such as elevation of the head of the bed and mild sedation, used in addition to the aggressive means outlined, may also be

Table 11-1. Options in management of cerebral edema and increased ICP

General measures	Fluids		
Elevate head of bed	Minimize free water (do not use D_5W)		
Minimize stimulation	Relative fluid restriction to 1,000 ml/m² body surface area/day		

Medical Agent	Onset of Action	Duration	Comments
Hyperventilation to PCO_2 25–35 mm Hg	Immediate	24 hr	
Hyperosmolar agents			
Mannitol, 20% solution, 1 g/kg IV during 5–30 min; repeat 0.25–0.5 g/kg every 2–6 hr[a]	30 min	Dose: hours Overall: 24–48 hr	Monitor serum osmolarity (maintain 300–320 mOsm/L), electrolytes, blood urea nitrogen
Glycerol, 10% solution, 0.25–1.0 g/kg PO every 4–6 hr[a]	8–12 hr	Dose: hours Overall: 24–48 hr	Less potential for rebound increase in ICP at end of duration of action than with mannitol
Steroids			
Dexamethasone, 10 mg IV, then 4 mg IV, every 6 hr	4–6 hr	Days	Works better for vasogenic edema (brain tumor) than for cytotoxic edema (stroke)

Surgery: See text

Barbiturate coma: In severe, life-threatening, increased ICP that is unresponsive to other treatment, barbiturate coma may be used. ICP monitoring is typically used.

ICP = intracranial pressure; IV = intravenous.

[a]Diuretics such as furosemide may be given with hyperosmolar agents, particularly if congestive heart failure is occurring as a side effect.

of some benefit in reducing an elevated ICP. If all other measures fail, barbiturate coma may be considered. If repeated doses of hyperosmolar or other diuretic agents are provided, serum osmolality should be monitored as a guide to therapy (serum osmolality should be maintained in the 300- to 320-mOsm per L range; acute elevation of the serum osmolality of >20 mOsm above the patient's usual level may result in an encephalopathy and should be avoided). However, the stable patient who remains awake and alert requires no antiedema therapy.

In patients with **cerebral infarction** and signs of increased ICP, such as a decreased level of consciousness, loss of spontaneous venous pulsations on ophthalmoscopic examination, or clinical features of herniation (pupillary enlargement ipsilateral to the infarcted hemisphere or pathologic corticospinal signs contralateral or ipsilateral to the hemispheric lesion), emergency measures to control the edema should be initiated (Table 11-1). Options include osmotic diuresis with hyperosmolar agents such as glycerol (administered orally, 10% solution in 0.4% normal saline at a dosage of 0.25 to 1.0 g per kg every 4 to 6 hours), 20% mannitol (administered intravenously at a dosage of 1 g per kg during a 30-minute period initially and then 0.25 to 0.5 g per kg every 2 to 6 hours as needed for acute ICP elevation, depending on the patient's ICP, cerebral perfusion pressure, serum osmolarity, and clinical findings), and free water restriction. Replacement fluids should be administered with attention to maintaining serum osmolality in the range of 300 to 320 mOsm per L; hypotonic and glucose-containing solutions should be avoided. A combination of osmotic agents and renal-loop diuretics such as furosemide (20 to 80 mg every 4 to 12 hours intravenously) or ethacrynic acid can reduce ICP in some patients when osmotic diuretics alone are inadequate or produce dangerous side effects (especially in patients with congestive heart failure). In addition, hyperventilation may be considered for patients whose condition is deteriorating as a result of increased ICP, including those with herniation syndromes. If clinical or radiographic deterioration continues in patients with large hemispheric infarction, then hemicraniectomy and decompression may be life saving and should be considered for selected patients.

In patients with **ICH** and an altered level of consciousness or evidence of herniation, ICP should be lowered emergently with intubation and mechanical hyperventilation, maintaining the PCO_2 at 25 to 30 mm Hg. Glycerol or mannitol (in the dosages discussed above) may also be used until emergency neurosurgical consultation is available. Dexamethasone, administered intravenously or intramuscularly in an initial bolus of 10 mg followed by 4 mg every 4 to 6 hours, has a more prolonged action but usually does not provide significant benefit during the initial 4 to 6 hours after administration. The benefit is generally greater in vasogenic edema, such as that associated with brain tumor, than with cytotoxic edema, which is the predominant edema subtype associated with stroke. Therefore, glucocorticoids are not routinely administered in the setting of

ICH but are used only in selected patients with evolving ICH-related cerebral edema.

Cerebellar hemorrhage (or infarction) with any evidence of brainstem compression constitutes a neurosurgical emergency. Immediate neurosurgical consultation should be obtained, and rapid consideration should be given to decompression, the alternative to which is often precipitous death.

In patients with **SAH**, increased ICP is often caused by hydrocephalus and typically is treated by external ventricular drainage, with gradual pressure reduction. Other patients may have increased ICP without hydrocephalus as a result of diffuse cerebral edema. In this subgroup, pressure reduction may often be achieved by hyperventilation, administration of mannitol or glycerol (as discussed above), or external ventricular drainage.

NURSING CARE

Patients with impaired consciousness require special attention to nutritional status; bowel and bladder function; and care of the skin, eyes, and mouth.

In comatose patients or in patients with swallowing problems, nutrition may be provided initially by intravenous solutions, but feeding by a nasogastric tube should be considered when the patient is neurologically stable. A diet of 1300 to 1400 calories per day with vitamin supplements or liquid feeding systems (Ensure or Osmolite) by constant drip at a rate of 75 to 100 ml per hour (1 to 1.5 calories per ml) or bolus feedings may be used. Fluid replacement should be 2 L per day; urine output should be monitored closely for balance with intake and, in general, should be at least 500 to 1000 ml per day. If the patient is alert and able to swallow, then oral feeding should be started with a liquid diet, followed by mechanical soft, bland, and regular diets. (Full liquid and soft diets may be easier to swallow without aspiration than clear liquids for patients with various degrees of dysphagia.) Percutaneous gastrostomy feeding should be considered in patients with a poor prognosis for regaining an adequate and safe swallowing mechanism.

For stool softening and prevention of straining with bowel movements, stool softeners such as docusate sodium, 100 mg orally twice daily, or laxatives may be used, especially in patients with SAH. An indwelling catheter should not be used in patients who are awake and able to cooperate with a voluntary voiding program. In comatose patients, the bladder should be emptied by catheterization at regular intervals of every 4 to 6 hours. If the patient is unconscious for >48 hours, then an indwelling Foley catheter may be required to monitor the patient's urine output, but this method is associated with higher risk for urinary bacterial colonization and infection.

Comatose patients should be turned in bed every 1 to 2 hours on an air mattress with tightly drawn sheets and sponge padding of body prominences to prevent pressure neuropathy and decubitus ulcers. Deep vein thromboses may be prevented by using subcutaneously administered heparin (unfractionated heparin 5,000 U twice daily or low-molecular-weight heparin), antiembolism stockings, or intermittent pneumatic compression devices. The patient's skin should be kept dry and powdered, with daily inspections over pressure points for erythema or ulcers. Ophthalmic ointments, methylcellulose eyedrops, and eye patching help to prevent corneal ulceration and abrasion.

Transient Ischemic Attack and Minor Cerebral Infarction

General Evaluation and Treatment

A **transient ischemic attack** (TIA) is defined as an episode of loss of brain function caused by cerebral ischemia that is localized to a limited region of the brain, with symptoms lasting <24 hours. **Minor cerebral infarction** (MCI) may be defined as a persistent loss of brain function attributed to brain ischemia, again localized to a limited region of the brain. The residual deficit is nondisabling; affected individuals are able to perform most of their usual activities and can ambulate without assistance. In general, for patients who present with a TIA or an MCI treatment may be initiated before determination of a definitive mechanism. The physician must choose from various therapeutic options while carefully considering the risk–benefit ratio as it applies to the specific circumstances involved. A systematic evaluation then should be undertaken to determine the specific mechanism for the cerebrovascular event(s) (see Appendix E-2).

SHOULD A PATIENT BE HOSPITALIZED?

Although in years past most patients with TIA or minor stroke were hospitalized, not all patients with TIA or minor stroke require inpatient evaluation. For patients with TIA or MCI, hospitalization should be directed toward those who are at higher risk for early recurrent ischemic events and include those who may have favorable results with short-term anticoagulation with intravenously administered heparin. In general, the following patients usually are the best candidates for **hospitalization**: (1) those with more than four ischemic episodes within the 2 weeks preceding the initial presentation (particularly those without transient monocular blindness in isolation); (2) those with a probable cardiac source of emboli (Tables 12-1 and 12-2), including atrial fibrillation, mechanical valve, dilated cardiomyopathy, known intracardiac thrombus, or recent myocardial infarction (MI); (3) symptomatic carotid artery stenosis or dissection; and (4) known hypercoagulable state. In patients with fewer than five TIAs, the most recent of which occurred within 2 weeks before presentation, and without probable cardiac source of embolus, symptomatic carotid artery stenosis, or hypercoagulable state, the issue of hospitalization is less clear. However, in general, if the deficit that is associated with the event was marked; if the events are increasing in frequency, severity, or duration; or if there are other factors that suggest a high risk for further events, including a carotid bruit ipsilateral to probable carotid symptoms, then a patient is often hospitalized for assessment. For patients with TIA that occurred >2 weeks before the

Table 12-1.   Proven cardiac risks for transient ischemic attack or minor stroke

Persistent atrial fibrillation
Paroxysmal atrial fibrillation
Sustained atrial flutter

Mechanical valve
Rheumatic valve disease

Dilated cardiomyopathy

Recent MI (within 1 mo)

Intracardiac thrombus

Intracardiac mass (atrial myxoma, papillary fibroelastoma)
Infectious endocarditis
Nonbacterial thrombotic endocarditis

MI = myocardial infarction.

Table 12-2.   Putative cardiac risks for transient ischemic attack or minor stroke

Sick sinus syndrome

Patent foramen ovale with or without atrial septal aneurysm

Atherosclerotic debris in the thoracic aorta

Spontaneous echocardiographic contrast

MI 2–6 mo earlier

Hypokinetic or akinetic left ventricular segment

MI = myocardial infarction.

current assessment or with symptoms involving only transient monocular blindness, an expedited outpatient workup may be indicated. Specific clinical syndromes, including stroke in the young, probable symptomatic carotid dissection, hypercoagulable state, inflammatory vasculopathies, stroke associated with illicit drug use, and cerebral venous thrombosis, usually lead to evaluation and treatment that is appropriate for the specific clinical entity.

In patients who are selected for hospitalization, antithrombotic therapy should be instituted. Aspirin, 75 to 325 mg per day, should be initiated in most patients. For those who are allergic to aspirin, clopidogrel, 75 mg per day, may be used in its place. In selected patients, short-term intravenous infusion of heparin may be considered, although the data supporting its use are limited. The rationale for use in this situation is based on theoretical and pharmacologic data, although there is evidence that patients with a cardiac source of emboli may benefit from heparin. The other clinical scenarios that are appropriate for hospitalization, including recurrent TIAs in the setting of a probable high-grade stenosis or crescendo TIAs, have not been subjected to a controlled trial of short-term heparin anticoagulation.

ANTICOAGULANTS

Heparin, a heterogeneous mixture of sulfate and muco-polysaccharides, activates antithrombin III and inhibits regulation factors II, IX, X, XI, and XII. It also blocks the conversion of fibrinogen to fibrin, exerts both proplatelet and antiplatelet aggregation actions, and accelerates fibrinolysis and inactivates thrombin through heparin cofactor II. Intravenous infusion of heparin in appropriate patients with TIA or MCI may be initiated with a bolus of 5,000 U followed by constant infusion of 800 to 1,000 U per hour. The anticoagulant effect of heparin is immediate and can be quantified from measurements of activated partial thromboplastin time. The therapeutic range is typically 1.5 to 2 times the normal control value. The patient's activated partial thromboplastin time should be monitored every 6 hours until the therapeutic value has been documented and then daily during the time of infusion.

Hemorrhagic complications are the most frequent side effects of heparin therapy. These complications are related to the dose and the duration of heparin therapy. They may be more common in patients with high systemic blood pressure, but this association has not been well documented. The frequency of intracerebral hemorrhage in patients who have had ischemic stroke is between 1% and 7%, but the risk is higher in patients with large ischemic stroke than in patients with TIA or MCI.

Another complication that is associated with heparin involves heparin-induced **thrombocytopenia**. This complication is usually mild and transient (related to increased platelet aggregation), but it may be more serious in 1% to 2% of patients. The more serious form is related to an immunoglobulin G– and immunoglobulin M–induced immune response that can be associated with "paradoxic" arterial occlusions, typically after 4 to 6 days of heparin treatment. For this reason, platelet counts should be determined every 2 days during heparin treatment. If heparin-induced thrombocytopenia develops and continued short-term parenteral anticoagulation is required, then treatment sometimes includes low-molecular-weight heparin (LMWH), which has less propensity for inducing thrombocytopenia than the usual unfractionated heparin. **LMWH** exerts its anticoagulation effect in a more selective pattern, affecting almost exclusively the intrinsic clotting pathway and having little effect on platelets and thrombin.

Recent data from the International Stroke Trial suggest that subcutaneous injections of unfractionated heparin offer no clinical advantage at 6 months after ischemic stroke. These data also do not support the routine use of subcutaneous heparin in acute cardioembolic stroke irrespective of the brain territory involved. In this situation, aspirin is the drug of choice. An alternative approach may be the use of warfarin as the first-choice drug. However, pending further evidence from clinical trials, the use of heparin or LMWH is still considered in selected patients with nonsurgical lesions, such as carotid artery dissection and progressive or recurrent ischemic symptoms, crescendo TIAs, recurrent cardiac embolism, acute cardioembolic stroke as a result of rheumatic atrial fibrillation (AF) and hypercoagulable states. The most recent American Stroke Association guidelines for the early treatment of patients with ischemic stroke recommend the subcutaneous administration of anticoagulants or the use of intermittent external compression stockings or aspirin for immobilized patients who cannot receive anticoagulants to prevent deep vein thrombosis.

INITIAL ASSESSMENT

The initial evaluation in an inpatient setting is relatively similar to that in an expedited outpatient setting. Computed tomography (CT) of the head without contrast should be performed to quickly distinguish nonhemorrhagic from hemorrhagic cerebrovascular disease. CT of the head with contrast or magnetic resonance imaging (MRI) of the head may be required if the initial scan indicates a possible arteriovenous malformation, meningioma, or other mass lesion. Other baseline studies include complete blood cell count, activated partial thromboplastin time and International Normalized Ratio (INR)/ prothrombin time, blood glucose, creatinine, liver function tests, electrolytes, erythrocyte sedimentation rate, and blood glucose. Lipid analyses, including high-density lipoprotein, low-density lipoprotein, and total cholesterol levels, should be performed but do not need to be performed acutely. Chest radiograph, electrogram, and rhythm strip should be obtained. Cardiac biomarkers such as troponin and creatine kinase also should be considered, particularly in circumstances in which any clinical suggestion of cardiac ischemia exists. Heparin may be indicated in selected patients (as noted above), but if contraindications to its use exist, then urgent evaluation without heparin is indicated. In patients who are selected for expedited outpatient evaluation and in patients who are hospitalized and do not have a specific indication for heparin, unless there is a contraindication to use of antiplatelet agents, aspirin 75 to 325 mg per day may be initiated during the evaluation as the mechanism is defined.

CARDIAC EVALUATION

The patient's baseline medical history and neurologic history already should have been obtained and a neurologic examination performed (Chapters 1 to 6). A minimal cardiac evaluation includes elicitation of cardiac history (with specific attention to both ischemic symptoms and previous arrhythmias) and cardiac examination that includes careful auscultation for cardiac murmurs. Minimal laboratory investigations include electrocardiography, rhythm strip, and chest radiography. Cardiac biomarkers, including troponin and creatine kinase, should be obtained. If one of the proven cardiac risks is identified (Table 12-1), then anticoagulation may be needed for long-term prophylaxis even if another potential mechanism for the TIA or MCI is identified. The putative cardiac risks (Table 12-2) also may require antiplatelet or anticoagulant therapy, but an alternative mechanism must be considered.

The remainder of the evaluation should be guided by the number and the character of ischemic events. If a patient has stereotyped spells, which indicate recurrent events in the same vascular distribution, then cardioembolic events are relatively less likely, although they are still part of the differential diagnosis.

Alternatively, nonstereotyped spells that implicate dissimilar symptoms during sequential spells and possible involvement of separate vascular territories lead to a different assessment.

SINGLE EVENT OR MULTIPLE SPELLS IN SAME VASCULAR DISTRIBUTION

In patients with multiple stereotyped spells or in those with only a single spell and no evidence of previous infarcts of large vessel distribution on CT or MRI, the evaluation should be tailored on the basis of the circulation implicated (Table 12-3).

Anterior Circulation

Clinical symptoms that are consistent with ischemia of the **carotid** distribution (Table 12-3) should lead to evaluation of the extracranial carotid artery with carotid ultrasonography, magnetic resonance angiography (MRA), or computed tomography angiography (CTA); these tests can detect a high-grade stenosis in the carotid system with a high degree of sensitivity. MRA is a subtype of MRI that can visualize noninvasively the extracranial and portions of the intracranial circulations. It has limited

Table 12-3.   Clinical symptoms associated with cerebral ischemia

Anterior circulation
  Motor dysfunction of contralateral extremities or face (or both)
    Clumsiness
    Weakness
    Paralysis
    Slurred speech
  Loss of vision in ipsilateral eye
  Homonymous hemianopia
  Aphasia if dominant hemisphere involved
  Sensory deficit of contralateral extremities or face (or both)
    Numbness or loss of sensation
    Paresthesias
Posterior circulation
  Motor dysfunction of any combination of extremities or face (or both)[a]
    Clumsiness
    Weakness
    Paralysis
  Loss of vision of one or both homonymous visual fields
  Sensory deficit of extremities or face (or both)[a]
    Numbness or loss of sensation
    Paresthesias
  The following typically occur but are nondiagnostic in isolation:
    Ataxic gait   Diplopia
    Ataxic extremities   Dysphagia
    Vertigo   Dysarthria

[a]Bilateral or alternating symptoms suggest involvement of the posterior circulation, and bilateral lower extremity symptoms may occur with unilateral carotid supply to both anterior cerebral arteries.

usefulness as a screening study, mainly because of its expense and its difficulty in delineating between high-grade vessel stenosis and occlusion.

If the results of the noninvasive studies suggest the presence of a high-grade stenosis in a surgically accessible artery that is appropriate for the distribution of TIA or MCI, then MRA or CTA should be considered if they have not been performed already and if the patient is a surgical candidate. If MRA or CTA verifies a high-grade stenosis, then **carotid endarterectomy (CEA)** should be strongly considered if there are no medical contraindications, because its benefit has been demonstrated clearly in this circumstance. If significant medical problems preclude CEA, then carotid angioplasty with stent placement (CAS) should be considered. Because MRA and CTA are noninvasive and carry a high degree of specificity and sensitivity in the evaluation of carotid occlusive disease, cerebral arteriography is not commonly needed for this indication. Even when arteriography is performed by experienced personnel, the associated risk for stroke is 0.5% to 1%.

For patients who are not surgical candidates, CAS typically is considered. In randomized CEA trials, the high rate of stroke in patients who are assigned to medical therapy with aspirin suggests that antiplatelet treatment with **aspirin** alone is relatively ineffective in those with high-grade stenosis of the extracranial internal carotid artery. In uncommon circumstances in which arteriography reveals thrombus in the extracranial carotid artery along with a carotid artery stenosis, short-term (1 to 2 months) anticoagulation with warfarin followed by CEA or carotid artery stenosis may be considered.

For patients with a single ischemic carotid distribution event and negative extracranial carotid screening study or evidence of only moderate stenosis, additional evaluation is indicated. Transesophageal echocardiography (TEE) is typically completed as the next step, with consideration for warfarin (see below) or surgical management depending on the delineation of a cardiac source of embolus. If the TEE also does not reveal a specific cause, then screening of intracranial vasculature with MRA or CTA may be considered. However, these additional studies may not change the antithrombotic agent selected in most patients given the clinical trial data that suggest that warfarin is not clearly better than aspirin in patients with symptomatic intracranial stenosis. Patients with intracranial stenosis in general will be treated with antiplatelet therapy (see below) and aggressive atherosclerosis risk factor control. In selected patients with intracranial stenosis and ongoing symptoms despite antiplatelet therapy, warfarin may be considered. Angioplasty with stent placement may also be considered in patients with ongoing ischemic symptoms despite maximal medical therapy. The medical management of cerebral ischemia is reviewed in Table 12-4.

The **coumarin anticoagulants** (warfarin and dicumarol) inhibit the clotting mechanism by interfering with synthesis of vitamin K–dependent factors II, VII, IX, and X. In addition, the coumarins deplete protein C and protein S, two indigenous anticoagulant proteins. The half-life of the inhibited clotting factors

Table 12-4.   Medical management of cerebral ischemia

Warfarin anticoagulation (INR 2.0–3.0)
    Short term (3 to 6 mo), followed by antiplatelet agent
        Symptomatic extracranial dissection of carotid or vertebral
        artery
    Consider longer term (at least 3 mo) (INR 2.0–3.0)
        Hypercoagulable state
        Cardiac source of emboli, level and duration of anticoagulation
        depending on cause
Aspirin (75–1,300 mg/day)
    Initial treatment in patients with TIA or cerebral infarction
    (clopidogrel or ticlopidine[a] if intolerant of or allergic to aspirin)
Clopidogrel (75 mg/day), aspirin in combination with extended-
    release dipyridamole, or ticlopidine (250 mg twice a day)[a]
    Recurrent symptoms with aspirin and no mechanism that may be
        better treated with warfarin or contraindication to warfarin
        detected
    Initial treatment in selected patients with TIA or cerebral
        infarction
    Use clopidogrel or ticlopidine in those who are allergic or
        sensitive to aspirin, requiring antiplatelet therapy

INR = International Normalized Ratio; TIA = transient ischemic attack.
[a]Monitor complete blood cell counts every 2 wk for 3 mo.

ranges from approximately 6 to 60 hours, which produces a 1- to 3-day delay between peak plasma concentration and maximal effect. In patients with embolic ischemic stroke and an established cardiac source of emboli, including atrial fibrillation, mechanical valve, dilated cardiomyopathy, known intracardiac thrombus, and recent MI, for which no contraindication to warfarin administration exists, consideration should be given to anticoagulation with warfarin, particularly if a good functional recovery from the index stroke has been achieved. In addition, there are selected other indications for warfarin, including defined hypercoagulable state, mobile aortic atheromatous debris, and symptomatic extracranial carotid or vertebral artery dissection.

Although in the past the usual therapeutic range of oral anticoagulation has been based on prothrombin time ratios, the intensity of coumarin anticoagulation is best measured by the **INR**. The INR is calculated by using the International Sensitivity Index (ISI) of the thromboplastin reagins, which are now supplied by most manufacturers, allowing calculation of an instrument-specific INR value for individual plasma samples. The formula for calculating the INR is INR = (prothrombin time ratio)^{ISI}.

Both warfarin and dicumarol are usually given once daily. The starting dosage varies according to size, age, and hepatic status of the patient as well as the urgency of the situation. In an average-sized adult with normal liver function, a starting dosage is dependent on the patient's age and previous experience with warfarin. Five milligrams per day is appropriate in most patients, although patients who are older than 80 years should not receive >3.5 mg per day. Exceptions include patients who are known to require more warfarin, on the basis of their previous experience with the medication. The dosage after the first day should be tailored on the basis of prothrombin time or INR response, which typically is minimal, if any, after the first day of therapy. If the first-day INR rise is ≥0.6, then the second-day warfarin dose should be less than half of that of the first day. For those with a first-day rise of ≥0.9, the INR should be rechecked in 6 hours and a decision made regarding subsequent warfarin dosing.

The **usual therapeutic range** for oral anticoagulation is an INR between 2.0 and 3.0. Higher intensity anticoagulation (such as that for mechanical heart valves) usually involves keeping the INR between 3.0 and 4.5 (Table 12-5). This INR level typically is checked in the morning, and the warfarin or dicumarol is taken in the evening. Dose levels are estimated on the basis of the assumption of an approximate 2-day delay until maximal effect on the INR or prothrombin time from a given dosage and little or no effect within the first 24 hours.

When therapy is switched to oral anticoagulation in the setting of intravenous heparin or LMWH use, the optimal timing for cessation of heparin is controversial. However, most experts advise that heparin should be used for at least 3 to 5 days after initiation of warfarin therapy or until the INR becomes therapeutic. The reason for the minimal delay of 3 to 5 days is that warfarin inhibits production of new clotting factors but does not eliminate clotting factors that are already present. The most important clotting factor for determining in vivo clotting is prothrombin, which has a half-life of approximately 2 days. It is necessary to go through at least 2 to 2.5 half-lives to reduce the existing level of prothrombin to an acceptable level of 25% to 35% or less.

Bleeding complications of the warfarin anticoagulants are related to the level of anticoagulation, with the risks particularly increasing above an INR of 3.0. Thus, it is important to check

Table 12-5.   Intensity level of anticoagulation for major disease categories

Indication	INR
Atrial fibrillation, atrial flutter	2–3
Ischemic heart disease	2–3
Deep vein thrombosis	2–3
Valvular heart disease	2–3
Dilated cardiomyopathy	2–3
Recent MI	2–3
Intracardiac thrombus	2.5–3.5
Mechanical heart valve	3.0–4.5
Extracranial carotid dissection	2.0–3.0
Mobile aortic atheromatous debris	2.0–3.0

MI = myocardial infarction.

the prothrombin time or INR regularly (usually daily) until the level has stabilized. After stabilization, levels are checked every 2 to 3 days for 1 week and eventually as infrequently as every 4 weeks if the patient has reached a maintenance dose and is otherwise stable. It is important to advise the patient not to take vitamin K, because it may interfere greatly with attempts at oral anticoagulation. Long-term anticoagulation has a complication rate from all bleeding episodes between 0.5% and 1% per 12 months. With careful monitoring in a controlled setting, such as in several recent atrial fibrillation trials, the bleeding complication rate is approximately 1.0% to 1.5% annually. In addition to a prothrombin time or INR higher than the therapeutic range, high systolic or diastolic blood pressure and age may be predictive features of an increased risk for hemorrhagic complications.

Antiplatelet therapy includes aspirin, aspirin combined with extended-release dipyridamole, clopidogrel, and ticlopidine. In patients who have TIA, MCI, or ischemic stroke and do not require warfarin, aspirin should be commenced unless contraindicated. For patients who are in sinus rhythm and have a history of TIA or ischemic stroke while on aspirin, consideration should be given to the addition of another antiplatelet agent, such as extended-release dipyridamole, or switch to clopidogrel. In patients who are to have CEA and are already taking aspirin, it is desirable for them to continue taking it up to and through the surgery unless contraindications exist. Patients who are to undergo carotid artery stenosis are treated with aspirin and clopidogrel before and after the procedure, with the clopidogrel then continued for 1 month and aspirin continued indefinitely.

Aspirin irreversibly limits platelet adhesion and aggregation, inhibiting production of cyclooxygenase and thromboxane A_2. Although aspirin has no effect on prothrombin time, partial thromboplastin time, or platelet count, it does prolong bleeding time with an effect that starts in 1 to 2 days and persists for 7 to 10 days.

The risk for nonfatal stroke is decreased by approximately 23% among patients who have had a previous stroke or TIA and are treated with aspirin. There is evidence that early aspirin is of benefit for a wide range of ischemic cerebrovascular events, and its prompt use should be routinely considered for all patients with suspected TIA or acute ischemic stroke, mainly to reduce the risk for early recurrence. The optimal dose of aspirin is controversial; the most common daily dosages range from 75 mg once daily to 325 mg twice daily.

Complications, including gastrointestinal irritation, ulceration, and bleeding, are clearly reduced with lower doses, and some theoretical considerations involving differential aspirin effects on prostacyclin (related to prostacyclinol) indicate that lower doses of aspirin could be more efficacious than higher doses. Although no randomized trials have documented clearly any differences in efficacy between low-dose and high-dose aspirin for prevention of stroke, most experts believe that higher doses of aspirin offer no added effectiveness but more adverse events. If the patient has another TIA or ischemic stroke on aspirin, then some experts recommend adding **extended-release dipyridamole** to aspirin or switching to clopidogrel or, less common, to ticlopidine.

As noted above, therapy with **clopidogrel** or **ticlopidine hydrochloride** could be considered, particularly for patients who are intolerant of or allergic to aspirin. Clopidogrel selectively inhibits the binding of adenosine diphosphate (ADP) to its platelet receptor and the subsequent ADP-mediated activation of the GPIIb/IIIa complex, thereby inhibiting platelet aggregation. Clopidogrel (75 mg per day) may be slightly more effective than aspirin alone but is far more expensive. Inhibition of platelet aggregation starts 2 hours after single oral doses of clopidogrel and reaches steady state between day 3 and day 7. Platelet aggregation and bleeding time gradually return to baseline values within 7 days after treatment is discontinued. The overall tolerance and side effects of clopidogrel are similar to aspirin (except gastrointestinal events, which are minimally lower on clopidogrel). Thrombocytopenia occurs very uncommonly on clopidogrel. Clopidogrel is contraindicated in patients who have severe liver impairment or active pathologic bleeding, such as peptic ulcer and intracranial hemorrhage, or are breast-feeding.

Ticlopidine is an antiplatelet agent that prohibits platelet deposition by suppressing ADP-induced platelet aggregation and aggregation as a result of various other factors. Like aspirin, it prolongs bleeding time but does not affect platelet count, partial thromboplastin time, or prothrombin time. With the usual dosage of 250 mg twice per day, its effect begins within 1 to 2 days and persists for 7 to 10 days. Because of the risk for adverse events, outlined below, and because of the availability of clopidogrel, ticlopidine is not commonly used.

Ticlopidine is also considerably more expensive than aspirin but also may be slightly more effective than aspirin in preventing future stroke among patients with TIA and ischemic stroke. **Side effects** from ticlopidine include severe neutropenia, which occurs in 0.5% to 1% of patients. This complication almost always occurs within the first 3 months of treatment and usually within the first 4 to 8 weeks. For this reason, patients who are given ticlopidine should have regular monitoring of complete blood cell counts every 2 weeks, especially during the first 3 months of therapy. Thrombotic thrombocytopenic purpura also has been reported occasionally, with a frequency of up to 1 in 2,000 to 1 in 4,000 patients. The peak occurrence is after 3 to 4 weeks of therapy, with some cases reported after >3 months of treatment. Other side effects of ticlopidine include abdominal pain, diarrhea, and rash.

Overall, indications for clopidogrel or ticlopidine use are similar. They are usually considered for aspirin-intolerant or aspirin-allergic patients and for those who have recurrent spells during aspirin therapy but did not have an event that may be more appropriately treated with warfarin. Combined aspirin and extended-release dipyridamole may be used for this same indication. Some authors have recommended the use of aspirin in combination with extended-release dipyridamole, clopidogrel, or ticlopidine as a first-line antiplatelet agent.

A recently developed orally administered fixed-dose thrombin inhibitor **Ximelagatran** demonstrated efficacy in clinical studies for ischemic stroke prevention in patients with nonrheumatic atrial fibrillation and might be an important alternative to warfarin if safety issues with long-term liver toxicity can be resolved in the future.

Posterior Circulation

Vertebrobasilar distribution ischemia often leads to symptoms that are related to brainstem, cerebellar, or occipital lobe dysfunction (Table 12-3). Further evaluation of the posterior circulation may be performed noninvasively. MRA, CTA, or transcranial Doppler (TCD) ultrasonography all are options for the noninvasive evaluation of the posterior circulation. MRA is sensitive and specific and allows evaluation of the vertebral and carotid arteries to the level of the aortic arch. TCD ultrasonography has a sensitivity of approximately 75% for detecting hemodynamically significant stenosis in the distal intracranial segments of the vertebral artery or the basilar artery. Cerebral arteriography may be performed to define the anatomy of the posterior circulation vasculature in selected cases with complex findings on the noninvasive imaging with MRA or CTA. However, the risk for arteriographic complication is 0.5% to 1%, and arteriography is not necessary in most patients with vertebrobasilar symptoms.

Should a stenosis be detected in the vertebral artery, initial treatment with antiplatelet therapy and aggressive atherosclerosis risk factor control is indicated. A similar approach is implemented for basilar artery stenosis. The use of **warfarin anticoagulation** in the setting of symptomatic intracranial stenosis continues to be somewhat controversial. However, the results of the Warfarin Aspirin Symptomatic Intracranial Disease (WASID) trial suggest that warfarin is not clearly more effective in preventing recurrent stroke and carries with it a higher risk for hemorrhagic complications. Patients with symptomatic high-grade stenosis in the basilar artery are sometimes still considered for warfarin anticoagulation, but there were no clear data that the benefit is greater than the risk in these patients. In selected patients with recurrent symptoms despite maximal medical therapy in the setting of a high-grade vertebral or basilar stenosis, angioplasty and stenting may be considered. The risk of such a procedure is higher if performed in the basilar artery, compared with the vertebral artery. In an occlusion of the vertebral or basilar artery with thromboembolic symptoms, a short course of warfarin anticoagulation (4 to 6 weeks) may be followed by antiplatelet therapy with aspirin, aspirin in combination with extended-release dipyridamole, clopidogrel, or ticlopidine. If the vertebrobasilar noninvasive studies are normal or fail to reveal a high-grade stenosis, then TEE may be considered. Depending on the results, warfarin may be indicated if a cardiac source of embolus is detected. If the TEE is also negative for embolic source, then treatment with **antiplatelet therapy** along with aggressive atherosclerosis risk factor control is indicated.

EVALUATION OF A PROBABLE EMBOLIC EVENT OR MULTIPLE EVENTS IN DIFFERENT VASCULAR DISTRIBUTIONS

In patients without a proven cardiac risk documented on the initial evaluation, certain clinical findings may suggest an **embolic event**, although they do not exclude a different mechanism. These include multiple areas of vascular involvement; abnormal CT or MRI findings indicative of a large vessel infarction in a vascular distribution that would not explain the current symptoms; and an embolic syndrome, suggested by various findings including ischemia of the posterior cerebral artery distribution with homonymous hemianopia, ischemia of the lower middle cerebral artery division and receptive aphasia, top of the basilar syndrome, rapidly resolving severe deficit of abrupt onset, and spontaneous hemorrhagic transformation.

Should the multiple symptoms be explained by a large vessel distribution in the anterior circulation, screening of the anterior circulation with carotid ultrasonography, MRA, or CTA should be performed because of the proven success of CEA in such cases. High-grade stenosis on a noninvasive study in the internal carotid artery should prompt surgical consideration if a patient is a surgical candidate or angioplasty/stenting consideration if the patient is not a surgical candidate. Because this is a subgroup of events that are not stereotyped or clearly associated with a proven cardiac risk (Table 12-1), TEE may need to be performed before CEA, because the potential for a cardioembolic source remains in this subgroup of patients.

If the noninvasive arterial studies do not reveal a cause for the events, then cardiac imaging with **TEE** is usually performed, providing superior resolution of the left atrium, left atrial appendage, aortic arch, and other cardiac basal structures. Although results of TEE prompt medical management changes in a relatively small number of patients overall, the proportion whose management is changed is higher among the subgroup of patients with no definite cause identified for their cerebrovascular symptoms by this point in the evaluation. **Holter monitoring** may also be useful in this setting. Patients with cerebral infarction of unknown cause may have underlying episodic arrhythmias that are known to be associated with an increased risk for systemic embolization, even in the presence of a normal electrocardiographic tracing.

If a **proven** cardiac risk factor (Table 12-1) is detected with these studies, then warfarin anticoagulation may be initiated depending on the specific finding (see Chapter 16). Detection of a **putative** cardiac risk factor (Table 12-2) may also necessitate warfarin anticoagulation or antiplatelet therapy if no other mechanism is noted. If TEE and Holter monitoring reveal normal findings and the other evaluation as outlined is normal, then a trial of an antiplatelet agent is indicated, along with aggressive atherosclerosis risk factor control.

RECURRENCE WITH ASPIRIN THERAPY

If spells recur with aspirin therapy, then the distribution of the symptoms will be a guide to the most appropriate therapy. Symptoms that recur in the **anterior circulation** should promote carotid ultrasonography if the original study was not of sufficient quality or if it was performed >3 months earlier. If carotid ultrasonography is normal or has already been performed then MRA, CTA, or TCD ultrasonography is the next appropriate step to evaluate the distal internal carotid artery, proximal middle and anterior cerebral arteries, vertebral arteries, and basilar. The use of aspirin (ASA) in combination with extended-release dipyridamole, clopidogrel, or ticlopidine is reasonable. If the noninvasive studies, including carotid ultrasonography, MRA or CTA, TCD ultrasonography, TEE, and possibly Holter monitoring, fail to reveal a cause for the event, then additional evaluation, including special coagulation studies, spinal fluid examination, and arteriography, may be required. If results are negative, empiric treatment with ASA combined with dipyridamole, clopidogrel, or ticlopidine is indicated. In selected patients in whom all other medical management fails, an empiric trial of warfarin may be considered, but there are limited data supporting such an approach. Increasing the aspirin dose theoretically also may be beneficial. In addition to the antithrombotic medications, aggressive atherosclerosis risk factor modification is indicated.

Recurrent symptoms in the distribution of the **posterior circulation** should prompt noninvasive imaging with either MRA or TCD ultrasonography, if this was not performed earlier. If results are negative, empiric treatment with ASA combined with extended-release dipyridamole, clopidogrel, or ticlopidine is indicated. In selected patients in whom all other medical management fails, an empiric trial of warfarin may be considered, but, again, there are limited data supporting such an approach. Increasing the aspirin dose theoretically also may be beneficial. If MRA, CTA, or TCD ultrasonography reveals a high-grade stenosis, as outlined above, then the overall efficacy of warfarin is not clearly defined in this context and antiplatelet therapy in combination with aggressive atherosclerosis risk factor control is indicated. If the MRA, CTA, or TCD ultrasonography is negative, then TEE is indicated and other evaluation to include Holter monitoring and special coagulation studies may follow if the cause is still unclear.

Recurrent clinical symptoms involving **multiple vascular territories** should prompt evaluation for a more proximal source of emboli. Evaluation might include TEE and Holter monitoring. One may also consider alternative diagnoses, including cerebral vasculitis and a hypercoagulable state, which may cause symptoms in multiple distributions. Treatment issues for specific causes that are delineated by this additional evaluation are reviewed in Chapter 16.

Major Cerebral Infarction

General Evaluation and Treatment

GENERAL MANAGEMENT CONSIDERATIONS

Patients with acute stroke should be treated with the same sense of urgency as patients with an acute myocardial infarction (MI). In the same sense that a heart attack indicates the need for emergency action because of a lack of blood supply to the heart muscle, an ischemic stroke (cerebral infarction) is a **brain attack** indicating an abrupt lack of blood supply to a region of the brain. Urgent medical or surgical intervention may be critical to long-term outcome. Most patients who present with cerebral infarction should be hospitalized for **urgent evaluation and treatment**.

The initial evaluation of a patient who presents with **cerebral infarction** is similar to that outlined for transient ischemic attack (TIA) and minor cerebral infarction (MCI) (see Chapter 12). Computed tomography (CT) without contrast or magnetic resonance imaging (MRI) examination is indicated to quickly distinguish between nonhemorrhagic and hemorrhagic cerebrovascular disease. If CT without contrast is performed initially, MRI or CT with contrast may be required if the initial scan indicates a possible arteriovenous malformation, meningioma, or other mass lesion. Other baseline studies should include complete blood cell count, activated partial thromboplastin time, International Normalized Ratio (INR), blood glucose, creatinine, liver function tests, electrolytes, and erythrocyte sedimentation rate. Lipid analyses, including high-density lipoprotein, low-density lipoprotein, and cholesterol levels, should be performed but do not need to be performed acutely. Cardiac biomarkers such as troponin and creatine kinase should be drawn acutely to rule out MI, given the frequent co-occurrence of coronary artery disease with cerebral infarction. A chest radiograph, an electrocardiogram, and a rhythm strip should also be obtained.

Treatment of patients with acute cerebral infarction differs somewhat from that of patients with TIA and minor stroke and includes (1) consideration of thrombolytic therapy or mechanical clot-dissolution techniques; (2) consideration of anticoagulants or antiplatelet agents; (3) intensive general medical care; (4) treatment of the neurologic deficit; (5) prevention of subsequent neurologic event; and (6) prevention and treatment of secondary complications such as bronchial pneumonia, urinary tract infection, and deep vein thrombosis (see Appendix E-3). As with TIA and MCI, cardiac evaluation should also include cardiac history (with special attention to ischemic symptoms, arrhythmia, and murmurs) and cardiac examination.

Subsequent evaluation is typically based on the magnitude of the deficit, the patient's age and medical status, and candidacy for therapeutic intervention, including either operation or medical intervention. Early after the onset of a severe deficit, it is not possible to classify the deficit as a TIA, an ischemic stroke, or a progressive stroke because if and when the deficit will clear is uncertain.

ACUTE THERAPEUTIC CONSIDERATIONS

The **initial therapeutic approach** to ischemic infarction is greatly dependent on the time from onset of symptoms to presentation for emergency medical care. If the history and examination verify that the probable cause of the symptoms is an ischemic stroke and if the onset of symptoms was <6 hours before the evaluation for anterior circulation ischemia or <12 hours before the evaluation for posterior circulation ischemia, then **emergent thrombolytic therapy or mechanical clot removal techniques** should be considered.

Thrombolytic agents such as recombinant tissue plasminogen activator (tPA), urokinase, prourokinase, and streptokinase given either intravenously or intra-arterially dissolve thrombi and are designed to reopen arteries that are occluded by emboli or a primary thrombus and induce reperfusion of an ischemic area of the brain. Although such reperfusion may be associated with a return in neurologic function of the affected area, clinical improvement may not occur, and administration may be complicated by intracerebral hemorrhage (ICH).

The time of onset of the infarction must be sought from the patient or the family; if a patient awakens from sleep with the deficit, intravenous (IV) thrombolytic therapy should not be considered unless the duration of the deficit is clearly <3 hours. The effectiveness and the safety of IV tPA use beyond 3 hours after symptom onset has not been demonstrated clearly but remains under study. The result of the CT head scan is very important in selecting patients for possible thrombolysis. The CT should not reveal any evidence of intracranial hemorrhage, mass effect, midline shift, significant early infarction, tumor, aneurysm, or vascular malformation. Clinical criteria that may exclude patients from IV tPA in addition to the 3-hour time cut-off are (1) rapidly improving or mild deficits, (2) obtundation or coma, (3) presentation with seizure, (4) history of intracranial hemorrhage or bleeding diathesis, (5) blood pressure (BP) increase persistently >185/110 mm Hg, (6) gastrointestinal hemorrhage or urinary tract hemorrhage within 21 days, and (7) recent large ischemic stroke within 14 days or small ischemic stroke within 4 days. Laboratory abnormalities that may preclude treatment are (1) heparin use within 48 hours with increased activated partial thromboplastin time, (2) warfarin use with INR >1.5, (3) serum glucose <50 or >400 mg per dl, and (4) platelet count <100,000 mm^3. Long-term aspirin, clopidogrel, or dipyridamole use is not a contraindication to use of IV tPA.

If the patient is a candidate for thrombolytic therapy, then the patient and the family should be counseled regarding the risks and benefits of such therapy. In the National Institutes of Health–funded treatment trial of IV tPA published in 1995, the efficacy in improving neurologic status at 3 months was defined for tPA compared with placebo, with the agent administered within 3 hours of symptom onset. There was a greater proportion

(12% absolute increase) of people with minimal or no deficit in the tPA group at 3 months after the event, and there was no increase in patients with severe deficits or disability. This finding is particularly important because there was a 6% occurrence of symptomatic hemorrhage within 36 hours of treatment in the tPA group compared with 0.6% in the placebo group. Data from acute stroke trials of streptokinase that were reported before the IV tPA trial suggested that any improvement in outcome in patients who receive thrombolytic therapy may be offset by an increase in poor outcomes caused by hemorrhage. In the IV tPA trial, despite the increased occurrence of symptomatic hemorrhage, the 90-day mortality rate was not different comparing those who were treated with IV tPA (17% mortality) and those who were treated with placebo (21% mortality).

An intracranial hemorrhage in the setting of thrombolytic therapy should be suspected if neurologic deterioration occurs or if there is new severe headache, acute hypertension, nausea, or vomiting. Use of tPA should be discontinued immediately if the infusion is ongoing, and a CT scan without contrast should be obtained. In the meantime, INR/prothrombin time, partial thromboplastin time, platelet count, hemoglobin, and fibrinogen value should be determined emergently, and platelets (6 to 8 units) and fibrinogen in the form of cryoprecipitate-containing factor VIII (6 to 8 units) should be prepared. If the CT scan confirms hemorrhage, then neurosurgical consultation should be obtained. A hematologist may aid in outlining optimal replacement therapy with platelets and cryoprecipitate. Another CT scan can be obtained 6 hours later, or sooner if the deficit worsens.

The tPA should be administered intravenously at a dose of 0.9 mg per kg (maximum 90 mg), with 10% given as a bolus and the remainder given over 60 minutes. Close monitoring in an intensive care unit should continue for 24 hours. Intravenous heparin, aspirin, other antiplatelet agents, and warfarin should not be used for 24 hours, and BP should be monitored closely, with the pressure kept at <180/105 mm Hg (see Chapter 11). A repeat CT head scan is typically performed 24 hours after treatment.

Although administering tPA (or other thrombolytic agents) intra-arterially may ultimately be more helpful than giving these agents intravenously, the procedures require more time and expertise tPA is considered for intra-arterial (IA) administration in selected patients with an acute major intracranial arterial occlusion. Emergency arteriography is performed by an interventionalist trained in use of intracranial catheters and thrombolytic agents. IA thrombolysis for anterior circulation ischemic stroke is typically not used beyond 6 hours after symptom onset. In the posterior circulation, because symptomatic basilar artery thrombosis is associated with a very high morbidity and mortality, IA tPA is occasionally recommended up to 12 hours or longer after symptom onset, but there is currently no robust evidence to recommend this treatment for routine practice.

Thrombolytic agents other than tPA are of unproven efficacy. Urokinase was evaluated in previous clinical trials, but the efficacy was never proved. A urokinase precursor, prourokinase, has been evaluated in a phase III prospective, placebo-controlled trial of IA administration for acute middle cerebral artery occlusion within 6 hours of symptom onset. The likelihood of having a good outcome at 90 days was higher in those who received prourokinase, with 40% of those treated having a good outcome compared with 25% of those who received placebo. Intracranial hemorrhage with neurologic symptoms was noted in 10% of those who received prourokinase, compared with 2% in control subjects. The overall mortality was similar. Because prourokinase has not been approved in the United States, tPA remains the most commonly used IA thrombolytic agent.

Combined use of IV and IA thrombolysis is under study but is of unproven benefit. This involves the use of a lower dose of IV tPA, followed by emergency arteriography and IA thrombolysis if an appropriate arterial occlusion is seen on the arteriogram.

Mechanical clot-removal techniques provide another potential management option for acute cerebral ischemia. There is some evidence that transcranial Doppler ultrasonography aimed at the site of intracranial arterial occlusion may accentuate the thrombolytic activity of tPA. This remains under study. Another technique that has been approved for use in acute cerebral infarction is the MERCI (Mechanical Embolus Removal in Cerebral Ischemia) Retriever device, approved in 2004 for use within 8 hours after onset of severe cerebral infarction. This tiny corkscrew-shaped device is implemented via an IA catheter. The goal is to remove a clot from within the artery, leading to an improvement in the blood flow to the area that had been blocked. In a nonrandomized, multicenter trial, the likelihood of opening the artery (recanalization) was higher in those who were treated with the device, 48%, compared with a historical control rate of 18%. Procedural complications occurred in 7.1%, and intracranial hemorrhage occurred in 7.8%. Those with successful recanalization had a better outcome, including a lower mortality. This device provides an alternative for patients who have severe acute cerebral infarction and are otherwise not a thrombolytic therapy candidate.

In patients who are not candidates for thrombolytic therapy or if 24 hours have passed since thrombolytic therapy, **antiplatelet therapy** with aspirin is typically initiated emergently. Clopidogrel may be considered in those with a clear aspirin allergy. Anticoagulation with heparin should be considered, but the data supporting its use are limited. Unfractionated **heparin** or low-molecular-weight heparin (LMWH) may be considered in patients with extracranial carotid artery dissection, probable cardiac source of embolus such as intracardiac thrombus or atrial fibrillation, or hypercoagulable states. The use of heparin in crescendo TIAs, symptomatic large artery stenosis, or progressive cerebral infarction (see later this chapter) is unproven. As described in Chapter 12, the rationale for heparin use in the setting of acute cerebral infarction is based on theoretical and pharmacologic data. The pharmacologic effect, complications, and dose initiation were described in Chapter 12. For patients with known or suspected ongoing sources for further embolization (for instance, cardiac embolic sources), the rationale for the use of heparin is strongest. In general, for patients with **small or moderate cerebral infarction** with one of the indications outlined above, treatment with heparin or a heparinoid may be initiated. Even though patients with embolic events are at greater risk for experiencing hemorrhagic transformation of an infarct, patients with small or moderate embolic infarcts may safely receive anticoagulation if the activated partial thromboplastin time is monitored closely, as described in Chapter 12. However, for patients with **large cardioembolic infarcts** involving the entire middle cerebral artery or internal carotid artery distribution, heparin is usually withheld for 7 days and a CT scan without contrast then is repeated. If there is no evidence of hemorrhagic transformation, treatment usually involves IV heparin with no bolus and close monitoring of the activated partial thromboplastin time.

Use of heparin anticoagulation assumes that the patient has no contraindications, such as bleeding peptic ulcer, uremia, hepatic failure, markedly increased BP ($\geq$200/120 mm Hg), or strong suspicion or evidence of bacterial endocarditis or sepsis. Heparin is typically administered as an initial bolus of 5,000 U, followed by a continuous drip of 1,000 U per hour to maintain the activated partial thromboplastin time at 1.5 to 2 times normal (see Chapter 12 for more information on heparin anticoagulation). If heparin-related **hemorrhagic side effects** occur, then protamine can be used to reverse the heparin anticoagulation at a dose of 5 ml of a 1% solution mixed with 20 ml of saline administered slowly intravenously, with no more than 50 mg given over a 10-minute period or 200 mg during 2 hours.

LMWH (see Chapter 12) may also be efficacious if initiated within 24 hours after stroke onset. In one study, at 6 months, there was a 20% higher frequency of death or dependence outcomes in the placebo group compared with the group that received high-dose LMWH. In another study, there was some evidence of an improvement in overall outcomes at 90 days among patients who were treated with LMWH but only in the subgroup of patients with cerebral infarction as a result of large artery stenosis or occlusion.

Other therapies that are currently under investigation include several categories of neuroprotective agents designed to limit or reverse parenchymal damage and may prove effective if given very early in the course of an ischemic event. Some of these agents are given before the mechanism of the infarction is clarified. Although ischemia may convert to irreversible cerebral infarction over a matter of minutes, marginal ischemic zones may possibly be affected by acute treatment during a period of hours or even days. This has led to the consideration of initiating these therapies as soon as possible after the onset of the event. At centers that participate in treatment trials for acute stroke, a patient's candidacy for the trials should be considered as early as possible after the onset of symptoms. To date, these agents, including calcium channel blockers, N-methyl-D-aspartate antagonists, and free radical scavengers, have not been shown to be efficacious.

Other agents, including **gangliosides**, **naloxone**, **clofibrate**, **hyperbaric oxygen**, **barbiturates**, **vasodilators** such as pentoxifylline, and various **hemodiluting agents** and **hypothermia**, also thus far have not been shown to be of practical benefit in clinical situations involving humans. Other urgent medical therapies that have been evaluated with clinical trials include isovolemic hemodilution and the lowering of hematocrit to reduce the blood velocity. These measures have produced no convincing improvement in mortality or stroke severity. Hypervolemic hemodilution also has not been shown to be beneficial, and the mortality among patients who receive treatment is higher than that in control subjects, although some have questioned the design of the available studies. In patients with acute stroke, numerous randomized, clinical trials have demonstrated no overall beneficial effect of hemodilution on survival or neurologic outcome. There is some evidence that a continuous 72-hour IV infusion of the defibrinogenating agent Ancrod beginning within 3 hours of ischemic stroke onset is associated with improved functional status—but not with improved survival—at 90 days.

The efficacy of **emergency surgical therapy** with carotid endarterectomy (CEA) in patients with acute occlusion of the carotid artery or progressive cerebral infarction remains uncertain. Middle cerebral artery embolectomy also has been advocated by some, although the procedure has been performed in only a small subgroup of patients and has not been subjected to a clinical trial. The use of angioplasty with or without stenting in the setting of acute ischemic stroke is also unsupported at this time, although the procedure is undergoing further study.

ACUTE MEDICAL MANAGEMENT FOR CEREBRAL INFARCTION

As acute thrombolysis and antithrombotic therapies are being considered in the first minutes and hours after presentation, **aggressive supportive medical management strategies** should be initiated (see also Chapter 11). Issues to address include (1) BP, (2) blood glucose levels, (3) fluid status, (4) temperature, and (5) oxygenation. **BP** is typically allowed to remain elevated acutely. In general, for patients who are not thrombolytic candidates, elevated BP is not treated acutely unless it is >230 mm Hg systolic or 120 mm Hg diastolic or if there is evidence of acute MI, left ventricular failure, renal failure as a result of accelerated hypertension, aortic dissection, hemorrhage, or hypertensive encephalopathy. For those who are treated with thrombolytic therapy, the immediate goal is to keep the BP <185 mm Hg systolic and 105 mm Hg diastolic. Hypotension is a concern because of potential for worsening the ischemic penumbra surrounding the infarction. For those with mean arterial pressure <100 mm Hg, volume expansion with normal saline, 5% albumin solution, or other volume expanders should be initiated.

Elevated **blood glucose** after acute cerebral infarction is associated with an increased risk for adverse clinical and radiologic outcomes. There is no clear evidence that aggressive hyperglycemia management improves outcome. However, elevated blood glucose levels >200 mg per dl should be considered for aggressive management with insulin infusion and close glucose monitoring. The **fluid status** also should be considered carefully. If there is any evidence of dehydration, then euvolemia should be the goal, with initiation of normal saline solution at approximately 100 ml per hour. Fluids that contain dextrose and those that contain free water should be avoided.

Hyperthermia with temperature >38.5°C occurring early after cerebral infarction may also be associated with poorer outcomes. It is important to consider the possible causes of the increased temperature. As the cause is being clarified, acetaminophen should be instituted, up to 4 g per day. If that is not successful in bringing the temperature to normal, then a cooling blanket should be considered.

Patients with any evidence of poor **oxygenation** should be started on oxygen via nasal cannula or close-fitting mask, as outlined in Chapter 11.

PROGRESSIVE ISCHEMIC STROKE

Approximately 20% of patients with infarction in the distribution of the carotid system and approximately 30% to 40% of patients with infarction of the vertebrobasilar distribution have a progressive course **(progressive infarction)**. Low BP or perfusion pressure, recurrent emboli, propagation of IA thrombus, cerebral edema, and hemorrhagic infarction are the most common mechanisms of progression. Alternatively, other causes must also be considered, including tumor, subdural hematoma, demyelinating disease, toxic-metabolic encephalopathy, and infectious processes such as brain abscess or focal encephalitis. In patients with progression caused by evolving **cerebral edema**, treatment with mannitol, glycerol, hyperventilation, and dexamethasone (see Chapter 11) may be initiated, although these measures may be of limited value in this context.

If the intracranial process is still considered to be **ischemic**, resulting from either recurrent emboli or propagation of intra-arterial thrombus, and thrombolytic or mechanical techniques are not indicated and the lesion is nonhemorrhagic on CT, then IV heparin therapy (see Chapter 12 for initiation of therapy) should be considered. However, there is limited evidence suggesting efficacy of heparin in this circumstance. When instituted, heparin treatment is usually continued for 3 to 5 days after the course has stabilized. If the worsening of the deficit occurs within 3 to 6 hours of onset of the original anterior circulation symptoms or within 12 hours of the onset of basilar artery thrombosis–related symptoms, then IA tPA or a mechanical dissolution technique may be considered, as outlined earlier. For these patients who continue to have progression of neurologic deficit, cerebral arteriography may be considered to define the mechanism. A few patients in this group may be considered for emergency endovascular or neurovascular surgical intervention, although no surgical trial has documented the efficacy of either CEA or cerebral arterial embolectomy.

Particular attention should be paid to **hypotension** and any **metabolic abnormalities** that can accentuate the focal neurologic deficit. MRI or CT with contrast should be performed urgently, if not done earlier, to identify **other types of intracranial pathologic processes** as a cause for the symptoms.

TREATMENT OF EARLY COMPLICATIONS

Among the 20% of patients who die within 30 days of the first cerebral infarction, 50% die of potentially treatable medical causes. The frequency of **pneumonia, deep vein thrombosis,** or

pulmonary embolism after a stroke has been estimated at 30%, 10%, and 5%, respectively. Approximately 30% of patients have deterioration during the first week after stroke; 70% of complications result from cerebral causes such as intracranial bleeding or rapidly progressive cerebral edema (see Chapter 11), and 30% result from systemic causes such as **cardiopulmonary failure** (including neurogenic pulmonary edema, myocardial damage, serious cardiac arrhythmias, and pulmonary embolism), **systemic infection**, **hyponatremia** (with inappropriate antidiuretic hormone syndrome or salt-wasting syndrome), side effects of **drugs** such as oversedation from tranquilizers, and other **metabolic causes** (including renal and hepatic failure). Early diagnosis and appropriate treatment of the specific cause of deterioration are essential. Urgent CT or MRI should be performed in patients with clinical deterioration to identify the aforementioned cerebral causes.

NONNEUROLOGIC COMPLICATIONS

Patients who are bedridden have an increased risk for development of **deep vein thrombosis and pulmonary embolism**. Intermittent pneumatic compression devices, passive physical therapy, elevating the legs 6 to 10 degrees, compression stockings, and low-dose heparin therapy (5,000 U of unfractionated heparin subcutaneously every 12 hours or use of fractionated heparin) may help to prevent deep vein thrombosis. Early heparin treatment in acute ischemic stroke and use of intermittent pneumatic compression devices have been associated with substantial reductions in deep vein thrombosis and with decreased mortality in several randomized trials. Evidence from randomized trials also suggests that antiplatelet therapy either alone or in addition to subcutaneously administered heparin should be considered for patients who are at substantial risk for venous thromboembolism. Because of the high risk for pulmonary embolism, which is fatal in 25% of cases, patients with acute deep vein thrombosis should be treated with heparin. Endovascular placement of an inferior vena cava filter should be performed in patients with contraindications to anticoagulant therapy.

Because **pulmonary embolism** is responsible for approximately 10% of the deaths in cases of ischemic stroke, patients should be questioned daily about the occurrence of chest pain and dyspnea. For patients in whom pulmonary embolism is strongly suspected, initial IV therapy with heparin, given in a dose of approximately 5,000 to 10,000 U, should be instituted immediately, even before diagnostic studies are completed if a patient is hemodynamically unstable. Arterial blood gas studies, chest radiography, electrocardiography, ventilation-perfusion scanning, and, in some patients, chest CT should be performed promptly to confirm the diagnosis. If the diagnosis is equivocal and the clinical suspicion is high, pulmonary angiography may be needed.

Pneumonia is also an important cause of death after ischemic stroke. Vigorous tracheobronchial toilet, deep-breathing exercises, and early mobilization are helpful preventive measures. For preventing aspiration pneumonia, swallowing should be tested before oral feeding is permitted. If there is any question about the safety of the patient's swallowing, then a formal study with fluoroscopy may clarify the potential for aspiration and consistency of food that is necessary to prevent aspiration. Antibiotic therapy is used only for clinical infection and is not used prophylactically. In cases of infection, empiric antibiotic therapy should be instituted until the specific infectious agent and antibiotic sensitivities are established.

Urinary tract infection may be complicated by secondary septicemia in approximately 5% of patients. Indwelling catheters should be avoided; the alternative approach used is frequent, intermittent catheterization to minimize bladder distention. In patients with incontinence or urinary retention, anticholinergic drugs may help in the recovery of bladder function.

Cardiovascular complications after stroke, such as cardiac arrhythmias, various types of myocardial damage (for example, contraction bands, focal myocardial necrosis, subendocardial ischemia), and electrocardiographic abnormalities (ST- and T-segment changes, U-wave abnormalities, QT prolongation, and sinus arrhythmias) should be treated whenever possible, with attention given to the underlying disease according to a cardiologist's suggestions. The treatment of cardiac ventricular arrhythmias after acute stroke often begins with beta-adrenergic blocking agents such as propranolol. IV antiarrhythmic agents may be necessary in cases of malignant arrhythmias that are not controlled by oral agents.

Gastrointestinal alterations after an acute cerebrovascular event include nausea and vomiting, acute peptic ulceration, and fecal incontinence or impaction. Proton pump inhibitors or histamine receptor blockers may be used for ulcer prophylaxis. Patients who are on anticoagulants and those who are on mechanical ventilation are at higher risk for hemorrhage and should be particularly considered for prophylaxis. Stool softeners, laxatives, and suppositories lessen the risk for impaction.

Decubitus ulcers are common and should be prevented with use of an air mattress on the bed, position adjustment every 1 to 2 hours, tight bed sheets, dry skin surfaces, and prevention of urinary and fecal incontinence.

For patients who are unable to close fully one or both eyes, artificial tears or blepharoplasty may be needed to maintain adequate corneal moisture and to prevent corneal clouding and ulceration.

NEUROLOGIC COMPLICATIONS

Seizures occur in approximately 10% of patients with cerebral infarction; 30% occur within the first 2 weeks and 75% within the first year after stroke onset. ICHs and embolic cortical infarcts are more frequently associated with seizures. Anticonvulsants are not routinely given as prophylactic agents in this situation.

Initially, seizures that result from an acute cerebrovascular event are treated with intravenously administered diazepam (5 to 10 mg, at a rate as high as 2 mg per minute, which may be repeated once in 5 to 15 minutes) followed by a loading dose of phenytoin given orally (15 to 20 mg per kg, given in a single dose, or split in three doses given every 8 hours) or IV fosphenytoin may be used. Fosphenytoin, which is rapidly metabolized to phenytoin, is given intravenously (15 to 20 mg per kg phenytoin equivalents at a rate as high as 150 mg of phenytoin equivalents per minute) or intramuscularly.

Electrocardiographic and BP monitoring should be used during and after acute IV administration of anticonvulsants because of concern about bradycardia and hypotension. If the duration of ventricular electrical activities (QT interval) widens, bradyarrhythmias occur, or hypotension appears, the infusion rate should be slowed.

Subarachnoid Hemorrhage

General Evaluation and Treatment

PATIENT EVALUATION

The diagnosis of subarachnoid hemorrhage (SAH) requires suspicion on the part of medical personnel in initial contact with the patient. Although the abrupt onset of a severe headache is a common presentation, less severe headache with or without an associated brief loss of consciousness, nausea, or vomiting may also signal SAH, and an initial, mild hemorrhage sometimes is missed. In any patient with new onset of an unusually severe or atypical headache, particularly if associated with a brief loss of consciousness, nausea, vomiting, stiff neck, or any focal neurologic findings, **computed tomography (CT) of the head** without contrast should be performed to determine whether intracranial hemorrhage is present (see algorithm for the management of SAH in Appendix E-4).

If obtained within 24 hours, the CT scan is abnormal in approximately 98% of cases of SAH and reveals the increased attenuation caused by hemorrhage in the subarachnoid space (Fig. 14-1). If the CT scan is negative, including no evidence of subtle SAH in the posterior horns of the lateral ventricles or over the sulci, then a **lumbar puncture** (**LP**) should be performed if there are no contraindications for the procedure (see Chapter 7 for details). If the CT scan shows evidence for SAH or intraparenchymal hemorrhage, an LP will not contribute significant additional diagnostic information and sometimes can be dangerous, especially if parenchymal blood is present. MRI is nearly as reliable as CT in demonstrating subarachnoid blood in the first few days after SAH but is often impractical. After a few days, MRI becomes increasingly superior to CT in demonstrating subarachnoid blood up to approximately 40 days after a hemorrhage.

The typical patient with SAH has grossly bloody spinal fluid. However, **traumatic LP** must be differentiated from true SAH. Three or four successive tubes of cerebrospinal fluid (CSF) are collected, and, if the specimens show progressively less blood, a traumatic LP is suggested. Clotting of the specimen virtually never occurs with true SAH. Xanthochromia, or the yellow-tinging of CSF caused by hemoglobin breakdown products, is present in the supernatant as early as 6 hours after SAH and remains in the spinal fluid for an average of 2 to 3 weeks. Erythrocytes often disappear within several days after SAH. The CSF may not show xanthochromia if small numbers of erythrocytes are present from SAH (approximately ≤400), and xanthochromia has been reported in rare instances with traumatic LP if the erythrocyte count is >200,000 per μl. Spectrophotometry of CSF for detection of oxyhemoglobin or bilirubin may also be of value in distinguishing between traumatic LP and true SAH, although that has not been fully evaluated.

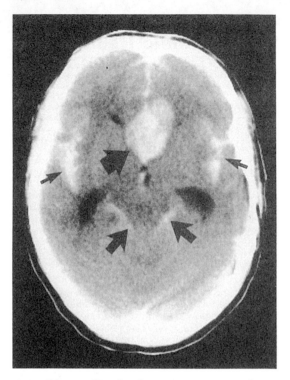

Figure 14-1.   CT scan of head without contrast: areas of increased attenuation consistent with SAH in the sylvian fissures (small arrows) and interhemispheric fissure (large arrow) and surrounding the brainstem (medium arrows). Hemorrhage was caused by an aneurysm of the anterior communicating artery.

In addition to a headache that varies from the classic severe, striking, generalized headache with meningismus to a much milder headache that resolves within 24 to 48 hours, other aspects of the neurologic history and examination are important in clarifying the potential presence of SAH. Because aneurysms may cause a mass effect on adjacent structures, including the cranial nerves and brainstem, symptoms that precede SAH may include diplopia, facial weakness, extremity weakness, and unsteadiness. In addition, aneurysms can occasionally present with transient symptoms caused by ischemia or seizures. Ischemic spells typically are thought to be caused by thrombus formation within or adjacent to the aneurysm and lead to distal embolization and ischemia. In addition to focal symptoms, more generalized symptoms, including transient loss of consciousness caused by a sudden increase in intracranial pressure (ICP), may occur at the time of the hemorrhage. Approximately one third of patients develop focal signs at or around the time of headache onset, and almost half develop unresponsiveness that lasts an hour or more.

A comprehensive neurologic examination should be performed in the patient with SAH, but profound muscle testing should be avoided because of the potential increased risk for rebleeding. On neurologic examination, the presence of any focal findings is important and may aid in localizing the aneurysm. Particular findings that may be useful include monocular visual deficits, which may indicate an ophthalmic artery aneurysm with optic nerve compression. Extraocular muscle abnormalities may indicate internal carotid artery, basilar artery, or ophthalmic aneurysms. A unilateral third cranial nerve palsy early in the course of the SAH strongly suggests an aneurysm of the posterior communicating artery. Sixth cranial nerve palsy may result from increased ICP or from a basilar artery aneurysm. Hemorrhage or mass effect from a middle cerebral artery aneurysm may cause aphasia and hemiparesis. Leg weakness and changes in behavior may be associated with rupture or mass effect from an anterior communicating artery or anterior cerebral artery aneurysm that affects the frontal lobe(s).

Initial CT scan may reveal the location of the hemorrhage as well as the possible source for the event, although standard CT imaging without contrast is unlikely to detect an uncalcified aneurysm, especially one that is <7 mm in size. An aneurysmal cause must be suspected in all cases of SAH or intracerebral hemorrhage (ICH) that cannot be clearly explained by an alternative cause. MRI and magnetic resonance angiography (MRA) are more likely to show the underlying cause, including relatively small aneurysms. After SAH is diagnosed and the patient is initially stabilized, urgent cerebral arteriography typically is indicated to attempt to define the cause of the SAH. Cerebral arteriography is the most sensitive study available; it reveals small saccular aneurysms and arteriovenous malformations (AVMs) as well as the associated morphology and anatomic characteristics. MRA and CT angiography are noninvasive means of detecting small aneurysms with a relatively high sensitivity, especially if the lesion is >3 mm in maximal diameter, but these studies alone are usually insufficient for surgical planning and typically are not used in isolation in the circumstance of acute SAH. If the initial arteriogram performed for SAH fails to reveal an aneurysm, a repeat study is usually performed 1 to 3 weeks later in an attempt to detect an aneurysm that was not visible on the early study. An exception to this recommendation for repeat arteriogram may be an SAH that is localized solely to a small clot anterior to the brainstem, the so-called perimesencephalic or pretruncal SAH. Posterior circulation aneurysms can cause such a CT appearance in some cases, so the issue of repeat arteriography in these patients is somewhat controversial. Other studies (Table 14-1) are also typically undertaken to identify other potential underlying factors that are causing or exacerbating SAH, such as hypocoagulable states.

TREATMENT

Early treatment of patients with SAH is directed toward the prevention and management of major **neurologic complications**, including rebleeding, vasospasm and cerebral ischemia, hydrocephalus, and seizures. Early treatment of SAH also involves the

Table 14-1.   Laboratory investigations for patients with SAH

Complete blood cell count
Prothrombin time, aPTT
Erythrocyte sedimentation rate
Blood glucose
Serum electrolytes
Urinalysis
Chest radiography
Electrocardiography
Head CT or MRI; consider LP (if hemorrhage is suspected and
   CT or MRI is negative)
Consider inpatient cardiac monitoring
Consider TCD (e.g., if vasospasm suspected)
Consider cerebral arteriography
Consider electroencephalography (if seizure is suspected)
Determination of arterial blood gas levels (if hypoxia is suspected)
Consider special coagulation studies (if cause is unclear despite
   arteriography)

aPTT = activated partial thromboplastin time; CT = computed tomography;
LP = lumbar puncture; MRI = magnetic resonance imaging; SAH = subarachnoid hemorrhage; TCD = transcranial Doppler ultrasonography.

management of various relatively common **systemic complications**, including electrolyte disturbances such as hyponatremia,
cardiac arrhythmia and myocardial damage, and neurogenic pulmonary edema. The overall general treatment strategy is summarized in Table 14-2 and Appendix E-4. Specific management of
aneurysms, AVMs, and other underlying conditions such as
hypocoagulable states is described in Chapter 17.

Prevention and Management of Neurologic Complications
Rebleeding
   The likelihood of **rebleeding** after SAH is greatest during the
first few days after initial hemorrhage, particularly the first
24 hours. This time sequence and the associated mortality rate of
approximately 50% make the prevention of rebleeding a major
priority in the early treatment of patients with SAH. Early surgical, endovascular, and medical intervention can prevent recurrent
hemorrhages. Results of the recently completed International
Subarachnoid Aneurysm Trial showed that endovascular ablation
(coiling) of ruptured aneurysms produces less periprocedural morbidity in a selected group of patients with aneurysmal SAH, but
the long-term risk for rebleeding from the treated aneurysms and
the risk for repeat procedures may be higher in this group (see
Chapter 17).
   Patients should be placed on **bed rest** in a **quiet room** and
kept under **close observation** either in an intensive care unit or
at least in a hospital room close to a nursing station. The head

Table 14-2. General management measures for SAH

1. Place patient on bed rest in quiet room
2. Provide ongoing monitoring of neurologic status (level of consciousness, focal deficit, Glasgow Coma Scale [see Appendix B])
3. Consider cardiac monitoring
4. Elevate head of bed 30 degrees
5. Prevent straining (stool softeners and antitussive agents as needed)
6. Provide oral nutrition for alert patients with intact gag reflex
7. Provide enteral nutrition with nasogastric tube for patients with decreased level of consciousness or impaired gag reflex
8. Maintain normovolemia and normal sodium level by starting with administration of 2–3 L/day D_5W and 0.9% normal saline and adjusting accordingly (see Table 14-5)
9. Mildly sedate patient if agitated: phenobarbital (30–60 mg two times a day) or chloral hydrate (500 mg three times a day)
10. Control mild pain with acetaminophen or propoxyphene and severe pain with codeine (60 mg, intramuscularly or orally, every 3–4 hr); use morphine (1- to 2-mg increments intravenously) only as last resort
11. Reduce BP conservatively and with careful monitoring if patient has extremely increased BP or evidence of acute end organ damage

BP = blood pressure; SAH = subarachnoid hemorrhage.

of the patient's bed should be elevated approximately 30 degrees to lower the patient's ICP. Straining should be prevented with stool softeners; coughing may be prevented with antitussive agents, such as codeine, as needed.

Serial assessments of level of consciousness by an experienced nursing staff are of great importance. The Glasgow Coma Scale (see Appendix B) may be used for this purpose. In addition, the Glasgow Coma Scale serves as a basis for the World Federation of Neurosurgeons Grading Scale, a commonly used prognostic scale in the setting of SAH (see Appendix C-4).

If the patient is **agitated**, a sedative, phenobarbital (30 to 60 mg twice daily) or chloral hydrate (500 mg three times daily), is recommended. The patient should not be oversedated, because the effect of medication may be indistinguishable from a depressed level of consciousness caused by rehemorrhage or other complications of SAH.

Analgesia should be provided for pain relief, because extra pain often leads to agitation and an increased likelihood of additional hemorrhage. Mild pain can be managed with acetaminophen or propoxyphene. For severe pain, codeine (60 mg, intramuscularly or orally, every 3 to 4 hours) may be used as needed. Morphine should be used only as a last resort for otherwise uncontrollable pain (given in small increments of 1 to 2 mg intravenously), because it may depress respiration and level of consciousness.

The use of **antifibrinolytic agents** such as ϵ-aminocaproic acid (Amicar [24 to 36 g per day in 1,000 ml of 5% dextrose solution]) or tranexamic acid (1 g intravenously or 1.5 g orally 4 to 6 times daily) have been shown to decrease rebleeding of aneurysms but do not seem to improve the overall outcome after SAH. In addition, these agents are associated with thrombotic side effects, including cerebral infarction, deep vein thrombosis, and pulmonary embolism. Consequently, administration of these antifibrinolytic agents does not seem to be warranted after a single SAH. However, the risk–benefit ratio is more likely to favor use of these agents if there is evidence of continued or recurrent hemorrhage after initial hemorrhage.

Deterioration of neurologic status, including level of consciousness, in patients with SAH may signify an episode of rebleeding, especially early after the original SAH. However, several other possible causes of neurologic deterioration are (1) delayed ischemic neurologic deficits that may be related to vasospasm (most commonly 4 to 14 days after SAH), (2) acute hydrocephalus, (3) cerebral edema, (4) electrolyte imbalances, (5) neurogenic pulmonary edema, (6) seizures, and (7) severe cardiac dysrhythmia or ischemia. CT of the head should be performed in patients with deterioration of neurologic status as soon as possible to attempt to confirm the existence of rebleeding or acute hydrocephalus. In some cases, the appearance of acute hydrocephalus or intraparenchymal clot with mass effect may warrant emergency surgical intervention (Table 14-3). Repeated LPs generally are not of value in confirming the cause of neurologic deterioration and may be hazardous.

Many patients who rebleed experience a sudden respiratory arrest at the onset of the rebleeding episode. In general, vigorous attempts should be made to resuscitate these patients, because recovery of complete neurologic function is possible in these circumstances, even after respiratory arrest.

After rebleeding, if the patient stabilizes and recovers, identification and clipping of an underlying aneurysm become even more urgent because further rebleeding episodes are common and associated with high mortality.

Vasospasm and Cerebral Ischemia

Another common and potentially serious complication of SAH hemorrhage is **cerebral vasospasm,** a narrowing of arteries in the intracranial segments of the carotid and vertebrobasilar

Table 14-3.   Indications for emergency surgical intervention in patients with SAH

1. Acute hydrocephalus causing substantial or progressive neurologic deficit
2. Large, surgically accessible intracerebral hematoma with significant mass effect
3. Rebleeding followed by partial or total recovery of neurologic function from a known aneurysm or AVM previously untreated or partially treated

AVM = arteriovenous malformation, SAH = subarachnoid hemorrhage.

circulations, typically most severe in areas of maximal hemorrhage. Vasospasm occurs in approximately 30% of patients with SAH, typically beginning about 3 to 5 days after the hemorrhage; maximal effect is at 5 to 14 days, and resolution occurs over 2 to 3 weeks.

Patients with suspected **cerebral ischemia** (a decrease in the level of consciousness, focal cerebral deficits, or both) should undergo CT, which may show evidence of cerebral infarction or evidence of other conditions that may mimic cerebral ischemia, including acute hydrocephalus, recurrent subarachnoid or intracerebral bleeding, or cerebral edema. Cerebral arteriography is the most sensitive means to evaluate vasospasm, although transcranial Doppler (TCD) ultrasonographic examination often provides noninvasive detection of vasospasm and is a much more practical way to provide ongoing monitoring of the condition. The arteriographic or TCD findings may not be associated with any clinical change because only approximately 50% of cases are associated with focal symptoms.

Several findings may be associated with an increased occurrence of vasospasm, such as an aneurysmal cause for the SAH; a significant amount of subarachnoid blood, particularly at the base of the brain; and intraventricular hemorrhage. Measures that can help **prevent** cerebral ischemia include (1) maintenance of a normal fluid and sodium balance, (2) conservative use or avoidance of antihypertensive agents, and (3) the use of calcium channel blocking agents (Table 14-4).

Fluid management should seek to maintain normovolemia and a normal sodium level. Hypovolemia is associated with the development of vasospasm and cerebral ischemia, whereas hypervolemia may be associated with cerebral edema and increased ICP. In general, most patients should be started on approximately 2 to 3 L per day of D_5W and 0.9% normal saline, with adjustments as needed, depending on body size, serial

---

Table 14-4.   Management of vasospasm and cerebral ischemia associated with SAH

1. Apply preventive measures, including adequate fluid and sodium intake and conservative use of antihypertensive agents and calcium channel blocking agents (nimodipine, 60 mg, orally, every 4 hr for 21 days)
2. Provide volume expansion with 5% albumin (e.g., 250 ml 4–6 times daily), colloid, or packed erythrocytes
3. Maintain central venous pressure at 8–12 mm Hg and pulmonary wedge pressure at 16–20 mm Hg
4. Consider induction of hypertension with phenylephrine and/or dopamine
5. Consider balloon angioplasty, surgical drainage of clot, and administration of tissue-plasminogen activator or other investigational therapy, preferably in the context of a randomized, clinical trial

SAH = subarachnoid hemorrhage.

weights, intake and output measurements, central hemodynamic measurements, serum electrolyte levels, and general nutrition status. However, there is a paucity of information on the efficacy of either hypervolemia alone or in combination with hypertension and hemodilution therapy (so-called triple-H therapy) for prevention or treatment of delayed ischemic neurologic deficits associated with SAH. **Hyponatremia** is common in patients with SAH; its management is discussed later in the section Hyponatremia.

One must be cautious about the use of **antihypertensive agents** in patients with SAH because they may precipitate or accentuate cerebral ischemic complications. At least part of the hypertension observed is often the result of Cushing's reflex, in which intracranial hypertension leads to peripheral hypertension to maintain cerebral perfusion. Alternatively, excessive hypertension may be associated with an increased risk for rebleeding. Treatment of hypertension is usually confined to careful, well-monitored, modest reductions in blood pressure (BP) for patients with evidence of organ damage or very high BP (see Chapter 11). In general, a mean arterial BP

$$\left(\frac{2 \times \text{diastolic} + \text{systolic}}{3} \right)$$

of 130 to 140 mm Hg or more or systolic pressure of 180 to 200 mm Hg or more may be treated with intermittent or continuous, intravenous (IV) administration of antihypertensive agents such as labetalol or sodium nitroprusside. The most appropriate goal BPs are controversial, although a mean arterial BP of ≤ 130 to 140 mm Hg is reasonable.

Calcium channel blocking agents, such as nimodipine, seem to be beneficial in improving outcomes after SAH, likely via a neuroprotective effect. Arteriogram studies do not demonstrate that occurrence of vasospasm on imaging is altered by nimodipine use, suggesting an alternative mechanism for its benefit. Nimodipine reduces the frequency of cerebral infarction and poor outcomes in aneurysmal SAH and therefore should be administered in a dosage of 60 mg orally every 4 hours for 21 days after SAH. IV administration of calcium antagonists, which is more expensive, may be reserved for patients who cannot take nimodipine orally.

Tirilazad, a 21-amino steroid neuroprotective agent, has been studied extensively in clinical trials and has not proved to be effective in preventing vasospasm or delayed ischemia. Other treatment strategies, including the use of antiplatelet agents, magnesium sulfate, calcitonin gene-related peptide, intrathecal injection of tissue-type plasminogen activator, and prophylactic transluminal angioplasty, are currently under investigation.

In patients with **confirmed symptomatic vasospasm**, despite the described preventive measures, **blood volume expansion** is indicated and may be accomplished by the administration of albumin solution (for instance, 5% albumin, 250 ml 4 to 6 times daily), colloid, or packed erythrocytes. Central venous pressures should be maintained between 8 and 12 mm Hg, capillary wedge pressures between 16 and 20 mm Hg, and the hematocrit value at approximately 40%. If treatment with calcium channel–blocking agents has not already been started, then it should be instituted (nimodipine, 60 mg, orally every 6 hours or nicardipine, 0.01 to 0.15 mg/kg/hour, intravenously), and nimodipine should be continued for 21 days. If these measures are ineffective, pressor agents such as dopamine (starting at 3 to 6 μg/kg/minute and titrating on the basis of BP response) or phenylephrine are sometimes given while maintaining the systolic BP at or less than a value of approximately 20 to 50 mm Hg above baseline.

Monitoring of cardiac output and serial TCD ultrasonographic examinations are often helpful for following patients. If clinically significant vasospasm persists despite the described measures, intracranial balloon angioplasty or catheter-directed intra-arterial infusion of a vasodilator, such as papaverine, can be considered in centers with experience in these techniques, preferably in the setting of an ongoing randomized, controlled trial, because the efficacy and the safety of these techniques have not been well established.

Acute Hydrocephalus

Subarachnoid blood may lead to ventricular enlargement and obstructive hydrocephalus. **Acute hydrocephalus** occurs in approximately 20% of patients with SAH, often presenting with either obtundation at the time of admission or increasing drowsiness within a few days of the SAH after an initial recovery. Paralysis of upward gaze and pupillary abnormalities may also be present. The diagnosis is confirmed by CT. Predictors of hydrocephalus include poor Glasgow Coma Score at admission, ICH in combination with SAH, and aneurysm in the posterior circulation.

In patients who have small to moderate amounts of subarachnoid blood and who stabilize and remain alert, an attempt at **conservative management** is reasonable because approximately half of these patients improve spontaneously without further intervention. In patients with neurologic impairment or deterioration resulting from the hydrocephalus, **neurosurgical intervention** should be urgently considered; this usually includes placement of an external ventricular drain. The amount of CSF drainage should be monitored carefully because excessive decompression may be associated with rebleeding of an underlying aneurysm. This risk is minimized by keeping the drainage at a moderate pressure level.

Seizures

Approximately 3% to 5% of patients with SAH have associated **seizures.** A single initial seizure at the time of hemorrhage does not predict the likelihood of future seizures, but patients with associated ICH are more likely to have early seizures. Patients with early seizures are usually treated with intravenously administered benzodiazepines, either diazepam (5 to 10 mg at a rate as high as 2 mg per minute, which may be repeated once in 5 to 15 minutes) or lorazepam, followed by an IV or oral loading dose of phenytoin in normal saline (15 to 20 mg per kg at a rate as high as 50 mg per minute) or fosphenytoin (15 to 20 mg per kg phenytoin equivalents at a rate as high as 150 mg phenytoin equivalents per minute). Electrocardiographic and BP monitoring should be used during and after acute administration. Phenytoin, fosphenytoin, or other agents may be used for maintenance therapy.

Prevention and Management of Nonneurologic Complications

Various systemic complications arise in patients with SAH, the identification and treatment of which may substantially alter long- and short-term outcomes.

Hyponatremia

By far the most common electrolyte disturbance associated with SAH is **hyponatremia**, which is present to some extent in up to 30% to 35% of cases and to a severe extent in approximately 5% of cases. Clinical manifestations, including minor alterations in level of consciousness, seizures, asterixis, and coma, usually do not develop until the sodium value is 120 mmol per L or less, a level of hyponatremia that is extremely uncommon after SAH. Hyponatremia usually develops between 2 and 10 days after SAH.

Treatment of the hyponatremia is based on identification of the underlying mechanism of the disorder, which may vary from patient to patient. Many cases of mild hyponatremia associated with SAH are the result of overhydration with hypotonic fluids and may be corrected by switching to smaller amounts of isotonic fluids without major manipulations in therapy (Table 14-5).

In many patients with substantial hyponatremia after SAH, the underlying cause is a **cerebral salt-wasting syndrome**. These patients tend to have a negative fluid balance, low central venous and pulmonary wedge pressures, decreasing weight, negative sodium balance, and excessive natriuresis. In these patients, hyponatremia is best corrected with isotonic saline, Ringer's lactate, or colloid while keeping the central venous pressure between

Table 14-5.   Management of hyponatremia

1. Avoid overhydration with hypotonic fluids
2. Look for evidence of salt-wasting syndrome or SIADH
3. If salt-wasting syndrome is associated with hypovolemia, then give isotonic saline, Ringer's lactate, or colloid to correct hyponatremia
4. If SIADH is present, then manage with fluid restriction (<1 L/day) and furosemide (40 mg/day); demeclocycline (300–600 mg, orally, twice a day) is uncommonly used in acute hyponatremia
5. Consider adding fludrocortisone acetate (1 mg twice a day) In rare instances of symptomatic, severe hyponatremia (<120 mEq/L), consider infusion of 3% saline at rate of 25–50 ml/hr
6. Avoid excessively rapid correction or overcorrection of sodium levels (≤20 mEq/L during 24 hr or 1.5–2 mEq/L/hr)

SIADH = syndrome of inappropriate antidiuretic hormone.

8 and 12 mm Hg. It may also be helpful to use fludrocortisone acetate (1 mg twice a day) to help reduce or eliminate a negative sodium balance. Previously, it was considered that patients with hyponatremia after SAH often have a **syndrome of inappropriate antidiuretic hormone (SIADH)**. Most recent studies suggest that this is rarely the case. When the syndrome does occur, these patients have a stable or positive fluid balance with normal to high central venous and pulmonary wedge pressures and stable to increasing body weight. These patients also have increased urine sodium and osmolality levels. For patients with SIADH, treatment usually involves fluid restriction (<1 L per day) and a loop diuretic such as furosemide (40 mg per day) or a drug that inhibits the ability of ADH to increase water reabsorption, such as demeclocycline (300 to 600 mg twice daily).

Regardless of the cause of the hyponatremia, it is generally advised that the abnormality be corrected slowly, not exceeding 20 mEq per L within 24 hours or 1.5 to 2 mEq/L/hour. In rare cases of severe, symptomatic hyponatremia and a sodium level <120 mEq per L, it is necessary to administer a 3% saline solution (25 to 50 ml per hour) with or without a loop diuretic to increase the plasma sodium concentration by approximately 10%.

Cardiac Dysfunction

SAH is also associated with various **cardiac arrhythmias** and other electrocardiographic changes resulting from **myocardial ischemia, infarction,** or other mechanical damage. Patients with known or suspected cardiac arrhythmias, other ongoing cardiac dysfunction, a history of cardiac disease, or intracranial hemorrhages causing significant or progressive neurologic deficits should be considered for continuous cardiac monitoring.

The treatment of cardiac ventricular arrhythmia often involves β-adrenergic blocking agents such as propranolol. Intravenously administered antiarrhythmic agents may be required in cases of malignant arrhythmias or those that are uncontrolled by oral agents. However, one must be careful because of the propensity of these agents to decrease BP. Life-threatening arrhythmias, such as ventricular fibrillation, are rare and usually of short duration. Patients with arrhythmias require ongoing cardiac monitoring and should be questioned daily about the occurrence of chest pain and dyspnea.

Other Nonneurologic Complications

Another less common complication of SAH is **neurogenic pulmonary edema**, which may present with sudden or subacute onset of dyspnea, cyanosis, and pink, frothy sputum. Treatment usually involves positive end-expiratory pressure ventilation and diuretics.

The most common **acid-base disorders** associated with SAH are **metabolic alkalosis and respiratory alkalosis**, the former caused by excessive vomiting, diuretics, and bicarbonate administration and the latter caused by hyperventilation. Potassium depletion is common in patients with metabolic acidosis and requires replacement with potassium chloride.

Adequate **nutrition** is important and is often accomplished by means of a nasogastric tube for patients who cannot be fed orally because of a decreased level of consciousness or impaired gag reflex. The caloric intake should be maintained at approximately 2,000 to 3,000 calories per day, or more in the setting of fever. Enteric feeding can be accomplished with various commercially available preparations (Ensure, Ensure Plus), which are usually given at half strength or full strength and better tolerated with a continuous-infusion feeding pump, if available. To avoid **aspiration**, patients are usually fed with the head elevated 30 degrees; hourly checks should be made for gastric residue. For intubated patients, the endotracheal cuff should be inflated during feeding. Oral medications may be crushed and given through the enteral tube.

Prophylaxis for **deep vein thrombosis and pulmonary embolism** can be accomplished by intermittent pneumatic compression devices applied to the legs, compression stockings, or mild range-of-motion foot exercises for patients who are awake and alert.

Intracerebral Hemorrhage

General Evaluation and Treatment

As noted in Chapter 1, patients with **intracerebral (intra-parenchymal) hemorrhage (ICH)** typically present with relatively abrupt onset of focal neurologic symptoms and signs that may be associated with early decreased level of alertness, headache, nausea, and vomiting. In patients with this abrupt onset of symptoms, clinically suspected intracranial hemorrhage should prompt urgent computed tomography (CT) or magnetic resonance imaging (MRI) to determine the location and the size of the hemorrhage (Fig. 15-1) and possibly to reveal other intracranial disease processes (see algorithm for management of ICH in Appendix E-5). The location of the hemorrhage may guide further evaluation that is necessary to define the mechanism. In addition to the five main locations for **intracranial hemorrhage** outlined in Chapter 8, the specific location of an intracerebral (intraparenchymal) hemorrhage may further define the likely mechanism of the hemorrhage. Given that the volume of the hemorrhage is such a strong predictor of outcome, the volume should be estimated from the CT scan using the ellipsoid method. The volume is estimated by measuring the width, length, and height of the hematoma, with multiplication of these measurements in centimeters and division by 2 to provide the very approximate volume in cubic centimeters.

Lobar ICHs are characterized by bleeding into the cortex or subcortical white matter. Common features at the onset include vomiting and localized headache (frontal hemorrhage usually afflicts the forehead area; temporal hemorrhage, the area around or anterior to the ipsilateral ear; parietal hemorrhage, the temple area; and occipital hemorrhage, the area around or over the ipsilateral eye).

In lobar ICHs, unlike deep supratentorial hemorrhages, the neurologic deficits are often more restricted and variable (frontal hematoma usually produces contralateral arm weakness; left temporal hematoma, aphasia and delirium; parietal hematoma, contralateral hemisensory loss; and occipital hematoma, contralateral homonymous hemianopia). Disturbances of the level of consciousness occur later in the clinical course, and a history of hypertension is less frequent. The neurologic deficit appears rapidly, within 1 to several minutes, but not instantaneously as it usually does with an embolus. Stiff neck or seizures at the onset are uncommon, and more than half of the patients are drowsy. However, a large lobar ICH may affect two or more lobes and may produce stupor or coma associated with severe neurologic deficit.

Most patients with **lobar hematoma** require further evaluation with arteriography because of the potential for underlying intracranial aneurysm or arteriovenous malformation (AVM). If aneurysm or AVM is highly suspected, arteriography is

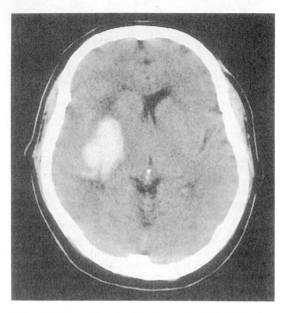

Figure 15-1.   CT scan of head without contrast: right basal ganglia hemorrhage.

necessary; if aneurysm is not detected, MRI with gadolinium may further clarify a cause for the hemorrhage. Amyloid angiopathy, underlying neoplasm, arteriographically occult vascular malformation, bleeding diathesis, and anticoagulant use are other primary considerations for hemorrhage at that site. Magnetic resonance angiography (MRA) and MRI may aid in revealing an underlying cause, including aneurysm, AVM or other vascular malformation, neoplasm, or multiple infarcts consistent with an inflammatory vascular disorder. There has been an ongoing debate regarding whether surgical therapy should be considered for lobar hemorrhages. In the International Surgical Therapy for Intracerebral Hemorrhage Trial (STICH), 1,033 patients with supratentorial ICH were randomly assigned to early surgery or medical management. The overall outcomes were similar, suggesting that surgery is not indicated for all ICHs. In the subgroup analysis, patients with lobar hemorrhage also were not benefited by surgery. However, hemorrhages that were ≤1 cm from the cortical surface did better with early surgery compared with conservative management. Whether selected patients with superficial hemorrhages should be treated surgically with craniotomy remains to be established.

Supratentorial deep hemorrhages into the basal ganglia and internal capsule are usually characterized by sudden onset of headache followed by acute or subacute (as long as 48 hours) loss of consciousness associated with contralateral hemiparesis, hemisensory loss, homonymous hemianopia, and, if the dominant hemisphere is involved, aphasia. Vomiting is common. In comatose patients, signs of uncal herniation (ipsilateral third cranial nerve palsy) or upper brainstem compression may appear (deep, irregular, or intermittent respiration; ipsilaterally dilated and fixed pupil; and decerebrate posturing).

The presence of upward gaze palsy with unreactive miotic pupils, sometimes associated with convergence paralysis, is characteristic of **thalamic hemorrhage** and helps to differentiate it from putaminal hemorrhage. Besides characteristic oculomotor abnormalities, thalamic hemorrhage often produces contralateral eye deviation, aphasia (dominant hemisphere involvement), neglect (nondominant hemisphere involvement), unilateral hemiplegia or hemiparesis, and unusual sensory syndromes (distressing dysesthesias and spontaneous pain occurring with a latency of days to weeks from onset).

In **putaminal hemorrhage**, the eyes are conjugately deviated to the side of the lesion, the pupillary size and reactivity are normal unless uncal herniation has occurred, and focal neurologic signs (dense, flaccid hemiplegia or hemiparesis, hemisensory loss, homonymous hemianopia, global aphasia [dominant hemisphere involvement], or hemi-inattention [nondominant hemisphere involvement]) and level of consciousness tend to worsen gradually within minutes to hours.

Caudate hemorrhages are characterized by headache, nausea, vomiting, and various types of behavioral abnormalities (such as disorientation or confusion), occasionally accompanied by a prominent short-term memory loss, transient gaze paresis, and contralateral hemiparesis without language disorders.

Basal ganglia hemorrhage is typically caused by chronic hypertension with associated lipohyalinosis and Charcot-Bouchard aneurysms in the small, perforating vasculature. In the presence of chronic hypertension, MRI with gadolinium may be performed to be certain that there is no underlying neoplasm, vascular malformation, or alternative cause. If there is no history of hypertension, then it is more likely that an underlying neoplasm, vascular malformation, or other cause is present, and further evaluation with MRI and, in younger patients with arteriography, is indicated. Hematomas in the putamen with signs of deterioration or progressive neurologic deficit may be amenable to surgical therapy; those in the thalamus and caudate are rarely operable. When the deficit is stable, hemorrhage into these subcortical locations is typically treated medically.

Primary brainstem hemorrhage usually occurs in the **pons** and results in early coma, quadriplegia, prominent decerebrate rigidity, pinpoint (1 mm) pupils that react to light, and the locked-in syndrome with some persistent ability to move the eyelids and eyes up and down. The eyes are often in midposition and have an impaired or absent response to caloric tests. Hyperpnea, hyperhidrosis, and hyperthermia are common. Primary **midbrain and medullary hemorrhages** are rare. When midbrain hemorrhage occurs, it often results in homolateral oculomotor paralysis with crossed hemiplegia (Weber's syndrome). When the hemorrhage enlarges, quadriplegia and coma often occur. Medullary hemorrhage usually produces early coma and rapid death.

Cerebellar hemorrhage usually develops in one of the cerebellar hemispheres (origination in the region of the dentate nucleus is common) within a period of several hours; loss of consciousness at the onset is uncommon. Repeated vomiting, nausea, severe occipital headache, and vertigo with inability to walk or stand (dysequilibrium, limb ataxia) are common early features. Often, some combination of the following signs or symptoms occur: mild peripheral facial palsy; dizziness; nystagmus; miosis; decreased corneal reflex; paresis of conjugate lateral gaze of the eyes to the side of the hemorrhage; forced deviation of the eyes to the side opposite the lesion; and ipsilateral abducens palsy, which indicates both cerebellar and pontine dysfunction (hemiplegia usually does not occur).

Pontine and cerebellar hemorrhage are also commonly a result of chronic hypertension. If the patient does not have a history of hypertension, MRI of the head with gadolinium should be performed. In younger patients and in those in whom a vascular malformation or other vascular lesion is suggested on the MRI, arteriography may need to be performed to clarify an underlying AVM. Hematomas in the brainstem are usually inoperable, but evacuation is occasionally attempted when there is evidence of neurologic deterioration in an otherwise healthy patient with a good life expectancy.

Because moderate to large cerebellar hematomas (2 to 3 cm or more in diameter) often lead to a life-threatening, downhill course with unpredictable deterioration caused by brainstem compression, it is important to monitor patients closely and to remove the hematoma before compression causes alteration in the level of consciousness and an unstable clinical situation. Often, immediate surgical intervention is indicated. However, alert patients who have smaller lesions and no signs of brainstem compression may be treated medically under close observation in the neurologic intensive care unit. The same treatment approach applies to a patient who has a stable neurologic course and unimpaired consciousness and is seen later than 1 week after the cerebellar hemorrhage. However, once a patient shows signs of brainstem compression or deterioration, such as a diminution in the level of consciousness, immediate evacuation of the clot is indicated as a potentially life-saving treatment, even if the patient is in a deep coma.

Patients with **subarachnoid hemorrhage (SAH) and ICH** are likely to have an underlying structural abnormality, such as a saccular aneurysm, and should have cerebral arteriography. Lumbar puncture (LP) should not be performed in patients who are suspected of having ICH because CT or MRI yields much more information; LP, in the presence of a central nervous system mass lesion, may lead to herniation.

Other laboratory tests are usually performed (as listed for SAH in Table 14-1) to assess further for underlying causes of the hemorrhage and associated complications. In severely impaired patients, the laboratory evaluation is usually not extensive, because 80% to 90% of such patients have a progressive and ultimately fatal clinical course. Specific treatment options relating to identified underlying causes are discussed in Chapter 17.

SURGICAL INTERVENTIONS

After initial medical and neurologic stabilization of the patient (see Chapter 11), the first general treatment consideration involves whether to undertake surgical intervention. A decision regarding immediate surgical intervention should be made on the basis of the size and the location of the hemorrhage and the condition of the patient (see Appendix E-5). As outlined earlier, the findings from STICH, a randomized trial of patients with ICH, did not demonstrate that early surgery was effective in improving outcome compared with conservative management.

In general, when clinical and CT criteria are considered in combination, **three categories** of patients emerge:

1.   those who have a profound neurologic deficit with associated brainstem involvement and a large hemorrhage noted on CT
2.   those who have a focal neurologic deficit with little or no evidence of brainstem compression or increased intracranial pressure (ICP) and a small, well-localized hemorrhage on CT
3.   those who have a focal deficit referable to their hemorrhage with minimal to mild signs of brainstem dysfunction but a moderate to large lesion on CT

Patients in the **first category** have a nearly uniform fatal course and, with the exception of patients with cerebellar hematomas, generally are not considered to be surgical candidates. The few patients who survive the initial days of their illness and who show stabilization and improvement with supportive medical treatment may be considered for surgical evacuation of the hemorrhage.

Patients in the **second category** are treated medically with appropriate attention to ventilation, fluid intake, electrolyte balance, and blood pressure (BP), as delineated below. Most patients in this category stabilize, and their neurologic deficit improves without surgical intervention.

Patients in the **third category** frequently have progressive deterioration and worsening during their clinical course and therefore should be considered for surgical therapy.

The location of the lesion is also an important determinant in the decision regarding surgical evacuation of the hematoma. Patients in the third group and even in the first group with **cerebellar hemorrhages** and evidence of brainstem compression or deterioration usually have an operation as soon as the anatomic diagnosis is established. Some patients in the third group with **laterally situated lobar hemispheric lesions** may be surgical candidates, and some are operated on once the diagnosis is established. Patients with **supratentorial deep hemorrhage** (often with intraventricular extension) are less frequently considered to be operative candidates. Some patients with supratentorial deep hemorrhage in the third group undergo surgical evacuation, and although occasional dramatic results are noted, most do not survive or are left with severe, persistent deficits. As outlined earlier, results of a clinical trial showed no overall benefit from early surgery in patients with spontaneous supratentorial hemorrhage when compared with initial conservative treatment. These data do not preclude a benefit from surgery (especially craniotomy) among patients with superficial hematomas, but this beneficial effect remains to be established. Patients with **primary brainstem hemorrhage** usually have a devastating course and are seldom operative candidates.

MEDICAL TREATMENT

Intracranial Pressure and Cerebral Edema

The medical management of patients with ICH (Table 15-1) often includes measures to decrease **cerebral edema** and **ICP**, as described in Chapter 11. For comatose patients, an ICP monitor may be placed, aiming for a cerebral perfusion pressure of 60 to 80 mm Hg. In addition to osmotherapy with mannitol or glycerol, many patients are hyperventilated in an attempt to decrease ICP. Current evidence does not support the use of corticosteroids for management of cerebral edema in patients with either hemorrhagic or ischemic stroke.

Table 15-1.   General principles of caring for patients with ICH

1. Place patient on bed rest in quiet room
2. Provide ongoing monitoring of neurologic status (level of consciousness, focal deficit, Glasgow Coma Scale)
3. Consider cardiac monitoring
4. Elevate head of bed 30 degrees
5. Prevent straining (stool softeners and antitussive agents as needed)
6. Provide oral nutrition for alert patients with intact gag reflex
7. Provide enteral nutrition with nasogastric tube for patients with decreased level of consciousness or impaired gag reflex
8. Maintain normovolemia and normal sodium level by starting with administration of 2–3 L/day D_5W and 0.9% normal saline and adjusting accordingly (see Table 14-5 and pages 194–195)
9. Mildly sedate patient if agitated: phenobarbital (30–60 mg two times a day) or chloral hydrate (500 mg three times a day)
10. Control mild pain with acetaminophen or propoxyphene and severe pain with codeine (60 mg, intramuscularly or orally, every 3–4 hr); use morphine (1- to 2-mg increments, intravenously) only as last resort
12. Reduce BP conservatively and with careful monitoring if patient has extremely increased BP or evidence of acute end organ damage
13. Treat increased ICP as needed (see Table 11-1)

BP = blood pressure; ICH = intracerebral hemorrhage; ICP = intracranial pressure.

Blood Pressure

It is important to stabilize and control BP in patients with ICH. As seen with SAH, BP is often increased, at least partly in response to increased ICP. Unlike SAH, isolated ICH does not have the same propensity to induce cerebral vasospasm; consequently, the lowering of BP can be somewhat more aggressive without undue concern about precipitating vasospasm. However, substantial overcorrection could result in decreased cerebral perfusion.

Target BP in this situation is a mean arterial pressure of <130 mm Hg. In general, antihypertensive medications are not used, but BPs higher than this can be controlled with labetalol or enalapril intravenously (see Chapter 11). The intravenous infusion subsequently can be tapered in conjunction with intravenous or oral medications.

In some patients, hypotension is a problem, and this can be controlled by a constant infusion of dopamine (starting at 3 to 6 μg/kg/minute and titrating on the basis of BP response) or phenylephrine to reach target levels of 120 to 140/80 to 90 mm Hg.

Anticonvulsants

Patients with evidence of seizure activity are treated with anticonvulsants. Patients with ongoing seizures are usually treated with intravenously administered diazepam (5 to 10 mg, at a rate as high as 2 mg per minute, which may be repeated once in 5 to 15 minutes) or lorazepam followed by a loading dose of phenytoin given orally (15 to 20 mg per kg, given in a single dose, or split in three doses given every 8 hours) or fosphenytoin (15 to 20 mg per kg phenytoin equivalents at a rate as high as 150 mg phenytoin equivalents per minute) or phenobarbital (20 mg per kg at a rate as high as 100 mg per minute). Maintenance therapy with phenytoin, fosphenytoin, or other agent can be given either orally through a nasogastric tube or intravenously. Prophylactic anticonvulsant use is not indicated in all patients with ICH but may be used in selected patients. Basal ganglia, thalamic, cerebellar, and pontine hemorrhages are associated with such a low occurrence of seizures that routine use of anticonvulsants is not indicated. Given the higher occurrence with lobar hemorrhages, some do advocate use of prophylactic medications in this subgroup of patients, often using phenytoin.

Fluid Management

The goal of fluid management is to maintain euvolemia. Free water–containing solutions should be avoided. Isotonic saline, 2 L per day, is reasonable in most patients.

Anticoagulation Reversal

In patients who have ICH and are on anticoagulation, it is imperative that the anticoagulation be discontinued, and the anticoagulation should be emergently reversed. For patients who are on warfarin, vitamin K, 1 to 2 mg, should be given intravenously. In addition, fresh frozen plasma (FFP) should be given, starting with 2 units. Complete replacement of coagulation factors is provided by 15 ml per kg FFP. Protamine sulfate is given to patients who are on heparin anticoagulation.

Hematoma Expansion

Clinical deterioration after presentation with ICH is not uncommonly caused by hemorrhage enlargement. CT evidence of ICH expansion occurs in 26% of patients within the first hour of admission, and an additional 12% show expansion within 20 hours. Large-volume hemorrhages are more likely to enlarge. A clinical trial suggests that recombinant activated factor VII may be of benefit in patients with ICH when treated for 4 hours. In the trial, treatment limited the growth of the hemorrhage, and at 90 days, mortality was reduced and overall functional outcome was improved. There was a small increase in the occurrence of thromboembolic complications.

Other General Care

Patients with ICH require **close observation**, particularly those who have signs of ICP, high BP, or brainstem compression soon after the onset of hemorrhage. This is best accomplished in an **intensive care unit** with a nursing staff that is experienced in performing serial neurologic assessments, including assessment of level of consciousness and focal deficits, and a standardized coma scale, such as the Glasgow Coma Scale (see Appendix B).

The patient should be kept on **bed rest** until neurologically and medically stable and alert for 24 to 48 hours. Supplemental oxygen should be given to hypoxic patients, aiming to maintain oxygen saturation at ≥95%.

Most patients require an **indwelling urinary catheter** or intermittent catheterization every 4 to 6 hours, and all patients require careful assessment of **fluid balance** and **daily weights**.

The clinician should be alert to the possibility of serious **cardiac arrhythmias**, such as ventricular tachycardia and severe bradycardia. Patients with preexisting cardiac disease and those with hemorrhages that are causing significant or progressive clinical deficits should be monitored with a continuous cardiac monitoring system.

Nutrition should be provided orally if the patient is alert and has a normal gag reflex. Otherwise, feeding should be accomplished by means of a nasogastric tube (inserting a nasogastric tube is usually delayed during the first few days of stroke, during which hydration therapy is given). Evidence from the Feed or Ordinary Diet (FOOD) trial showed that early tube feeding tended to reduce the risk for dying but those who survived tended to remain severely disabled and dependent and that there was no benefit of routine use of food supplements in the trial. However, some experts believe that because of the association between undernutrition at the time of stroke and poor outcome, supplements might still be required for selected patients who are at nutritional risk. Caloric intake should be approximately 2,000 to 3,000 calories per day, or more if the patient is febrile. Feeding is usually begun with a full liquid diet or with a liquid feeding system (Ensure, Ensure Plus), as described in Chapter 11.

Prevention of deep vein thrombosis and pulmonary emboli is assisted by the use of lower-extremity intermittent pneumatic compression devices, compression stockings, and range-of-motion exercises.

Pain control is accomplished with acetaminophen or propoxyphene. Salicylates and nonsteroidal anti-inflammatory drugs should be avoided, as for other types of intracranial hemorrhage, because of their inhibitory effect on coagulation. More severe pain can be controlled with codeine, 60 mg orally or intravenously every 4 to 6 hours. **Agitation** is controlled with phenobarbital, 30 to 60 mg twice a day, or chloral hydrate, 500 mg three times a day, but the clinician must be careful not to oversedate the patient. **Nausea and vomiting** are controlled with prochlorperazine, 10 mg intramuscularly or orally every 4 to 6 hours as needed.

Skin care is also important in the general care of patients with ICH, particularly those who are not alert. Patients should be turned at least once each hour, and their skin should be kept dry and powdered and be inspected regularly for erythema.

SUGGESTED READING FOR PART III

A randomized, blinded trial of clopidogrel versus aspirin in patients at risk of ischaemic events (CAPRIE). CAPRIE Steering Committee. *Lancet.* 1996;348:1329–1338.

Adams HP Jr, Adams RJ, Brott T, et al. Stroke Council of the American Stroke Association. Guidelines for the early management of patients with ischemic stroke: a scientific statement from the Stroke Council of the American Stroke Association. *Stroke.* 2003;34:1056–1083 .

Adams HP Jr, Brott TG, Furlan AJ, et al. Guidelines for thrombolytic therapy for acute stroke: a supplement to the guidelines for the management of patients with acute ischemic stroke. A statement for healthcare professionals from a special writing group of the Stroke Council, American Heart Association. *Stroke.* 1996;27:1711–1718.

Albers GW, Hart RG, Lutsep HL, et al. AHA Scientific Statement. Supplement to the guidelines for the management of transient ischemic attacks: a statement from the Ad Hoc Committee on Guidelines for the Management of Transient Ischemic Attacks. Stroke Council, American Heart Association. *Stroke.* 1999; 30:2502–2511.

Alberts MJ, Hademenos G, Latchaw RE, et al., for the Brain Attack Coalition. Recommendations for the establishment of primary stroke centers. *JAMA.* 2000;283:3102–3109.

Alexandrov AV, Molina CA, Grotta JC, et al. Ultrasound-enhanced systemic thrombolysis for acute ischemic stroke. *N Engl J Med.* 2004;351:2170–2178.

Berge E, Abdelnoor M, Nakstad PH, et al. Low molecular-weight heparin versus aspirin in patients with acute ischaemic stroke and atrial fibrillation: a double-blind randomised study. HAEST Study Group. Heparin in Acute Embolic Stroke Trial. *Lancet.* 2000;355:1205–1210.

Brilstra EH, Rinkel GJE, Algra A, et al. Rebleeding, secondary ischemia, and timing of operation in patients with subarachnoid hemorrhage. *Neurology.* 2000;55:1656–1660.

Brott TG, Brown RD Jr, Meyer FB, et al. Carotid revascularization for prevention of stroke: carotid endarterectomy and carotid artery stenting. *Mayo Clin Proc.* 2004;79:1197–1208.

Brown RD Jr, Flemming KD, Meyer FB, et al. Natural history, evaluation, and management of intracranial vascular malformations. *Mayo Clin Proc.* 2005;80:269–281.

Brown RD Jr, Wiebers DO. Subarachnoid hemorrhage and unruptured intracranial aneurysms. In: Ginsberg M, Bogousslavsky J, eds. *Cerebrovascular disease: pathophysiology, diagnosis, and management.* Vol 2. Malden: Blackwell Science; 1998:1502–1531.

Brown RD Jr, Wiebers DO, Piepgras DG. Intracranial vascular malformations. In: Yanagihara T, Piepgras DG, eds. *Subarachnoid hemorrhage.* New York: Marcel Dekker; 1997:113–138.

CAST: randomized placebo-controlled trial of early aspirin use in 20,000 patients with acute ischaemic stroke. CAST (Chinese Acute Stroke Trial) Collaborative Group. *Lancet.* 1997;349:1641–1649.

Chang HS, Hongo K, Nakagawa H. Adverse effects of limited hypotensive anesthesia on the outcome of patients with subarachnoid hemorrhage. *J Neurosurg.* 2000;92:971–975.

Chen ZM, Sandercock P, Pan HC, et al. Indications for early aspirin use in acute ischemic stroke: a combined analysis of 40,000 randomized patients from the chinese acute stroke trial and the international stroke trial. On behalf of the CAST and IST collaborative groups. *Stroke.* 2000;31:1240–1249.

Chimowitz MI, Lynn MJ, Howlett-Smith H, et al. Comparison of warfarin and aspirin for symptomatic intracranial arterial stenosis. *N Engl J Med.* 2005;352:1305–1316.

Chobanian A, Bakris G, Black H, et al. The Seventh Report of the Joint National Committee on Prevention, Detection, Evaluation, and Treatment of High Blood Pressure. The JNC 7 Report. *JAMA.* 2003;289:2560–2572.

Clagget GP, Salzman EW, Wheeler HB, et al. Prevention of venous thromboembolism. *Chest.* 1992;102[Suppl]:391S–407S.

Clark WM, Wissman S, Albers GW, et al. Recombinant tissue-type plasminogen activator (alteplase) for ischemic stroke 3 to 5 hours after symptom onset. The ATLANTIS study: a randomized controlled trial. Alteplase thrombolysis for acute non-interventional therapy in ischemic stroke. *JAMA.* 1999;282:2019–2026.

Cloft HJ, Joseph GJ, Dion JE. Risk of cerebral angiography in patients with subarachnoid hemorrhage, cerebral aneurysm, and arteriovenous malformation—a meta-analysis. *Stroke.* 1999;30:317–320.

Coletta EM, Murphy JB. The complications of immobility in the elderly stroke patient. *J Am Board Fam Pract.* 1992;5:389–397.

Cruickshank AM. CSF spectrophotometry in the diagnosis of subarachnoid haemorrhage. *J Clin Pathol.* 2001;54: 827–830.

Diener HC, Bogousslavsky J, Brass LM, et al., on behalf of the MATCH Investigators. Aspirin and clopidogrel compared with clopidogrel alone after recent ischaemic stroke or transient ischaemic attack in high-risk patients (MATCH): randomised, double-blind, placebo-controlled trial. *Lancet.* 2004;364:331–337.

Diener HC, Cunha L, Forbes C, et al. European Stroke Prevention Study 2: dipyridamole and acetylsalicylic acid in the secondary prevention of stroke. *J Neurol Sci.* 1996;143:1–13.

Dodick DW, Meissner I, Meyer FB, et al. Evaluation and management of asymptomatic carotid artery stenosis. *Mayo Clin Proc.* 2004;79:937–944.

Dorhout Mees SM, Rinkel GJE, Hop JW, et al. Antiplatelet therapy in aneurysmal subarachnoid hemorrhage: a systemic review. *Stroke.* 2003;34:2285–2289.

Dromerick A, Reding M. Medical and neurological complications during inpatient stroke rehabilitation. *Stroke.* 1994;25:358–361.

Emergency Cardiac Care Committee and Subcommittees, American Heart Association. Guidelines for cardiopulmonary resuscitation and emergency cardiac care. Part IV. Special resuscitation situations. *JAMA.* 1992;268:2242–2250.

Feigin VL, Rinkel GJ, Algra A, et al. Calcium antagonists in patients with aneurysmal subarachnoid hemorrhage: a systematic review. *Neurology.* 1998;50:4 876–883.

Feigin VL, Rinkel GJ, Algra A, et al. Calcium antagonists for aneurysmal subarachnoid hemorrhage *Cochrane Database Syst Rev.* 2000;(2):CD000483.

Flemming KD, Brown RD Jr. Secondary prevention strategies in ischemic stroke: identification and optimal management of modifiable risk factors. *Mayo Clin Proc.* 2004;79:1330–1340.

Flemming KD, Brown RD Jr, Petty GW, et al. Evaluation and management of transient ischemic attack and minor cerebral infarction. *Mayo Clin Proc.* 2004;79:1071–1086.

Flemming KD, Wiebers DO. Optimizing antiplatelet therapy to prevent ischemic stroke. *Emerg Med.* 2002;34:28–37.

FOOD Trial Collaboration. Poor nutritional status on admission predicts poor outcomes after stroke: observational data from the FOOD trial. *Stroke.* 2003;34:1450–1456.

Fulgham JR, Ingall TJ, Stead LG, et al. Management of acute ischemic stroke. *Mayo Clin Proc.* 2004;79:1459–1469.

Furlan A, Higashida R, Wechsler L, et al. Intra-arterial prourokinase for acute ischemic stroke. The PROACT II study: a randomized controlled trial. Prolyse in Acute Cerebral Thromboembolism. *JAMA.* 1999;282:2003–2011.

Gladman JR, Lomas S, Lincoln NB. Provision of physiotherapy and occupational therapy in outpatient departments and day hospitals for stroke patients in Nottingham. *Int Disabil Stud.* 1991;13:38–41.

Gobin YP, Starkman S, Duckwiler GR, et al. A phase I study of mechanical embolus removal in cerebral ischemia. *Stroke.* 2004;35:2848–2854.

Gorelick PB, Richardson D, Kelly M, et al. Aspirin and ticlopidine for prevention of recurrent stroke in black patients. A randomized trial. *JAMA.* 2003;289:2947–2957.

Grubb R, Derdeyn C, Fritsch S, et al. Importance of hemodynamic factors in the prognosis of symptomatic carotid occlusion. *JAMA.* 1998;280:1055–1060.

Hacke W, Kaste M, Fieschi C, et al. Randomised double-blind placebo-controlled trial of thrombolytic therapy with intravenous alteplase in acute ischaemic stroke (ECASS II). Second European-Australasian Acute Stroke Study Investigators. *Lancet.* 1998;352:1245–1251.

Halperin JL, Executive Steering Committee. Ximelagatran compared with warfarin for prevention of thromboembolism in patients with nonvalvular atrial fibrillation: rationale, objectives, and design of a pair of clinical studies and baseline patient characteristics (SPORTIF III and V). *Am Heart J.* 2003;146:431–438.

Horner J, Brazer SR, Massey EW. Aspiration in bilateral stroke patients: a validation study. *Neurology.* 1993;43:430–433.

IMS trial investigators. Combined intravenous and intra-arterial recanalization for acute ischemic stroke: the Interventional Management of Stroke Study. *Stroke.* 2004;35:904–911.

Kay R, Wong KS, Yu YL, et al. Low-molecular-weight heparin for the treatment of acute ischemic stroke. *N Engl J Med.* 1995;333:1588–1593.

Kennedy J, Newcommon NJ, Cole-Kaskayne A, et al. Organised stroke care increases the number and the speed with which patients with acute ischemic stroke are thrombolysed. *Stroke.* 2002;33:354.

Kilpatrick CJ, Davis SM, Tress BM, et al. Epileptic seizures in acute stroke. *Arch Neurol.* 1990;47:157–160.

Kothari R, Sauerbeck L, Jauch E, et al. Patient's awareness of stroke signs, symptoms, and risk factors. *Stroke*. 1997;28: 1871–1875.

Kothari RU, Brott T, Broderick JP, et al. The ABCs of measuring intracerebral hemorrhage volumes. *Stroke*. 1996;27:1304–1305.

Leahy NM. Complications in the acute stages of stroke: nursing's pivotal role. *Nurs Clin North Am*. 1991;26:971–983.

Lisk DR, Grotta JC, Lamki LM, et al. Should hypertension be treated after acute stroke? A randomized controlled trial using single photon emission computed tomography. *Arch Neurol*. 1993;50:855–862.

Manno EM, Atkinson JL, Fulgham JR, et al. Emerging medical and surgical management strategies in the evaluation and treatment of intracerebral hemorrhage. *Mayo Clin Proc*. 2005;80:420–433.

Marler JR, Brott T, Broderick J, et al. Tissue plasminogen activator for acute ischemic stroke. *N Engl J Med*. 1995;333:1581–1587.

Marler JR, Tilley BC, Lu M, et al. Early stroke treatment associated with better outcome: the NINDS rt-PA stroke study. *Neurology*. 2000;55:1649–1655.

Mayer SA, Brun NC, Begtrup K, et al. Recombinant activated factor VII for acute intracerebral hemorrhage. *N Engl J Med*. 2005;352:777–785.

Mendelow AD, Gregson BA, Fernandes HM, et al., STICH investigators. Early surgery versus initial conservative treatment in patients with spontaneous supratentorial intracerebral haematomas in the International Surgical Trial in Intracerebral Haemorrhage (STICH): a randomised trial. *Lancet*. 2005;365:387–397.

Mohr J, Thompson J, Lazar R, et al. W-ARSS: a comparison of warfarin and aspirin for the prevention of recurrent ischemic stroke. *N Engl J Med*. 2001;345:1444–1451

Muizelaar JP, Zwienenberg M, Rudisill NA, et al. The prophylactic use of transluminal balloon angioplasty in patients with Fisher grade 3 subarachnoid hemorrhage: a pilot study. *J Neurosurg*. 1999;91:51–58.

Patel RV, Kertland HR, Jahns BE, et al. Labetalol: response and safety in critically ill hemorrhagic stroke patients. *Ann Pharmacother*. 1993;27:180–181.

Petty GW, Brown RD Jr, Whisnant JP, et al. Frequency of major complications of aspirin, warfarin, and intravenous heparin for secondary stroke prevention: a population-based study. *Ann Intern Med*. 1999;130:14–22.

Petty GW, Brown RD Jr, Whisnant JP, et al. Survival and recurrence after first cerebral infarction: a population-based study in Rochester, Minnesota, 1975 through 1989. *Neurology*. 1998;50:208–216.

Qureshi AL, Tuhrim S, Broderick JP, et al. Spontaneous intracerebral hemorrhage. *N Engl J Med*. 2001;344:1450–1460.

Rinkel GJE, Djibuti M, Algra A, et al. Prevalence and risk of rupture of intracranial aneurysms—a systematic review. *Stroke*. 1998;29:251–256.

Rothwell PM, Giles MF, Flossmann E, et al. A simple score (ABCD) to identify individuals at high early risk of stroke after transient ischemic attack. *Lancet*. 2005;366:29–36.

Saxena R, Koudstaal PJ. Anticoagulants versus antiplatelet therapy for preventing stroke in patients with nonrheumatic atrial fibrillation and a history of stroke or transient ischemic attack. *Stroke*. 2005;36:914–915.

Sherman DG, Atkinson RP, Chippendale T, et al. Intravenous ancrod for treatment of acute ischemic stroke: the STAT study: a randomized controlled trial. Stroke Treatment with Ancrod Trial. *JAMA*. 2000;283:18 2395–2403.

Stone SP, Whincup P. Standards for the hospital management of stroke patients. *J R Coll Physicians Load*. 1994;28:52–58.

Stroke Unit Trialists' Collaboration. Organised inpatient (stroke unit) care for stroke. *Cochrane Database Syst Rev*. 2001;(1):CD000197.

The International Stroke Trial (IST): a randomised trial of aspirin, subcutaneous heparin, both, or neither among 19435 patients with acute ischaemic stroke. International Stroke Trial Collaborative Group. *Lancet*. 1997;349:1569–1581.

Treggiari MM, Walder B, Suter PM, et al. Systematic review of the prevention of delayed ischemic neurological deficits with hypertension, hypervolemia, and hemodilution therapy following subarachnoid hemorrhage. *J Neurosurg*. 98(5):978–984.

Vermeij FH, Hasan D, Bijvoet HWC, et al. Impact of medical treatment on the outcome of patients after aneurysmal subarachnoid hemorrhage. *Stroke*. 1998;29:924–930.

White PM, Wardlaw JM, Easton V. Can noninvasive imaging accurately depict intracranial aneurysms? A systematic review. *Radiology*. 2000;217:361–370.

Wiebers DO, Piepgras DG, Meyer FB, et al. Pathogenesis, natural history, and treatment of unruptured intracranial aneurysms. *Mayo Clin Proc*. 2004;79:1572–1583.

Wiebers DO, Whisnant JP, Huston J III, et al.; International Study of Unruptured Intracranial Aneurysms Investigators. Unruptured intracranial aneurysms: natural history, clinical outcome, and risks of surgical and endovascular treatment. *Lancet*. 2003;362:103–110.

Wiesmann M, Mayer TE, Yousry I, et al. Detection of hyperacute subarachnoid hemorrhage of the brain by using magnetic resonance imaging. *J Neurosurg*. 2002;96:684–689.

Wijdicks EFM, Kallmes DF, Manno EM, et al. Subarachnoid hemorrhage: neurointensive care and aneurysm repair. *Mayo Clin Proc*. 2005;80:550–559.

Wolf PA, Clagett GP, Easton JD, et al. Preventing ischemic stroke in patients with prior stroke and transient ischemic attack: a statement for healthcare professionals from the stroke council of the American Heart Association. *Stroke*. 1999;30:1991–1994.

Yadav JS, Wholey MK, Kuntz RE, et al. Protected carotid-artery stenting versus endarterectomy in high-risk patients. *N Engl J Med*. 2004;351:1493–1501.

Medical and Surgical Management Based on Specific Mechanisms of Cerebrovascular Disease

Whenever possible, management of a patient is based on precise definition of the underlying pathophysiologic mechanism for the cerebrovascular condition. After general medical and neurologic examinations, certain diagnostic studies are usually performed to help identify the underlying pathophysiologic mechanism for the cerebrovascular symptoms. If the responsible pathophysiologic mechanism can be identified, appropriate treatment is established. One way of categorizing the various **ischemic pathophysiologic mechanisms** is by four major groupings, progressing from proximal to distal in the vascular system, as follows: (1) cardiac disease, (2) large vessel disease, (3) small vessel disease, and (4) hematologic disease. **Hemorrhagic mechanisms** can be categorized best according to location of the hemorrhage.

Four Major Categories of Ischemic Cerebrovascular Disease

Identification and Treatment

CARDIAC DISEASE

Cerebrovascular conditions that result from cardiac disorders include cerebral infarction, transient ischemic attack (TIA), syncope, and global anoxia. Heart disease may produce cerebral ischemic symptoms by means of several mechanisms. It is useful to group these into

1. disturbances that are associated with **pump failure** and result in generalized cerebral ischemia (syncope) or infarction (anoxic encephalopathy)
2. conditions that more frequently predispose to **thromboembolism** associated with focal cerebral ischemic events

Disturbances that are associated with pump failure consist primarily of cardiac arrhythmias, including cardiac arrest and congestive heart failure. **Embolic cerebral infarction or TIA** from a cardiac source (Fig. 16-1) may result from any of three basic mechanisms:

1. generation of embolic fragments from heart valves
2. production of intracardiac thrombi from local stagnation and endocardial alterations
3. shunting of systemic venous thrombi into the arterial circulation

Patients with ischemic cerebrovascular disease or retinal ischemic events should be examined for evidence of cardiac rhythm disorders (such as atrial fibrillation, paroxysmal atrial fibrillation, chronic atrial flutter, and sick sinus syndrome), valvular lesions (such as rheumatic valve disease, prosthetic valves, papillary fibroelastoma, nonbacterial thrombotic endocarditis, mitral stenosis, mitral valve prolapse, mitral annular calcification, and subacute bacterial endocarditis), and lesions of the myocardium (such as recent infarction, old infarction with segmental akinesia or aneurysmal dilation, markedly reduced ejection fraction, and dilated cardiomyopathy), lesions of the atrium (atrial myxoma), or other cardiac structural disorders (left atrial thrombus or left ventricular thrombus) (see Table 8-1).

The most common cardiac disorders that are implicated in cerebrovascular ischemia can be divided into **proven and putative cardiac risks** on the basis of the available epidemiologic and clinical evidence substantiating the role of these disorders in cerebrovascular disease (Table 16-1).

Cardioembolic infarction is the cause of approximately 20% to 25% of all ischemic strokes. The onset of focal neurologic deficit

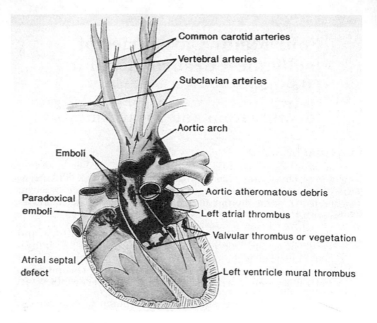

Figure 16-1.   Emboli originating from the heart.

Table 16-1.   Cardiac risks for cerebrovascular ischemia

Proven cardiac risks
    Persistent atrial fibrillation
    Paroxysmal atrial fibrillation
    Sustained atrial flutter
    Mechanical valve
    Rheumatic valve disease
    Dilated cardiomyopathy
    Recent MI (within 1 month)
    Intracardiac thrombus
    Intracardiac mass (i.e., atrial myxoma, papillary fibroelastoma)
    Infectious endocarditis
    Nonbacterial thrombotic endocarditis
Putative or uncertain cardiac risks
    Sick sinus syndrome
    Patent foramen ovale with or without atrial septal aneurysm
    Atherosclerotic debris in the thoracic aorta
    Spontaneous echocardiographic contrast
    MI 2–6 mo earlier
    Hypokinetic or akinetic left ventricular segment
    Calcification of mitral annulus

MI = myocardial infarction.

typically is very sudden and most often maximal at onset, but sometimes the neurologic deficit may be incomplete or may worsen significantly after onset. Focal or generalized seizures tend to occur early after embolic cerebral infarction with cortical involvement but may also commence many months after the acute ischemic episode. Some cases of "idiopathic" epilepsy in the elderly may result from this kind of clinically silent cortical cerebral infarction.

The basis for clinical diagnosis is the demonstration of a cardiac source of embolus or right-to-left shunt with a venous source of emboli and no evidence for other causes of ischemic stroke. Evidence of emboli in other locations such as the retina, kidney, or spleen and multiple cerebral infarctions in different vascular distributions make the diagnosis even more certain. In addition, certain clinical syndromes and radiographic findings may suggest embolism as the underlying mechanism, although they are not specific for an embolic cause.

Most cardioembolic infarcts involve the cortex and are commonly in the distribution of the cortical branches of the middle cerebral artery. They produce symptoms such as unilateral lower facial weakness associated with severe dysphasia, contralateral brachial or hand monoplegia or paresis with or without cortical sensory loss, and relatively isolated Broca's aphasia or motor speech apraxia or Wernicke's aphasia. A sudden, isolated homonymous hemianopia that is apparent to the patient may occur with a posterior cerebral territory embolus; sudden unilateral foot weakness or incoordination may be caused by an anterior cerebral territory embolus. Cardioembolic ischemic strokes may also involve the cerebellar hemispheres but relatively uncommonly affect the brainstem.

Septic cerebral embolism with bacterial endocarditis often produces a focal neurologic deficit associated with nonfocal symptoms such as confusion, agitation, or delirium caused by tiny septic infarcts with microscopic abscesses. However, depression of consciousness caused by a large arterial embolus may also occur. Computed tomography (CT) or magnetic resonance imaging (MRI) often reveals some degree of hemorrhagic transformation, and multiple brain or systemic infarcts typically are present.

The **differential diagnosis** of embolic ischemic events includes other subtypes of cerebral infarction as well as primary intracerebral hemorrhage (ICH), primary seizure disorder with postictal focal deficit, metabolic disorders (such as hypoglycemia), and functional disorders. Noncardiac causes of cerebral embolism include atherosclerosis of the aorta and craniocervical arteries and, in the presence of right-to-left cardiac shunting, pulmonary or peripheral venous thrombosis or tumor, fat (after major fractures), or air (after neck or chest injury or operation) emboli.

Valve-Related Cerebral Emboli

Valve-related cerebral emboli may result from various conditions, including rheumatic heart disease, other aortic and mitral valvular diseases, prosthetic valves, cardiac procedures, and infective and noninfective endocarditis. Cerebral embolization in **rheumatic heart disease** may occur during the acute illness, when inflammatory vegetations on the heart valves may detach and embolize, or, more common, during the chronic phase of the disease, when valvular deformity, atrial enlargement, and abnormal cardiac rhythm have developed. The greatest risk for cerebral infarction from chronic rheumatic heart disease occurs within 1 year after the onset of atrial fibrillation. In clinical series, the brain is the site of emboli in roughly 30% of patients, but in autopsy series, nearly 50% of patients show cerebral infarction presumably related to emboli. Mitral stenosis has been present in most of these patients.

Anticoagulation treatment with intravenously administered heparin or subcutaneous low molecular weight heparin (LMWH) followed by warfarin anticoagulation or valve repair is recommended for all embolic cerebral events associated with rheumatic heart disease, particularly in patients with an audible murmur or those in whom surgical therapy is to be delayed or cannot be done.

Spontaneous calcium embolization uncommonly occurs with **calcific aortic stenosis**, but more commonly such embolization produces symptomatic retinal rather than cerebral ischemia. Cerebral ischemic events without some other clear cause have been noted in patients with **mitral valve prolapse**. However, available data suggest that mitral valve prolapse plays a limited role in cerebral ischemia. Embolic material may uncommonly arise from the surface of the prolapsed, degenerated mitral valve. **Mitral annulus calcification** is another possible risk factor for cardioembolic events, but the overall association with cerebral ischemia is unproved.

Prosthetic and porcine heart valves are associated with an increased occurrence of cerebral and systemic emboli. The risk is higher with prosthetic valves, and chronic anticoagulation is used in this setting. Even with therapeutic warfarin (International Normalized Ratio [INR], 3.0 to 4.5), the rate of stroke is 2% to 4% per year, and the risk is higher with prosthetic mitral valves than with prosthetic aortic valves. In addition to warfarin, some advocate concurrent use of extended-release dipyridamole because of some evidence suggesting a potential reduction in the risk for stroke.

Cardiac catheterization and arteriography, performed in nearly all patients before cardiac surgery, are associated with a low risk for cerebrovascular complications (approximately 0.2%). Such complications may occur from direct displacement of clot or atheromatous material or from trauma to the arterial intima, which causes subsequent embolization.

Cardiac operations of all types are associated with an increased risk for cerebral ischemia. This may be caused by manipulation that leads to clot formation and embolization; nonfocal encephalopathic syndromes caused by either hypotension or anoxia; or multifocal ischemic syndromes caused by embolization of air, fibrin, calcium, or fat globules. Focal ischemic deficits are observed more frequently after valve operations than they are after coronary bypass procedures. Late embolization is a complication of valve replacement and is more common with mitral valve replacement than it is with aortic valve prostheses.

Cerebral embolization occurs in approximately 20% of patients with **infective endocarditis** and may be the presenting symptom of the disorder. The probability of embolization is highest in patients with mitral valve involvement. Four distinct clinical and pathologic syndromes are observed: (1) focal cerebral infarction (the most common) that results from embolic occlusion of large arteries, (2) multiple small areas of cerebral infarction that produce a diffuse encephalopathy with or without alteration in consciousness, (3) meningitis from small infected emboli that lodge in meningeal arteries, and (4) mycotic aneurysm formation that results from septic embolization with subsequent aneurysmal rupture and intracranial hemorrhage.

Treatment of patients with **infective endocarditis** includes appropriate antimicrobial therapy for at least 4 weeks (blood culture analysis should be repeated 5 to 7 days after the treatment to confirm eradication of the infection), usually guided by culture results. Anticoagulants are not used, at least during the period of active infection, because of the increased risk for hemorrhagic infarction. If mycotic aneurysm is detected on cerebral arteriography, then repeat arteriography is necessary after antimicrobial therapy, and surgical intervention may be necessary if an aneurysm persists.

Nonbacterial thrombotic endocarditis, also called marantic endocarditis, usually occurs in cachectic, debilitated elderly patients with some underlying systemic disease, most commonly carcinoma. Pathologically, nonbacterial thrombotic endocarditis vegetations consist of amorphous, acellular material composed of a mixture of fibrin and platelets. Fewer than half of the patients with this condition have heart murmurs. As with infective endocarditis, many patients show signs of diffuse cerebral dysfunction, either alone or in association with recognizable focal deficits.

Although the value of antithrombotic therapy is still undetermined in patients with **marantic (nonbacterial thrombotic) endocarditis**, the use of anticoagulants followed by antiplatelet therapy is usually advised for patients with focal cerebral ischemic events. Disseminated intravascular coagulation, often associated with nonbacterial endocarditis, may independently produce multiple small areas of cerebral infarction.

Noninfectious valvular deposits called **Libman-Sacks endocarditis** may occur in patients with systemic lupus erythematosus. Patients with cerebral or systemic emboli in this context typically are treated with at least short-term warfarin anticoagulation. Therapy is often switched to an antiplatelet agent, especially when serial echocardiographic studies demonstrate lesion resolution.

A papillary fibroelastoma is an uncommon, histologically benign tumor, most commonly found on the cardiac valves and rarely seen on the endocardium. They can serve as a source of emboli, causing sudden death as a result of coronary artery occlusion, or cerebral infarction. When detected, they are usually treated with surgical resection, often performed without the need for valve replacement. If surgery cannot be performed, then warfarin should be initiated.

Intracardiac Thrombi

Atrial fibrillation is the cardiac arrhythmia most frequently associated with embolic brain infarction. In this condition, the atria do not contract effectively, and the resultant stagnation of blood predisposes to intraluminal thrombi. The risk for cerebral embolization increases with longer duration of the dysrhythmia; an enlarged left atrium; previous systemic thromboembolism; history of hypertension or congestive heart failure; and associated valvular heart disease, especially mitral stenosis.

If atrial fibrillation is a **new finding** at the time of presentation with an ischemic event, conversion to normal sinus rhythm with either electrical or chemical cardioversion may be indicated. Conversion of atrial fibrillation to a normal rhythm is associated with a risk for embolization, which often occurs within 48 hours. Anticoagulant therapy should precede conversion, especially in high-risk patients (those with recent or recurrent embolization, cardiac enlargement, heart failure, or associated mitral valve disease) and patients in whom the absence of left atrium thrombus is not documented by transesophageal echocardiography (TEE).

In patients with **chronic atrial fibrillation**, medical therapy is indicated to prevent systemic embolic events. Long-term oral anticoagulation is recommended (INR, 2.0 to 3.0; a lower range of 1.8 to 2.5 may also be efficacious), except in patients who are younger than 60 years and have no associated cardiovascular disease, including hypertension, recent congestive heart failure, left atrial enlargement, left ventricular dysfunction, or previous thromboembolic events. The recommendation for anticoagulation becomes even stronger for patients who have had focal cerebrovascular ischemic events within the previous 2 years. Aspirin or other antiplatelet drug (for example, clopidogrel) may be a useful prophylactic agent in patients with a contraindication to warfarin or in elderly patients.

Sick sinus syndrome is a common dysrhythmia among the elderly, occurring in 2% to 3% of people older than 75 years. The risk for cerebral ischemia in individuals with sick sinus syndrome is controversial. Although some investigators believe that this is a relatively benign condition, others have documented an increased risk for cerebral embolism, particularly among those with a bradycardia-tachycardia syndrome.

The most appropriate therapy for primary prevention of stroke in sick sinus syndrome is unknown. Some have advocated dual-chamber pacing, whereas others believe that long-term anticoagulation is necessary. Further study is necessary to define better the risk for stroke and clarify the most efficacious prophylactic treatment approach. In patients with cerebral ischemic events related to sick sinus syndrome, a pacemaker should be implanted.

Atrial flutter may also be associated with an increased risk for thromboembolic events. Population-based data have demonstrated that the risk is at least as high as in those with lone atrial fibrillation. They also are at increased risk for future atrial fibrillation. Although specific guidelines do not exist, these patients likely should be treated similar to those with lone atrial fibrillation, including the use of anticoagulation in all patients who have atrial flutter and are older than 65 years or among those with previous thromboembolic events.

Patients who experience transient loss of consciousness and syncopal events associated with **other serious rhythm disorders**, such as complete heart block or serious paroxysmal ventricular rhythm disturbances, usually do not require antithrombotic therapy because of the relatively low risk for thromboembolism.

Brain infarction occurs in approximately 10% of patients with **myocardial infarction (MI)**, with a particularly increased risk in the first 30 days after MI. Although systemic hypotension may be responsible for some ischemic brain deficits, clinical and autopsy studies have shown that most focal brain lesions are caused by the formation of mural thrombus and subsequent embolization. Autopsy studies reveal that left ventricular thrombus may occur in up to 44% of patients after MI, especially in those with large areas of infarcted tissue and congestive heart failure. When cerebral embolization occurs, it is often within the first 30 days after acute MI and may be the presenting symptom. In addition, because a ventricular aneurysm develops as an additional source of thrombus formation in 5% to 20% of patients with MI, cerebral events that occur later should be evaluated carefully for a possible cardiac source. In this situation, long-term anticoagulant therapy should be instituted unless contraindications exist. After MI, patients who receive warfarin may have a reduction in recurrent MI and cerebrovascular events compared with those who are treated with placebo. After a patient has had MI, anticoagulation may begin with intravenously administered heparin (or subcutaneous LMWH) followed by oral anticoagulant therapy (warfarin) alone, and use of heparin may be discontinued when the INR is therapeutic (2.0 to 3.0; see Chapter 12). Although the most efficacious duration of therapy is not known, warfarin therapy is usually continued for several months and then an antiplatelet agent alone is continued.

Congestive heart failure is characterized by cardiac enlargement, poor myocardial contractility, and decreased cardiac output that predisposes to blood stagnation and intracardiac thrombi. Any pathologic condition that interferes with cardiac filling or emptying may be associated with congestive heart failure. Although occasionally congestive heart failure is the only identifiable cause of intracardiac or pulmonary venous thrombus formation, other identifiable cardiac disorders, such as MI, generalized cardiomyopathy, valvular disease, or arrhythmia, may also contribute to thrombus at these sites.

In patients who have focal cerebral ischemic events associated with **cardiomyopathy and** in whom the ejection fraction is <30% or if definite mural thrombi are seen on echocardiography, then anticoagulants are used. Among these patients, as well as in patients with various **congenital heart diseases**, decisions regarding long-term anticoagulant therapy should be considered on an individual basis.

Systemic Venous Thrombi

The foramen ovale is anatomically patent in 15% of individuals and retains the functional capacity of patency in an additional 15%. In these situations, venous emboli can occasionally enter the cerebral circulation (paradoxical embolism), especially after pulmonary embolization with an associated increase in pulmonary and right atrial pressures. The clinical syndrome is uncommon, but the diagnosis should be suspected in patients who have deep venous thrombosis, pulmonary embolism, or recent prolonged sedentary period and in whom acute focal cerebral deficit subsequently develops. Other cardiac deficits that produce right-to-left shunts also may cause paradoxical emboli. Approximately 5% of children with cyanotic congenital heart disease have cerebral infarction. In most cases, these infarcts are embolic, occurring in the first 2 years of life. Associated hematologic deficits may also predispose these children to cerebral ischemia.

Patients with embolic cerebral infarction or TIA that results from **systemic venous thrombi**, including patients with **interatrial or interventricular septal defects**, should receive warfarin for at least 3 months, even if the primary cardiac disorder is surgically corrected. If the defect is not surgically corrected, then chronic therapy with warfarin should be considered. Recurrent embolic cerebrovascular events after cessation of anticoagulation or hemodynamic evidence of pulmonary hypertension indicates the need for longer term warfarin therapy. If **pulmonary vein thrombosis** is suspected as the cause of a cerebrovascular ischemic event, then heparin therapy should be given, followed by warfarin for 3 months.

Approximately 25% of patients who have stroke and have a cardioembolic source have another potential cause of the ischemic event. If one of the proven cardiac risks (Table 16-1) is identified in a patient with an ischemic cerebrovascular event, then long-term anticoagulation with warfarin may be needed for prophylaxis even if another potential mechanism for the current ischemic event is identified. In patients with cardioembolic stroke, heparin typically is given in the acute stage, followed by warfarin therapy in nonhypertensive patients with small or moderate strokes. In patients with a small cerebral infarct, use of heparin is usually not delayed, but use of heparin should be delayed in those with a moderate stroke until CT that is performed 24 to 48 hours after the event reveals no significant hemorrhagic transformation. Anticoagulant therapy may be postponed (a few days to 2 weeks) or not used if the stroke is large or if a patient is severely hypertensive.

LARGE VESSEL DISEASE

Atherosclerosis

The most commonly identified disease process that produces retinal or cerebral ischemia is atherosclerosis. Atherosclerosis may produce cerebral symptoms through a hemodynamic or thromboembolic mechanism or both (Fig. 16-2). The lumen of an involved artery may become progressively narrowed and eventually occluded by atherosclerotic deposits. Blood flow across the stenotic area becomes impaired when >75% of the luminal area becomes compromised. This process usually progresses slowly during years or decades, often allowing time to establish collateral blood flow distal to the lesion. Consequently, not uncommonly, asymptomatic patients have occlusion of one or

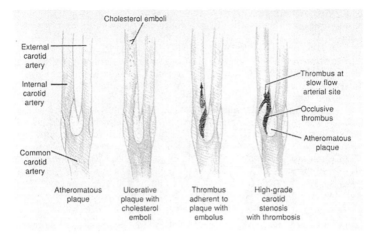

Figure 16-2.   Thrombus formation in atherosclerosis.

more major cranial cervical arteries. When collateral circulation distal to the lesion is insufficient, **hemodynamic** compromise occurs and produces symptoms of cerebral ischemia. The terminal branches (watershed areas) of the anterior, middle, and posterior cerebral arteries are most frequently involved.

Thromboembolism is another mechanism whereby atherosclerosis may produce cerebral ischemic symptoms. Atherosclerotic deposits in the process of evolution tend to ulcerate and form necrotic areas that are capable of attracting blood products, and clot formation results. This atherothrombotic material may either stenose or occlude the vessel lumen, or it may break off to embolize distally in the arterial tree. When either mechanism is combined with systemic factors such as hypotension, hypoxia, anemia, abnormal blood viscosity, and hypoglycemia, focal or multifocal cerebral ischemia may result.

Pathologic changes of atherosclerosis are characterized by focal proliferation of smooth muscle cells within the intima of medium-sized to large arteries and associated deposits of lipids (including cholesterol), blood products, calcium, and fibrous tissue. Although atherosclerosis is usually found diffusely in multiple areas of the body, the primary sources of cerebrovascular symptoms are atherosclerotic deposits, usually localized at cervical artery bifurcations. The most commonly affected areas (Fig. 16-3) in the neck are (1) the proximal portions of the internal carotid arteries and (2) the proximal portions of the vertebral arteries. Intracranially, the circle of Willis and the basilar artery are the areas of maximal involvement. With the increasing use of TEE, aortic arch atherosclerosis has become recognized as a frequent finding in association with cerebral ischemia. Although this finding is a marker for systemic atherosclerosis, the primary association with cerebral ischemia is unproven and still under study.

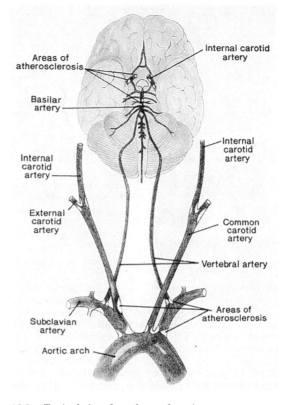

Figure 16-3.   Typical sites for atherosclerosis in the craniocervical arteries.

Epidemiologic studies have identified several factors that seem to contribute to the formation of atherosclerosis. Among these risk factors, cigarette smoking and hypertension are the most clearly implicated. Diabetes mellitus and elevated serum total cholesterol, low-density lipoprotein cholesterol, triglyceride levels, homocysteine, and chronic inflammation have also been implicated. Atherosclerosis and its complications are especially likely to develop in patients with combinations of these risk factors (see Chapters 23 and 25 to 27).

Cerebral infarction that is caused by atherosclerosis is the cause of 15% to 30% of all ischemic strokes, resulting from primary arterial occlusion by atherosclerotic plaque enlargement, thrombus formation at a site of stenosis, or embolism of thrombus or plaque fragments. Artery-to-artery emboli may cause infarcts that are indistinguishable from cardiac embolic infarcts.

Extracranial vertebral artery occlusive disease that results from atherosclerosis or other causes uncommonly causes brainstem or posterior circulation strokes because of compensatory flow from the contralateral vertebral artery or rostral cervical arteries and retrograde flow down the basilar artery from the carotid-posterior communicating artery system. More often, atherosclerosis causes a syndrome of vertebrobasilar insufficiency or may result in TIAs, including symptoms such as dizziness, presyncopal sensation, blurred vision, diplopia, vertigo, dysarthria, extremity weakness, incoordination, sensory loss, facial weakness or loss of sensation, and imbalance.

A history of TIAs and cervical bruit is more frequent in patients with atherothrombotic infarction than it is in those with other types of stroke. In addition to atherosclerosis, causes of craniocervical occlusive disease with associated thrombosis include arteritis; hematologic disorders; carotid, vertebrobasilar, or cerebral arterial dissection; and systemic or central nervous system (CNS) infections (see Table 8-1). Many patients with thrombotic infarction have sudden or stepwise (stuttering) onset of their neurologic deficits. The clinical diagnosis is established by evidence of arterial stenosis or occlusion at one or more sites (see Chapters 12 and 13).

Laboratory evaluation of patients with possible atherosclerotic carotid artery occlusive disease must include tests that define the presence, location, and severity of the lesion. The evaluation approach for patients with TIA and ischemic stroke is outlined in Chapters 12 and 13. Initial noninvasive screening for the presence of "pressure-significant" or "hemodynamically significant" stenoses in the carotid system is usually performed with carotid ultrasonographic/duplex studies. Oculopneumoplethysmography is also used occasionally. Other studies that further define the location and the severity of carotid lesions include magnetic resonance angiography (MRA), CT angiography (CTA), and cerebral arteriography. Intracranial arterial lesions may be identified by transcranial Doppler (TCD) ultrasonography, MRA, CTA, and cerebral arteriography. Ophthalmic and intracranial carotid artery hemodynamics may be evaluated with oculopneumoplethysmography and TCD ultrasonography.

If an appropriate, surgically correctable atherosclerotic lesion is defined, **carotid endarterectomy (CEA)** is considered (Fig. 16-4). The surgery is highly beneficial for patients with 70% to 99% (as measured using the methods of the North American Symptomatic Carotid Endarterectomy Trial—NASCET) recently symptomatic stenosis: the number needed to treat is approximately 8 for any stroke or surgical death; on average, surgery for patients with 50% to 69% stenosis is only modestly effective: the number needed to treat is approximately 14, and the effect is not felt until several years after surgery; surgery confers no benefit at all if the stenosis is <50%. However, the severity of stenosis alone cannot be enough to decide surgery. CEA is performed with the goal of preventing cerebral ischemia in the territory of the artery that is subjected to the procedure and generally should be considered only by surgeons whose combined stroke morbidity and mortality from arteriography and the surgical procedure is <3% for asymptomatic patients and <6% for symptomatic patients. Medical management becomes more of a consideration in the presence of one or more of the following conditions, in the setting of asymptomatic carotid disease: (1) evidence of severe or progressive renal, hepatic, pulmonary, or cardiac failure; (2) uncontrolled diabetes mellitus or unregulated hypertension;

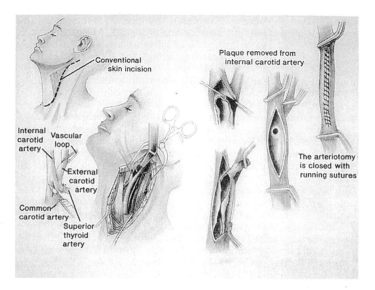

Figure 16-4. Basic techniques of CEA.

(3) cancer that confers a low 5-year survival rate; (4) the coexistence of other (such as cardiac) sources for cerebral emboli; or (5) the presence of a tandem lesion distally in the same arterial distribution of equal or greater severity compared with the carotid bifurcation area lesion. CEA generally is not considered in the circumstance of known carotid occlusion, except in rare instances of acute occlusion, when CEA can be performed immediately (for instance, an occlusion that occurs during arteriography in a hospital setting).

The overall effect of CEA on the immediate and subsequent risk for stroke is influenced by patient selection and the availability of a surgeon who is able to perform the procedure with low morbidity and mortality. Patients who have undergone successful CEA for TIA or minor stroke continue to be at risk for subsequent ipsilateral hemispheric stroke with a cumulative risk of approximately 9.5% over the first 4 years after the operation.

Symptomatic carotid artery stenosis that reduces the diameter of the artery **70% or more** and is associated with single or multiple TIAs or minor cerebral infarction (within a 6-month interval) are **proven indications** for CEA (Table 16-2). Antiplatelet therapy should not be discontinued preoperatively if it is already being given. Patients with cerebral infarction and moderate to severe deficit were not eligible for the major trials that evaluated CEA in symptomatic patients. In general, a surgeon will wait 2 to 6 weeks after the patient has had a significant cerebral infarction to decrease the risk for hemorrhagic transformation. In this subgroup, the procedure typically is reserved for patients who have a reasonable functional recovery.

Table 16-2.   Indications for CEA

Symptomatic
  Proven
    Symptomatic carotid stenosis, >70%
    Symptomatic carotid stenosis, 50% to 69%
  Unproven but acceptable
    Stroke in evolution
    Simultaneous coronary artery bypass grafting
  Uncertain
    Acute carotid occlusion, symptomatic
  Unacceptable
    Symptomatic carotid stenosis, ≤50%, unless thrombus
      demonstrated
    Long-standing carotid occlusion
Asymptomatic
  Proven
    Selected patients with carotid stenosis, ≥60%[a]
  Unproven but acceptable
    Selected patients with carotid stenosis ≥60%, who are mild to
      moderate surgical risks, are women, or have multiple or
      diffuse atherosclerotic lesions
  Unacceptable
    Asymptomatic carotid stenosis, ≥60%
    Long-standing carotid occlusion
    Carotid dissection (asymptomatic or asymptomatic after
      initiation of medical treatment)
    Patients with carotid stenosis, ≥60%, who are moderately
      high or high surgical risks

CEA = carotid endarterectomy.
[a]Patients who seem to benefit the most: (1) men seem to benefit more than women; (2) patients with no major organ failure, including cardiac, pulmonary, or renal disease; (3) patients with no other relative or absolute contraindications to operation; (4) patients with relatively isolated, high-grade, easily accessible lesions in area of the carotid bifurcation; and (5) patients aged 80 years or younger.

For **symptomatic patients** with TIAs or minor cerebral infarction associated with a moderate carotid artery stenosis of **50% to 69%**, CEA should be considered **acceptable but of lower overall efficacy** for the prevention of stroke compared with CEA for symptomatic stenosis >70% (Table 16-2). Whether CEA is indicated in the setting of progressing stroke related to carotid artery stenosis is controversial and has not been studied adequately. At this time, many investigators consider the procedure to be **acceptable but not of proven value** for patients with **progressive ischemic stroke** related to carotid artery stenosis of 70% or more, with or without ulceration.

CAROTID ANGIOPLASTY WITH STENT PLACEMENT

Another treatment option for patients with carotid occlusive disease is carotid angioplasty with stent placement (CAS) (Fig. 16-5). The procedure is performed in a similar manner to a carotid arteriography, via a groin artery access. Most interventionalists

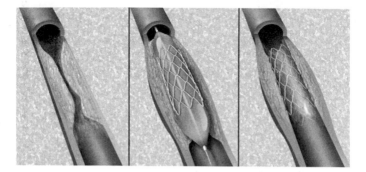

Figure 16-5.   **Basic technique of carotid angioplasty with stent placement.**

also typically use a distal protection device in the distal internal carotid artery. This is a small umbrella-shaped filtering device that is deployed temporarily before the angioplasty and stent placement. Aspirin and clopidogrel are initiated before a CAS procedure. Clopidogrel is used for 1 month, and aspirin is continued indefinitely.

The risk and durability of CAS compared with CEA is being defined in a large, randomized trial. Available data suggest that the risks may be relatively similar, but the long-term durability and stenosis recurrence risks are not proved. CAS typically is used for symptomatic patients with a carotid stenosis >70% in severity, who are at high risk for CEA. The high-risk factors may include surgical factors such as previous radiation to the neck, previous ipsilateral radical neck dissection, recurrent stenosis after CEA, high cervical internal carotid artery lesions, common carotid artery lesions below the clavicle, and severe tandem lesions. Medical factors that place the patient at high risk include severe coronary artery disease, significant angina, recent MI and the need for carotid artery revascularization, placement on the list for major organ transplantation, concurrent requirement for aortocoronary bypass, ejection fraction <30%, severe pulmonary disease, and uncontrolled diabetes.

In patients who are at high risk for CEA and have a high-grade symptomatic stenosis, CAS is the preferred treatment, particularly given the risk with medical management. Asymptomatic patients who have severe carotid stenosis and are at high risk for CEA because of the surgical or medical factors outlined above are also sometimes considered for CAS.

Patients with symptomatic stenosis in the distal internal carotid artery, middle cerebral artery, vertebral artery, or basilar artery typically are treated with antiplatelet therapy and aggressive risk factor control. Warfarin is infrequently used for this indication. The Warfarin Aspirin Symptomatic Intracranial Disease (WASID) trial data suggest that warfarin is not better than aspirin therapy for symptomatic intracranial stenosis but carries with it a somewhat higher likelihood of hemorrhagic complication. Whether warfarin is more effective for very severe intracranial stenosis, particularly in the basilar artery, with recent ischemic symptoms is uncertain from the WASID data. Transluminal balloon angioplasty of the vertebral and basilar arteries may be considered in selected patients who have symptomatic stenotic lesions of a vertebral artery, severe narrowing of the basilar artery, severe narrowing of the distal internal carotid artery or middle cerebral artery, or long segments of stenosis with irregularity and evidence of thromboemboli and who fail medical therapy that consists of antiplatelet or anticoagulation therapy and aggressive risk factor control. Bypass procedures are also considered in some patients with stenosis or occlusion that is not amenable to CEA or angioplasty/stenting.

Ipsilateral CEA in **combination with coronary artery bypass grafting** is also generally considered to be **acceptable but not yet proven** in a symptomatic patient who experiences TIAs or minor cerebral infarction in the presence of unilateral or bilateral stenosis of 70% or more and who is in need of coronary artery bypass grafting. CAS may provide a better alternative in this patient group with severe coronary artery disease, with a strong indication for a carotid procedure.

Another surgical procedure, **extracranial-to-intracranial bypass**, has been found to be generally ineffective for preventing ischemic stroke among patients with focal cerebral ischemic symptoms and various underlying craniocervical occlusive lesions. However, rarely may patients be candidates for such a procedure, such as those with incapacitating recurrent, reproducible, hemodynamic (postural) cerebral ischemic events or progressive visual loss from venous stasis retinopathy in the setting of inoperable internal carotid system occlusive disease. Whether selected patients with carotid occlusion and severe hemodynamic compromise, as assessed by positron emission tomography scanning, may preferentially benefit from the bypass procedure is under investigation. (Chapter 24 and Table 16-2 address asymptomatic carotid stenosis.)

Fibromuscular Dysplasia

Fibromuscular dysplasia (FMD) is a noninflammatory disease that usually affects one or both internal carotid arteries above the carotid bifurcation. Cerebral arteriography (often performed for unrelated symptoms) usually shows a characteristic beaded-lumen appearance, with multiple stenoses, elongation and kinking, and, occasionally, intracranial aneurysm formation. The hyperplastic changes of the arterial intima and media may stenose or occlude the arterial lumen and predispose to thromboembolism. Dissection of the involved segments of the carotid artery may occur, leading to vessel stenosis or aneurysmal dilation with blood stagnation and thrombus formation.

In patients with cerebrovascular ischemia associated with FMD, aggressive intervention options such as CEA, endovascular arterial dilation, and angioplasty with stent placement are rarely necessary, unless the patient has ongoing symptoms despite medical therapy. On the basis of available information, treating these patients conservatively (antiplatelet therapy) is usually preferable because of the relatively benign natural history of the condition. Medical treatment with warfarin for

3 to 6 months may be considered in selected patients with hemo-dynamically significant carotid artery stenosis associated with ipsilateral TIA, minor cerebral infarction, or recurrent focal ischemic events, particularly if a dissection that is causing the stenosis has occurred. When FMD is complicated by dissection associated with ischemic cerebrovascular symptoms, anticoagulant therapy is often used, as least for a several-month course. Repeat imaging then is performed, and if the dissection has healed, then the anticoagulation may be discontinued, with ongoing aspirin use. The evidence supporting warfarin use in this situation is limited, so if the patient is not a good warfarin candidate, then antiplatelet therapy may be used. If the patient with FMD has a co-occurring intracranial aneurysm, that lesion requires a separate thoughtful review of the most appropriate management, whether it be conservative treatment, aneurysm coiling, or clipping.

CAROTID ARTERY DISSECTION

Carotid artery dissection may be related to trauma, FMD, or collagen disorders, or it may occur spontaneously. This disorder is noted primarily in young women. The clinical syndrome includes ocular pain, ipsilateral Horner's syndrome, and hemi-cranial discomfort with or without focal ischemic cerebrovascular deficits. MRA, CTA, or cerebral arteriography demonstrates an elongated narrowing, often with a conical tapering and sometimes with an accompanying "distal pouch." Some authors believe that FMD and spontaneous carotid artery dissection are part of the clinical spectrum of one disease process. However, the cause of each of these conditions remains unknown.

Anticoagulation therapy with heparin followed by approximately 3 to 6 months of warfarin therapy generally is recommended for **extracranial internal carotid artery dissection** associated with focal cerebral ischemic events. However, the use of warfarin is controversial if the disorder involves hemorrhage into the arterial wall but is often still considered given that the ischemic symptoms are caused by thrombotic and embolic complications. If warfarin therapy is contraindicated because of other medical problems, then antiplatelet therapy is considered. Surgical or endovascular treatment typically is not used for carotid artery dissection, because partial or complete resolution of the dissection and thrombosis with recanalization during a period of several months generally occurs. After medical management is initiated, the MRA or CTA typically is repeated in approximately 3 to 6 months, and if the lumen has improved or normalized, then the warfarin may be discontinued. Extracranial vertebral artery dissections that do not extend intracranially typically are treated in the same manner, with a course of warfarin anticoagulation.

Management of the uncommon **intracranial carotid artery dissection** is still controversial. Antiplatelet therapy is often recommended (especially in situations without focal cerebral ischemic symptoms or when such symptoms have not occurred within the past week). Although there is some risk for arterial rupture, early therapy with heparin and warfarin typically is given if cerebral ischemic symptoms have occurred within the past week, particularly if they are recurrent. If embolic symptoms recur during heparin therapy, surgical or endovascular options should be considered. Hemodynamic events often resolve with recanalization of the thrombosed vessel; thus, a delay in surgical intervention is prudent. Patients with brainstem ischemia caused by vertebral or basilar artery dissection should be treated medically with early heparin anticoagulation if they have no evidence of intracranial bleeding. Warfarin typically then is used for approximately 3 to 6 months. MRA or CTA then is repeated, and if the lumen has improved or normalized, antiplatelet therapy may be continued.

Radiation

Sometimes, intensive **brain or neck radiation** (for example, for brain tumors, lymphoma, and carcinoma of the larynx) may result in arterial, capillary, or venous vasculopathy and lead to ischemic or hemorrhagic stroke or TIA. In these patients, the time from radiation to cerebrovascular complications is usually 6 months to 2 years. Radiation may also promote premature and rapidly worsening atherosclerosis, which may lead to large vessel occlusive disease. This is managed as outlined above for large artery stenosis or occlusion, along with aggressive atherosclerosis risk factor control.

Homocystinuria

Homocystinuria is also associated with thromboembolic infarcts and should be considered in the differential diagnosis of stroke in the young. Although the usual mechanism is premature atherosclerotic narrowing of large vessels, occlusion without preceding stenosis may also occur. The administration of a low-methionine diet and large doses of pyridoxine, vitamin B_{12}, and folate may be helpful. In a trial of vitamin replacement therapy in patients with mild hyperhomocysteinemia presenting with a nondisabling cerebral infarction, the risk for recurrent stroke was no different in those who received high-dose vitamins, compared with a low dose. There was strong association of the level of homocysteine and overall risk in adverse vascular outcome, so the optimal treatment of these patients remains under study.

SMALL VESSEL DISEASE

Hypertension

Hypertension (systolic blood pressure [BP] of 140 mm Hg or more or diastolic BP of 90 mm Hg or more) may affect brain performance indirectly by contributing to the development of impaired cardiac function or directly by producing physiologic and pathologic changes in the cerebral circulation. Although atherosclerosis is regularly encountered in normotensive patients, it occurs with increased frequency and severity in patients with hypertension. Thus, atherosclerotic cerebrovascular disease causes many of the stroke syndromes that develop in patients with hypertension. However, the more specific cerebrovascular abnormality in patients with sustained hypertension consists of fibrinoid necrosis, lipohyalinosis, and miliary microaneurysms, resulting in a nonatherosclerotic segmental degeneration in the walls of penetrating arteries. These lesions, found almost exclusively in the brain of patients with hypertension, are located primarily in the basal ganglia, thalamus, pons, cerebellum, and subcortex—the same regions in which both lacunar infarction and ICH predominate.

Lacunar infarctions cause approximately 15% of all ischemic strokes and tend to be associated with certain clinical syndromes. Lacunar infarctions are small (<1.5 cm in greatest diameter) and result from involvement of deep, small, penetrating branches of the major intracranial arteries without involvement of the cortex. Because these arterial branches have poor collateral connections, obstruction of blood flow caused by fibrin deposition, lipohyalinosis, microatheroma, or thrombus leads to infarction in the limited distribution of one of these arteries. Other possible causes of these clinical syndromes are a small hemorrhage or a very small embolic infarct.

Lacunar infarcts are the single most frequent cerebrovascular lesion found in elderly patients with hypertension and may or may not be symptomatic, depending on their location. Lacunes typically do not cause deficits such as aphasia, homonymous hemianopia, coma, seizures, isolated memory impairment, monoplegia, or loss of consciousness. They may occur during sleep, and progression in a stepwise manner during 1 to 4 days is not uncommon. The **five most common recognizable syndromes** described are as follows:

1. **Pure motor hemiparesis** with weakness involving face, arm, and leg on one side of the body caused by a lesion in the contralateral internal capsule or base of the pons
2. **Pure sensory stroke** with numbness of the face, arm, and leg on one side of the body caused by a lesion in or near the contralateral thalamus
3. **Dysarthria clumsy hand syndrome** with severe dysarthria, mild hand weakness and clumsiness, facial weakness, and dysphagia caused by a lesion in the base of the pons
4. **Ataxic hemiparesis** with pure motor hemiparesis and ataxia in the affected limbs, caused by a lesion in the base of the upper pons
5. **Sensorimotor stroke**, with weakness and sensory loss involving the face, arm, and leg on one side of the body. This is caused by a lesion in the thalamus and adjacent posterior limb of the internal capsule.

Although all of these syndromes usually indicate lacunar disease, other ischemic mechanisms may be involved.

Lacunar infarction is suspected when the clinical symptoms correspond to one of the five syndromes. CT is positive in only approximately 50% of cases; MRI is often more useful for characterizing the topography of the lesion. When performed, electroencephalography typically is normal, and MRA, CTA, or cerebral arteriography shows no visible arterial occlusion consistent with the patient's findings. Sometimes these infarctions are asymptomatic, revealed incidentally by brain imaging or autopsy.

Lacunar infarction that occurs in the distribution of the anterior circulation should be evaluated with carotid duplex, MRA, or CTA. Lacunar infarctions in the posterior circulation may be

evaluated with MRA, CTA, or TCD ultrasonography of the vertebrobasilar system. The diagnostic evaluation of lacunar events
is somewhat controversial. Many studies support the concept
that up to 90% of lacunar infarcts occur in the setting of chronic
hypertension and its associated pathologic changes of the arterial
system, but others have reported a lower prevalence of hypertension in such patients, which makes a comprehensive evaluation for a thrombotic or embolic cause more likely to define an
alternative cause. If doubt exists about the nature of the cerebral infarction that is responsible for the symptoms because of a
clinical syndrome that is inconsistent with a classic lacunar
syndrome or tomography of the infarct on CT or MRI at a location or of a larger size than typically would be seen in a lacunar
stroke, then additional studies to include an MRA or CTA,
echocardiography, and blood tests may be necessary to help eliminate other causes of infarction.

Single lacunar infarction generally has a good prognosis, and
rehabilitation efforts are usually successful. Treatment should
be directed at gradual reduction of BP, smoking cessation, lipid
management, and diabetes control. Clinical trial data suggest
that lowering of BP in patients who present with TIA or cerebral
infarction results in a reduction in recurrent stroke risk. In the
PROGRESS trial of 6,000 patients with either recent cerebral
infarction or TIA, patients who received antihypertensive medications, achieving a mean reduction in BP of 12/5 mm Hg, had
a 43% reduction in recurrent stroke over 4 years of follow-up.
The reduction was noted irrespective of initial BP, suggesting
that BP reduction should be considered in most patients who
present with cerebral infarction. In addition to risk factor control, antiplatelet therapy with aspirin or aspirin in combination
with extended-release dipyridamole or clopidogrel is recommended. There is no evidence that warfarin anticoagulation is of
benefit in this setting.

Cerebrovascular diseases also may be associated with acute
elevation of BP, referred to as **hypertensive crises**. Clinical syndromes include hypertensive encephalopathy (see Chapter 19),
hypertensive hemorrhagic stroke (see Chapter 17), and severe
hypertension associated with pregnancy (see Chapter 22).

Arteritis

Intracranial arteritis may or may not be associated with an
identifiable infectious cause. **Infectious** conditions include those
in which the arteritis seems to be due to meningeal involvement
(bacterial, fungal, tuberculous, and syphilitic meningitis) and
those in which the arteritis occurs independent of meningitis
(aspergillosis, mucormycosis, herpes zoster, malaria, trichinosis,
rickettsial diseases, and schistosomiasis). The **noninfectious**
processes often involve the brain parenchyma in addition to
cerebral arteries of a given caliber.

Infectious Arteritis

Several different CNS infective processes result in a reactive
change in the cerebral blood vessels, known as **obliterative
endarteritis**. The condition is characterized by an inflammatory
cellular infiltrate and thickening of the arterial intima, which

may stenose or occlude the lumen or serve as a nidus for thromboembolism. Bacterial, fungal, and tuberculous meningitides that bathe the smaller leptomeningeal arteries in purulent or granulomatous exudate may lead to obliterative endarteritis in the vessels. The process may remain focal but usually becomes more generalized and causes numerous, small, superficial areas of cerebral infarction. With rare exception, the patient appears very ill and has clear-cut signs of meningeal irritation before any ischemic symptoms develop.

Once a common cause of ischemic stroke in young adults, **tertiary syphilis** now is rare. All forms of tertiary syphilis may be associated with vascular involvement, but clinical cerebrovascular symptoms are most prominent with meningovascular syphilis, which usually develops 5 to 10 years after the initial infection. The endarteritis is usually confined to the intracranial arteries, but the aorta and major cervical arteries also may be affected. Multifocal cerebral ischemic symptoms in the territories of the middle and posterior cerebral arteries are the most common.

Other rare infectious causes of cerebral endarteritis include **malaria** and **rickettsial diseases**, in which cerebral ischemic symptoms are often preceded by convulsions, psychosis, or depressed levels of consciousness. These infections include **aspergillosis**, which usually occurs in association with systemic disease, especially involving the respiratory system; **mucormycosis**, which occurs in patients who have diabetes mellitus and have periorbital and cavernous sinus infections; **herpes zoster**, which leads to involvement of the distal internal carotid artery and proximal cerebral arteries, with delayed contralateral hemiplegia being the most common syndrome; **trichinosis**, which is associated with an inflammatory myopathy and, less frequently, with meningoencephalitis; and **schistosomiasis mansoni**, with lymphadenopathy, hepatosplenomegaly, eosinophilia, gastrointestinal hemorrhages and obstructions, and transverse myelitis. Appropriate aggressive antimicrobial therapy should be provided for the treatment of cerebral vasculitis caused by any of these infectious entities.

Noninfectious Arteritis

The noninfectious inflammatory angiopathies include those that primarily affect the arterioles and capillaries (systemic lupus erythematosus), those that primarily affect small- or medium-sized arteries (polyarteritis nodosa and isolated CNS angiitis), and those that primarily affect medium-sized to large arteries (temporal arteritis and Takayasu's disease). Takayasu's disease is discussed here in the context of inflammatory angiopathies, but the primary site of involvement is near the origin of the major vessels of the aortic arch.

Systemic lupus erythematosus (SLE) is a diffuse, connective tissue disorder in which 50% to 75% of patients have CNS involvement sometime during the course of the disease. However, only approximately 2% of patients with SLE have neurologic manifestations when first examined. Most of these patients already have prominent clinical systemic involvement (skin, bone marrow, heart, liver, kidneys, lungs, muscle, and peripheral nerves). CNS findings are usually those of a diffuse encephalopathy with delirium, seizures, acute psychosis, and increased intracranial pressure. Focal or multifocal cerebral and brainstem infarcts occur, but they rarely produce recognizable arterial syndromes. The cause of the CNS findings in SLE may be multifactorial. Multifocal infarction with inflammatory vasculitis is uncommonly noted on histologic examination; small-vessel vasculopathy without inflammation typically is seen. When SLE is associated with hypertension, ICH or small vessel hypertensive occlusive changes may result. Treatment with high-dose corticosteroids is recommended for cerebrovascular disease caused by systemic lupus erythematosus (in pregnant patients, this treatment is advised throughout pregnancy and during the first 2 months postpartum to limit puerperal exacerbations). If SLE manifests as thromboembolic events, then antiphospholipid antibodies and TEE should be obtained.

From 10% to 20% of patients with **polyarteritis nodosa** have CNS involvement, almost invariably after systemic manifestation of the disease. The pathologic findings vary from multifocal infarction or (especially when associated with hypertension) ICH to isolated large cerebral infarction resulting from occlusion of a major cerebral artery. The clinical features, therefore, may be those of diffuse disease of the CNS, such as headache, dementia, psychosis, generalized seizures, or focal or multifocal disease with facial paralysis, deafness, ocular nerve palsies, cerebellar abnormalities, or focal seizures. Corticosteroids such as prednisone (1 mg/kg/day in three to four divided doses) with or without immunosuppressive agents, such as cyclophosphamide (2 to 4 mg/kg/day in a single morning dose followed by a generous amount of water to avoid hemorrhagic cystitis), seem to improve the survival of patients with polyarteritis nodosa.

A rare vasculitis, **isolated CNS angiitis (granulomatous angiitis)**, unlike SLE and periarteritis nodosa, is usually confined to the CNS. Symptoms result from widespread occlusion of small parenchymal and leptomeningeal arteries and veins. The condition is often heralded by a flu-like illness, with headache and generalized weakness, followed by confusion, seizures, or unifocal or multifocal neurologic deficits. MRI or CT may demonstrate single or multiple cerebral infarctions, meningeal enhancement, or subcortical enhancement with administration of contrast agent or, less common, show subarachnoid hemorrhage or ICH. Cerebrospinal fluid examination may reveal increased protein and lymphocytic pleocytosis. Findings on cerebral arteriography are usually abnormal and demonstrate alternating dilation and constriction (beading) of medium-sized and small intracranial arteries.

Meningeal and cortical biopsies are necessary in patients with equivocal or atypical arteriographic findings or in those who do not respond to treatment. There is no standard treatment of cerebrovascular disease associated with isolated CNS angiitis, although treatment with prednisone (60 to 100 mg per day orally) alone or in combination with cyclophosphamide in a single morning dose of 1 to 2 mg per kg orally (adjusted to avoid severe leukopenia) or monthly intravenous (IV) dose is the most common initial treatment approach. Patients who do not tolerate cyclophosphamide may be given azathioprine (2 mg/kg/day) or other immunomodulating agents such as mycophenolate mofetil.

A generalized granulomatous vascular disease, **temporal arteritis** (cranial arteritis, giant cell arteritis) usually involves the superficial temporal and extracranial scalp arteries and ophthalmic arteries in patients who are older than 55 years. The inflammatory reaction within the superficial temporal arteries often makes these arteries tender to palpation and gives them a swollen, erythematous, beaded appearance. An unremitting unilateral or bilateral temporal headache is common, but any distribution of head and face pain may occur. Painful chewing may be caused by jaw muscle ischemia with claudication or by contact between moving skin and temporalis muscles. Occlusion of the ophthalmic artery or its branches, which occurs in 20% to 25% of patients, results in ipsilateral eye pain and visual impairment that progresses to complete blindness. In 10% to 20% of patients, both eyes are affected. Cerebral infarction is a rare complication but may occur in both carotid and vertebrobasilar artery distributions.

Most patients also have features of a more generalized vasculitis, including fever, malaise, weight loss, and polymyalgia rheumatica. Laboratory findings show elevated erythrocyte sedimentation rate (ESR), slightly increased leukocyte count, and mild anemia. Temporal artery biopsy is indicated to make a definitive diagnosis. Clinical findings that are most strongly correlated with a positive biopsy include jaw claudication and abnormality of the superficial temporal arteries, including erythema, tenderness, and beading.

When temporal arteritis is suspected (age over 55 years, increased ESR, with common clinical symptoms include local [often pulsating] pain in the temporal region over the temporal artery [often enlarged and tender on palpation], ipsilateral blindness in one eye, polymyalgia, and fever), corticosteroid treatment (60 to 100 mg of prednisone daily) is initiated, even before the biopsy can be arranged. This dose typically is maintained for 1 month, with a slow reduction in dose, depending on the patient's clinical response and decrease in ESR. Daily low-dose corticosteroid therapy is usually required for 2 years or longer, depending on response to the treatment (repeated laboratory monitoring of ESR is required).

A chronic inflammatory arteriopathy of unknown origin, **Takayasu's arteritis** (pulseless disease) most commonly affects young women. Involvement of the aortic arch and its branches results in narrowing of major-vessel ostia and cerebral ischemic symptoms, including ischemic Takayasu's retinopathy. Clinically, there may be reduction or absence of subclavian, carotid, brachial, and radial pulses, with bruits over affected or collateral vessels and neurologic symptoms of cerebrovascular insufficiency such as blurred vision (especially with activity), dizziness, decreased visual acuity, memory loss, and hemiparetic and hemisensory syndromes. Systemic complications include secondary hypertension caused by renal artery involvement; systemic symptoms such as malaise, arthralgias, fever, anorexia, weight loss, and night sweats; aortic regurgitation; aortic aneurysm; and laboratory abnormalities (such as elevated ESR, anemia, leukocytosis, and elevated C-reactive protein level). MRA, CTA, or arteriography of the aortic arch demonstrates diffuse narrowing and occlusion of multiple large arteries as they originate from the aortic arch, with or without fusiform aortic dilation and calcification.

In the early stages of the disease, corticosteroid therapy with prednisone is recommended. Initial doses as large as 100 mg daily are continued until inflammatory factors are controlled, usually 2 to 4 weeks, with subsequent reduction of the dose. For chronic symptomatic lesions such as renovascular hypertension, cerebrovascular or limb ischemia, dilation of the ascending aorta with aortic insufficiency, or thoracic or abdominal aortic aneurysms, a reconstructive procedure on severely involved vessels may be necessary to restore flow and prevent further ischemia and infarction.

Behçet's disease is an uncommon, recurrent, inflammatory disorder that affects the CNS, occasionally complicated by ischemic stroke. Episodes characteristically resolve completely during several weeks and tend to involve the brainstem. Men are affected more often than women. Typical clinical features usually include recurrent aphthous or herpetiform oral ulceration, recurrent genital ulceration, anterior or posterior uveitis, retinal vasculitis, erythema nodosum, papulopustular lesions, recurrent (aseptic) meningoencephalitis, cranial nerve (particularly abducens) palsies, and cerebellar ataxia. Because the cause of the disease is assumed to be autoimmune, treatment with corticosteroids or other immunosuppressive agents has been recommended.

Other systemic vasculitic syndromes are uncommonly associated with cerebral ischemia or infarction. These include **Wegener's granulomatosis** with primary involvement of the lungs, kidneys, and upper respiratory tract. **Rheumatoid arthritis** is more commonly associated with neuropathy, but cerebral infarction has been described. **Sjögren's syndrome** may cause dementia; cranial neuropathies, especially of the trigeminal nerves; and, less common, cerebral ischemia. **Sarcoidosis** of the nervous system may cause a cerebral vasculitis with cerebral infarction. Aseptic meningitis, cranial nerve palsies (especially cranial nerve VII), and hypothalamic dysfunction also typically are present.

HEMATOLOGIC DISEASE

Abnormalities in blood cell constituents and plasma proteins may result in a hypercoagulable or hypocoagulable state, with corresponding abnormalities in blood viscosity and stasis, which predispose the patient to cerebral ischemia or cerebral hemorrhage.

Polycythemia

Patients with primary or secondary polycythemia may have neurologic symptoms on the basis of increased red blood cell mass with hyperviscosity and increased vascular resistance. Cerebral arterial or venous thrombosis involving both small and large vessels may occur with focal areas of infarction or hemorrhagic infarction. From 10% to 20% of patients have clear-cut focal cerebral ischemic events (usually TIAs) that correlate with the values of the hematocrit and regress partially or totally after adequate therapy. In contrast, the reduction in red blood cell

mass and oxygen-carrying capacity that occurs with various ane-
mic states is rarely associated with focal cerebral ischemia.

Treatment of patients with polycythemia is complex and typically includes reduction of blood volume with phlebotomy (especially with hematocrit value $\geq$55%), with a goal hematocrit
value of 40% to 45%. Thrombocytosis should be controlled with
myelosuppression (alkylating agents, hydroxyurea, or radioac-
tive phosphorus). Young patients may be treated with phlebotomy alone to avoid the long-term risk of myelosuppressive agents.

Thrombocythemia

Thrombocythemia also has been associated with focal ischemic
neurologic lesions. This disorder may be primary or secondary to
other forms of myeloproliferative disease, such as polycythemia
vera. Megakaryocyte hyperplasia and increased platelet production result in elevation of the platelet count. Even in the absence
of preexistent atherosclerosis, spontaneous platelet aggregation
occurs with thromboembolic ischemic manifestations. In symptomatic patients, maintained suppression of platelet counts to
lower than 500×10^9 per L may prevent recurrence of serious
events. Treatment of acute cerebrovascular events in patients
with thrombocythemia (essential thrombocytosis) should begin
with emergency plateletpheresis. Lowering the platelet count
also may be achieved by therapy with hydroxyurea, alkylating
agents, or ^{32}P radiotherapy followed by administration of
antiplatelet agents such as aspirin, clopidogrel, or extended-
release dipyridamole to reduce the risk for recurrent thromboses.

Thrombocytopenic Purpura

An uncommon disorder, thrombotic thrombocytopenic purpura,
is likely a multicentric vasculitis. The hematologic and
cerebrovascular manifestations are the result of secondary
mechanical damage to erythrocytes. The damage causes
hemolytic anemia, fever, and increased utilization of platelets to
form diffuse microvascular thrombotic occlusions. Occlusion of
terminal arterioles in the brain produces multiple small infarcts
and a fluctuating encephalopathy, focal neurologic signs and
symptoms, seizures, and coma; the neurologic findings are often
reversible. The clinical picture may also include intracerebral
(often multiple) hemorrhage. Systemic symptoms may include
abdominal pain, myalgias, arthralgias, and ecchymoses. In addition to brain involvement, other areas that may be involved
include the pancreas, adrenal glands, heart, and kidney.

Laboratory evaluation includes looking for evidence of
Coombs-negative hemolytic anemia with elevated lactate dehy-
drogenase, fragmented erythrocytes, decreased platelet count,
and erythroid hyperplasia with increased megakaryocytes in the
bone marrow. Proteinuria, hematuria, and abnormal results of
liver function studies also are found. The white blood cell count
typically is normal or slightly elevated, and the prothrombin
time and activated partial thromboplastin time (aPTT) are
normal in most patients.

No consistently effective treatment of thrombotic thrombocytopenic purpura is available, although high-dose corticosteroids
(prednisone, 1 to 2 mg/kg/day), plasmapheresis (1.5 plasma

volume removal in 4 days), and infusions of fresh frozen plasma are often recommended. In addition, splenectomy or use of vincristine sulfate (Oncovin, Vincasar PFS) after plasmapheresis may lessen the plasma dependency, which can become protracted in some patients. Platelet inhibitors (such as aspirin and dipyridamole) are of unclear benefit and generally are not used if a patient is severely thrombocytopenic.

Sickle Cell Disease

Occurring in approximately 1 in 600 black Americans at birth, sickle cell disease is inherited as an autosomal dominant trait. When red blood cells that contain hemoglobin SS are exposed to low oxygen tension, their structure is altered in a way that increases blood viscosity and leads to multiple small vessel occlusions. When large arteries are involved through vessel wall ischemia from occlusion of nutrient arteries, large focal cerebral infarctions may occur. Other cerebrovascular lesions that are associated with sickle cell disease include multiple small cortical and subcortical hemorrhages or hemorrhagic infarcts, cortical vein and venous sinus thrombosis, massive ICH, and, rarely, subarachnoid hemorrhage. A large artery vasculopathy may lead to infarcts in border zone areas as a result of hemodynamic factors or may form the nidus for clot formation, leading to distal emboli and cortical infarction. Sickle cell crises are often precipitated by stress, physical exertion, hypoxia, or acute infection and are rarely manifested as a thrombotic crisis associated with fever and abdominal, bone, or chest pain. Children who are younger than 15 years are at greater risk for cerebrovascular complications.

TCD studies are useful in selecting patients who would benefit from aggressive primary prevention strategies. In the Stroke Prevention Trial in Sickle Cell Anemia (STOP) study, children who were aged 2 to 16 years were evaluated with TCD. Those with velocities >200 cm per second were randomly assigned to either intermittent transfusions or standard care. The transfusion group, with its goal to keep the hemoglobin S level below 30%, was highly effective in reducing the risk for first stroke. In children in whom ischemic stroke has occurred, after acute evaluation with appropriate imaging, exchange transfusions and IV hydration should be initiated. On the basis of the results mentioned above, long-term intermittent transfusions typically are implemented. In adults who have sickle cell disease and have had cerebral infarction, a complete evaluation should be performed to determine whether there is any alternative cause of the cerebral infarction, and appropriate secondary prevention should be implemented on the basis of the findings. Chronic intermittent transfusions, as advocated in children, are often considered.

Dysproteinemia

The various dysproteinemias, including macroglobulinemia, cryoglobulinemia, and multiple myeloma, also may be associated with thrombotic cerebrovascular complications. The usual picture is that of a diffuse encephalopathic disorder caused by the disseminated vascular lesions that form at the capillary, arteriolar, and venous levels and produce multifocal microinfarction and hemorrhage. Large areas of focal infarction are less common and may be the result of dural sinus thrombosis. Plasma exchange (large-volume plasmapheresis) seems to be efficacious in the acute treatment of at least some dysproteinemia-related hyperviscosity syndromes, although persistent control may require more prolonged treatment with chemotherapeutic agents.

Antiphospholipid Antibody Syndromes

Antiphospholipid antibodies, including lupus anticoagulant and anticardiolipin antibodies, have been associated with an increased occurrence of cerebral infarction. A history of frequent miscarriages, previous ischemic stroke, or other recurrent arterial or venous thromboses may be detected. Arterial infarct patterns vary widely, including both cortical and subcortical locations. Venous sinus thrombosis may also occur. The diagnosis is made on the basis of the combination of clinical and laboratory findings. In addition to direct measurement of circulating lupus anticoagulant and anticardiolipin antibody levels, a prolonged aPTT or false-positive Venereal Disease Research Laboratory test may also indicate the presence of a circulating antiphospholipid antibody. Other laboratory findings that may be associated with these syndromes are hemolytic anemia, decreased serum complement (C4), thrombocytopenia, and positive antinuclear antibody level.

Treatment is controversial, and the benefits of various therapies remain unproven. For patients with focal cerebral ischemic symptoms, warfarin is commonly used, although aspirin, aspirin and extended-release dipyridamole in combination, clopidogrel, and ticlopidine are other options. Others have advocated high doses (60 to 100 mg per day) of prednisone, which sometimes can suppress antiphospholipid antibody levels, particularly those related to lupus anticoagulant. Prednisone (or other immunosuppressant) therapy sometimes has been added to anticoagulant or antiplatelet therapy in patients with continuing cerebral ischemic events. Rarely, plasmapheresis has been used in patients with acute encephalopathy or disseminated intravascular coagulation.

Sneddon's syndrome, characterized by recurrent strokes and livedo reticularis in younger patients, may be associated with antiphospholipid antibodies.

Deficiencies of protein C, protein S, and antithrombin III or resistance to activated protein C may also occur on either a hereditary or an acquired basis. Although venous occlusive disease of the extremities typically occurs, patients uncommonly may present with arterial occlusions, including cerebral vessels, causing infarction. Factor V Leiden positivity is mainly a risk factor for deep venous thrombosis and pulmonary emboli and is unlikely to play a primary role in arterial occlusions that lead to TIA or cerebral infarction.

Leukemia

Leukemia and its attendant leukocytosis and hyperviscosity may be accompanied by cerebral arterial or venous thrombosis. However, cerebral symptoms that develop during the course of the disease are more commonly the result of intracranial hemorrhage or infection. Treatment of myelogenous or lymphocytic leukemia involves different regimens for distinct phases and is directed toward complete eradication of the leukemic cells or control of cell counts by means of cytotoxic drugs and bone marrow transplantation from a human leukocyte antigen–compatible donor.

Disseminated Intravascular Coagulation

Disseminated intravascular coagulation may be associated with virtually any pathologic process that produces tissue damage (such as massive tissue trauma, obstetric complications, cardiothoracic operation, burns, severe infections, heat stroke, incompatible blood transfusions, disseminated malignancy, shock from many causes, massive brain damage including stroke) and results in the release of tissue thromboplastins into the circulation with subsequent activation of the coagulation process, thrombin formation, subsequent platelet and clotting factor consumption, and the formation of fibrin thrombi and emboli throughout the microvasculature. The early thrombotic phase of disseminated intravascular coagulation leads to widespread small infarctions in many organs (including the brain) followed by a phase of secondary fibrinolysis that results in petechial hemorrhages around small penetrating vessels. The mortality rate in patients with disseminated intravascular coagulation varies, depending on the underlying disorder.

The clinical presentation of disseminated intravascular coagulation is dependent on the stage and the severity of the syndrome. The neurologic complications include (1) a syndrome of acute encephalopathy characterized by fluctuating focal neurologic symptoms that usually are associated with altered levels of consciousness, (2) venous sinus thrombosis, (3) ICH (usually subcortical petechial hemorrhages), and (4) cerebral arterial occlusions (small- to medium-sized arteries are frequently involved). Extensive skin and mucous membrane bleeding are common. The diagnosis is confirmed by blood test results revealing thrombocytopenia; presence of schistocytes or fragmented red blood cells; prolonged prothrombin, partial thromboplastin, and thrombin times; reduced plasma fibrinogen level; and elevated fibrin degradation products.

Treatment of disseminated intravascular coagulation should include control of the underlying disease and maintenance of adequate oxygenation and BP. If significant hemorrhagic or ischemic complications are present, then treatment should be initiated. In patients with thrombosis, heparin therapy (IV bolus followed by continuous IV infusion and a target aPTT of two times control) is usually added, and hemorrhage is treated aggressively with platelets and fresh frozen plasma. (Disseminated intravascular coagulation associated with fulminant liver failure generally is considered a contraindication for heparin therapy.) The target platelet count during therapy generally is approximately 50×10^9 per L. Increasing fibrinogen and platelet levels indicate that the process is coming under control and often correlate with a reduction in hemorrhagic complications. In patients with ongoing hemorrhage and lack of platelet or fibrinogen response to the transfusions, addition of antithrombotic treatment with heparin should be considered to impede fibrin formation.

Five Major Categories of Hemorrhagic Disease

Treatment of Specific Underlying Mechanisms

Hemorrhagic cerebrovascular disorders cause 15% to 20% of all strokes. These conditions can be divided into five subgroups on the basis of the location of the primary hemorrhage: (from superficial to deep) epidural, subdural, subarachnoid, intracerebral, and intraventricular hemorrhage (see Fig. 1-1 and Table 8-2).

The clinical features of hemorrhagic cerebrovascular disease vary, depending on the site and the size of the hemorrhage, and occasionally may not be clinically distinguishable from other types of stroke. Computed tomography (CT) or magnetic resonance imaging (MRI) allows precise differentiation and localization of brain hemorrhage and also helps to determine the extent of damage. When performed, cerebral arteriography may show an avascular mass in the region of hemorrhage.

Deterioration of a patient with hemorrhagic stroke is usually attributed to rebleeding (most commonly with saccular aneurysms and arteriovenous malformations [AVMs]); progressive cerebral edema; or other systemic causes such as heart, renal, or hepatic failure, serious cardiac arrhythmias, recurrent cardiac emboli, acute myocardial infarction, pneumonia, pulmonary embolism, septicemia, drug effects, or electrolyte disturbances such as hyponatremia (associated with salt-wasting syndrome or inappropriate antidiuretic hormone syndrome).

EPIDURAL HEMATOMA

Epidural hematoma is a collection of blood between the skull and dura and commonly results from a parietal or temporal skull fracture with laceration of the middle meningeal artery and, occasionally, from a dural sinus tear. Because the dura becomes adherent to the skull with age, epidural hematoma rarely occurs in the elderly. A lucid interval, of several minutes to a few hours, followed by increasing severity of headache associated with nausea, vomiting, progressive impairment of consciousness, and contralateral hemiparesis is the classic clinical course. Pupillary dilation on the side of the hematoma is often an indication of transtentorial herniation. In this situation, the head injury and the hemorrhage are ipsilateral to the dilated pupil in 90% of patients, and the pulse is often <60 beats per minute, with a concomitant increase in systolic blood pressure (BP).

Radiography of the skull may reveal a fracture line that crosses the groove associated with the middle meningeal artery. CT or MRI reveals a lenticular-shaped (biconvex; Fig. 17-1) or, rarely, a crescent-shaped clot with a smooth inner margin, and cerebral arteriography shows inward displacement of the surface arteries. Lumbar puncture may precipitate transtentorial herniation

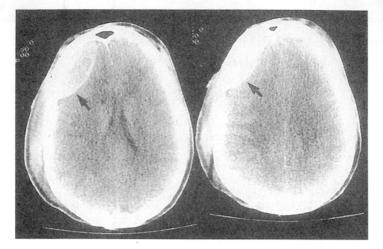

Figure 17-1.   CT scan of the head without contrast: lenticular-shaped clot consistent with an epidural hematoma (arrows).

and is contraindicated in this setting. Early diagnosis and immediate neurosurgical consultation may be lifesaving. Treatment typically involves placement of several burr holes, evacuation of the hematoma, and identification and ligation of the bleeding vessel.

SUBDURAL HEMATOMA

Subdural hematoma occurs 10 times more often than epidural hematoma. Subdural hematoma results from head trauma with a tear in a vein as it crosses the subdural space. Because the blood is collected between the dura and the underlying brain, nonfocal neurologic symptoms such as headache, nausea, vomiting, and altered consciousness are often more prominent than focal or lateralizing signs. Symptoms may fluctuate and, when focal, may (rarely) resemble transient ischemic attacks. A lucid interval between the trauma and comatose state is usually absent or brief. CT or MRI (Fig. 17-2) demonstrates a crescent-shaped (or, less common, lenticular-shaped) high-intensity mass consistent with hemorrhage, typically located over one or both (10% of cases) hemispheres. At 1 to 3 weeks after the appearance of subdural blood, the lesion changes from hyperdense to isodense on CT and thereafter becomes hypodense. Cerebral arteriography shows displacement of the brain away from the inner table of the skull.

Depending on the interval between the head injury and the onset of symptoms, subdural hematomas may be acute (within 24 hours), subacute (1 to 14 days), or chronic (>14 days). **Acute or subacute subdural hematoma** may be unilateral or bilateral and frequently results from a severe, high-speed head injury. A combination of subdural hematoma, cerebral contusion, and laceration is common. Urgent surgical treatment with placement of

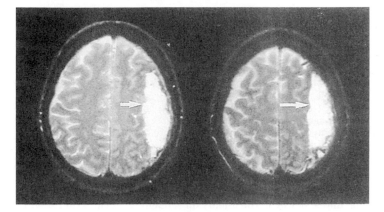

Figure 17-2.   MRI scan of the head: high-intensity mass consistent with a subdural hematoma (arrows).

burr holes and evacuation of the subdural hematoma is often indicated to prevent the development of deep coma.

In contrast to acute or subacute subdural hematoma, **chronic subdural hematoma** usually results from a less severe head injury, which may have been trivial or even forgotten. A gradual drift into drowsiness, inattentiveness, incoherence of thinking, confusion, stupor, and coma may be associated with increasing headache and, rarely, a seizure. Mental deterioration may be prominent, resembling dementia, brain tumor, drug intoxication, or depressive illness. Focal signs may include ipsilateral dilated pupil and hemiparesis, which may be contralateral, ipsilateral, or both. In infants and children, vomiting and seizures are prominent manifestations of chronic subdural hematoma. In these age groups, retinal hemorrhage in association with subdural hematoma may be manifestations of the so-called shaken infant syndrome.

Patients who have small, chronic subdural hematomas without severe or progressive deficit and in whom follow-up with serial neurologic examination and CT is possible can be managed conservatively. In cases of chronic subdural hematoma with severe or progressive deficit, surgical treatment is generally recommended.

SUBARACHNOID HEMORRHAGE

Subarachnoid hemorrhage (SAH) causes 5% to 10% of all strokes, affecting females more often than males (1.5 to 2:1). The disorder usually presents with the very sudden onset of a new, severe headache, which is commonly associated with vomiting and follows a rapid alteration of the level of consciousness, including unconsciousness with recovery in a few minutes. SAH may be caused by a ruptured intracranial saccular aneurysm (approximately 75% to 80% of all cases); AVM (approximately 5% of all cases); or other conditions, including mycotic, atherosclerotic, traumatic, dissecting, or neoplastic aneurysms or vasculitis (approximately 5% of all cases). SAH is of unknown cause in approximately 10% to 15% of all cases (see Table 8-2).

Intracranial Aneurysm

The most common cause of SAH is a ruptured **intracranial aneurysm** (Fig. 17-3). Saccular or berry aneurysms represent 80% to 90% of all intracranial aneurysms and normally appear as small, rounded, berry-like arterial outpouchings, but other shapes (sessile, pedunculated, multilobed) are also seen. The size of saccular aneurysms ranges from 2 mm to several centimeters in diameter, and most lesions are between 2 and 10 mm in greatest diameter.

Intracranial aneurysms usually go undetected until rupture results in a clinical picture of SAH, intracerebral hemorrhage (ICH), or both. The clinical features that are associated with SAH and ICH are described in detail in Chapters 14 and 15. In some instances, however, the aneurysm is diagnosed before rupture on the basis of SAH related to a separate aneurysm or clinical signs and symptoms unrelated to intracranial hemorrhage, including cranial nerve compression, compression of other central nervous system (CNS) structures, seizures, focal headaches, and cerebral ischemic events that result from embolism of thrombus within

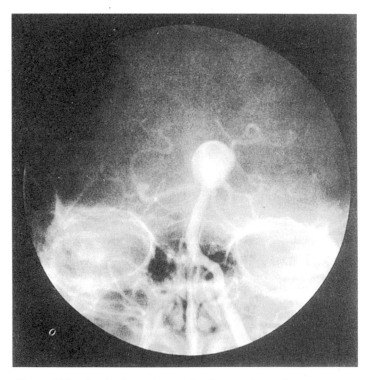

Figure 17-3.   Cerebral arteriogram: basilar caput saccular aneurysm.

large aneurysms. Alternatively, the diagnosis may be fortuitous after CT, MRI, or cerebral arteriographic studies that are performed for an unrelated disorder.

On the basis of existing evidence, it appears that most aneurysms probably form over a relatively short time (hours, days, or weeks) and attain a size allowed by the limits of elasticity in the elastic components of the walls of the aneurysm. At that point, either the aneurysm ruptures or, if the limits of elasticity are not exceeded and the aneurysm maintains itself intact, the walls undergo a process of compensatory hardening, similar to the process in other vascular walls that are subjected to arterial BPs, in which excessive amounts of collagen are formed. The tensile strength of collagen is several hundred times that of elastic fibers. With this added tensile strength, which continues to accumulate over time, the likelihood of rupture decreases unless the aneurysm is large at the time it initially stabilizes. Aneurysms that are 7 to 10 mm or more in size at the time of initial stabilization are much more likely to undergo subsequent growth and rupture, because the stress on the wall increases with the square of the diameter of the aneurysm. Therefore, it follows that the critical size for aneurysm rupture is lower if rupture occurs at the time of or soon after formation, as appears to be the case for most aneurysms that rupture. The mean size of aneurysms that are discovered after rupture is approximately 7.5 mm; the mean size of aneurysms discovered before rupture, which then go on to rupture, is approximately 20 mm.

It is important to recognize that ruptured and unruptured intracranial aneurysms constitute distinctly different clinical entities and need to be considered and managed as such. A more thorough discussion of the treatment of patients with unruptured intracranial aneurysms can be found in Chapter 29.

Intracranial aneurysms are typically located at large artery bifurcations involving the circle of Willis and its major branches (Fig. 17-4): internal carotid-posterior communicating artery junction, approximately 30%; anterior communicating artery, 30%; proximal middle cerebral artery, 20% to 25%; and posterior circulation, 10% to 15% among patients with aneurysms that are discovered subsequent to rupture. The locations of unruptured intracranial aneurysms (discovered before rupture) differ somewhat (Fig. 17-4): internal carotid-posterior communicating junction, approximately 45%; anterior communicating artery, 10% to 15%; proximal middle cerebral artery, 30% to 35%; and posterior circulation, 5% to 10%.

Intracranial aneurysms are rare in childhood, and the incidence of aneurysmal SAH is higher in women than in men (ratio, approximately 3:2). Approximately 20% to 30% of patients with saccular aneurysms have a family history of SAH or intracranial aneurysm, and 20% to 25% of patients have multiple aneurysms.

The pathogenesis of intracranial saccular aneurysms is controversial and may be multifactorial. There is convincing evidence that these are not congenital lesions but, rather, that they develop with increasing age. This possibility, however, does not preclude a genetic predisposition for these lesions to develop. Cigarette smoking and female gender appear to be associated with the development of unruptured intracranial aneurysms. Various

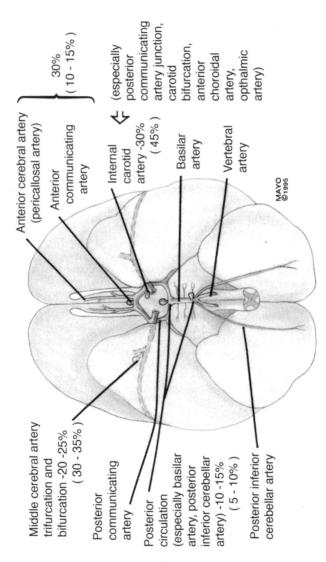

Anterior cerebral artery (pericallosal artery)

Anterior communicating artery

30% (10 - 15%)

Internal carotid artery -30% (45%)

(especially posterior communicating artery junction, carotid bifurcation, anterior choroidal artery, opthalmic artery)

Basilar artery

Vertebral artery

MAYO © 1995

Middle cerebral artery trifurcation and bifurcation -20 -25% (30 - 35%)

Posterior communicating artery

Posterior circulation (especially basilar artery, posterior inferior cerebellar artery) -10 -15% (5 - 10%)

Posterior inferior cerebellar artery

Figure 17-4.   Most common sites of ruptured and unruptured (in parentheses) saccular aneurysms.

other environmental factors (use of oral contraceptives, hypertension [particularly sudden increases in BP], use of stimulant drugs, physical stress, and alcohol consumption) may also have some role in the pathogenesis of ruptured and/or unruptured intracranial aneurysms. Medical conditions that have been associated with intracranial aneurysm include autosomal dominant polycystic kidney disease, intracranial AVM, coarctation ·of the aorta, Marfan's syndrome, Ehlers-Danlos syndrome, fibromuscular dysplasia, pseudoxanthoma elasticum, moyamoya disease, neurofibromatosis, and pituitary tumors.

Several large autopsy studies have shown a wide range in overall frequency (0.2% to 9.9%) of intracranial aneurysms in the general population. More recent prospective angiographic and autopsy studies suggest an overall frequency of approximately 2% to 4%. The incidence of aneurysmal SAH increases progressively with age, and the average annual incidence is approximately 6 to 10 per 100,000 population per year. These data suggest that most intracranial aneurysms never rupture.

Approximately 5% of all cerebral aneurysms are **mycotic cerebral aneurysms**. They commonly result from infected arterial emboli, primarily as a complication of acute or subacute bacterial endocarditis, and lead to septic degeneration of the elastic lamina and the muscular coats of the arterial wall. The most common sites of mycotic aneurysm formation are the distal middle cerebral artery branches, as seen in 2% of cases of bacterial endocarditis. The lesions often resolve with antibiotic treatment, although some symptomatic lesions require surgical clipping.

Dissecting and traumatic intracranial aneurysms are rare. The clinical presentation of **dissecting intracranial aneurysms** in a relatively young patient may consist of a focal and severe headache followed by progressive stroke, brain edema, and death. Typically, **traumatic intracranial aneurysms** develop after neck or head trauma (penetrating trauma, bony fractures), and occur most commonly in the internal carotid, middle cerebral, and anterior cerebral arteries.

Neoplastic cerebral aneurysms may be caused by arterial emboli from a cardiac (atrial) myxoma. Cerebral arteriography shows irregular filling defects in major and minor cerebral arterial branches, fusiform and saccular aneurysms, and arterial occlusions. Systemic emboli often occur.

Nonsaccular (fusiform) intracranial aneurysms may develop in patients with widespread atherosclerosis and hypertension and affect primarily the basilar, internal carotid, middle cerebral, and anterior cerebral arteries. Radiographic abnormalities include tortuosity, widening, and elongation of the affected arteries. Other terms such as dolichoectasia, ectasia, aneurysmal malformation, atherosclerotic aneurysm, and cirsoid aneurysm have also been applied to this category of lesions. In contrast to saccular or mycotic aneurysms, these aneurysms uncommonly present with SAH, but they may cause cerebral ischemia or mass effect. They typically are treated conservatively, although antiplatelet agents or even anticoagulants may be needed if thromboembolic events from the fusiform aneurysm occur.

Early **investigation and treatment** of intracranial aneurysms are important, particularly when the aneurysm has produced intracranial hemorrhage (see Appendix E-4). Even in pregnant patients, radiologic and therapeutic or surgical procedures should not be delayed or avoided, although special shielding during radiography is required (see Chapter 22). The clinical decisions that are involved in managing these patients vary with the type of aneurysm, but in patients who present with SAH, CT should be performed as soon as possible. CT may confirm the presence of subarachnoid blood, detect associated ICH and intraventricular hemorrhage, and, in some instances, demonstrate the aneurysm. If CT is nondiagnostic, then lumbar puncture may confirm the diagnosis of SAH (see Chapter 14). Magnetic resonance angiography (MRA) or CT angiography may also reveal the aneurysm, particularly if it is >3 mm in maximal diameter.

Arteriography of all intracranial vessels should be performed to identify the bleeding source as early as possible. In patients with SAH of unknown cause and initially negative arteriography, repeat arteriography to search for an occult intracranial aneurysm should be considered if the first arteriogram shows significant vasospasm or fails to demonstrate the entire vascular tree or if CT demonstrates a large amount of subarachnoid blood, especially when the blood is located diffusely or anteriorly. When the initial arteriogram performed for SAH fails to reveal an aneurysm, it is usually repeated 1 to 3 weeks later in an attempt to detect an aneurysm that was not visible on the earlier study. When the SAH is localized solely to a small clot anterior to the brainstem, this is called a perimesencephalic or pretruncal SAH. Posterior circulation aneurysms can cause such a CT appearance in some cases, so the issue of repeat arteriography in these patients is somewhat controversial. The initial arteriography may be delayed in patients who show a severe alteration in consciousness with or without focal neurologic deficits (Hunt and Hess clinical grade 4 or 5 [Appendix C-4]) because their prognosis is very poor (80% to 90% mortality rate in the first 30 days) and the early operative mortality rate is high (15% to 40%). In these patients, supportive treatment is generally indicated. If the patients improve with supportive treatment, then more aggressive diagnostic and therapeutic procedures are generally pursued. Alternatively, patients with little or no neurologic deficit (Hunt and Hess clinical grade 1, 2, or 3) have a more favorable prognosis (10% to 30% mortality rate during 30 days), but many of the deaths in this group result from rebleeding in the first 2 weeks after initial SAH. The potential advantages of early operation (including direct surgical clipping of the neck of the aneurysm [Fig. 17-5] or endovascular treatment of the aneurysm [Fig. 17-6]) must be weighed against the increased operative mortality rate during the first week after SAH. A recent large, randomized, controlled clinical trial (International Subarachnoid Aneurysm Trial [ISAT]) that compared surgical clipping to endovascular coiling for ruptured intracranial aneurysms documented significantly less early morbidity and mortality associated with endovascular repair, but the risk for subsequent rebleeding from the treated aneurysms and the risk for repeat procedures seem to be higher in this group. Long-term durability and effectiveness of these

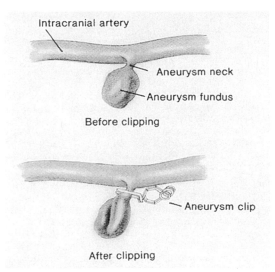

Figure 17-5. Basic technique of clipping of saccular aneurysm.

treatments is currently under investigation. Internal carotid artery ligation alone or in combination with extracranial-intracranial arterial bypass has become less popular because of high complication rates, but it is still used occasionally as treatment for large internal carotid system aneurysms. Management of patients with unruptured aneurysms is discussed in Chapter 29.

Early aneurysm operation (within the first 3 days after hemorrhage) is especially indicated for patients who are alert, have little or no neurologic deficit (a Hunt and Hess clinical grade of 1, 2, or 3), have no CT evidence of brain swelling, and are considered to be medically stable. Certain aneurysmal locations (notably basilar tip) favor endovascular procedures, whereas others (notably middle cerebral artery) may favor open surgery. After operation, the patient is usually followed in the neurointensive care unit until neurologically stable, with transcranial Doppler ultrasonography every 1 to 2 days. The patient should be kept well hydrated, be maintained on oxygen, and have central venous access for monitoring of central venous pressure. (Prevention and treatment of vasospasm are discussed in Chapter 14.)

Vascular Malformations

AVMs are the most common type of intracranial vascular malformation that causes neurologic symptoms. Other classifications of vascular malformations that may lead to neurologic disease include **cavernous malformations (cavernous hemangiomas)**, **venous malformations (venous angiomas)**, and **dural-based arteriovenous fistulae**. According to autopsy series, approximately 63% of supratentorial and 43% of infratentorial vascular malformations are arteriovenous in type. The

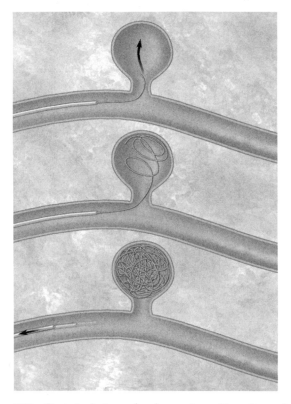

Figure 17-6.   Basic technique of endovascular coiling of saccular aneurysm. A tiny metallic coil or multiple coils, inserted into the aneurysm through a catheter, expand to fill the aneurysm. After the catheter is removed, the coil remains and allows clot to form in the aneurysm to isolate it from the circulation.

overall frequency of detection of intracranial vascular malformations is 2.75 per 100,000 person-years, whereas the prevalence of these lesions in one population-based study was 19.0 per 100,000 person-years.

AVMs most commonly present with intracranial hemorrhage or seizures. Other manifestations include headaches, which may mimic migraine, progressive neurologic deficit, pulsatile tinnitus, and transient cerebral ischemia. If a lesion is detected before hemorrhage, the risk for hemorrhage is approximately 2% to 3% per year, and the case fatality rate is 15% to 30%. The most frequent site for intracranial hemorrhage is intracerebral, followed by subarachnoid, intraventricular, and subdural. AVMs cause approximately 5% of all SAHs.

Cavernous malformations may also cause significant intracranial hemorrhage, but the hemorrhages are less common than AVM hemorrhages to be clinically relevant and typically are intracerebral in site. More common presentations include seizures, progressive neurologic deficit, and headache. **Venous malformations** are the most common vascular malformation detected at autopsy, but the clinical importance of these lesions is unclear. They are rarely associated with intracranial hemorrhage (both intracerebral and subarachnoid) and seizures. When hemorrhage is noted in association with a venous malformation, another type of vascular malformation, most typically a cavernous malformation, is usually found to have caused the hemorrhage at the time of surgery. **Dural-based arteriovenous fistulae** usually present with pulsatile tinnitus, headache, loss of visual acuity, and diplopia, although intracranial hemorrhage may also occur.

Radiologic imaging studies that are performed after a patient presents with ICH may suggest the presence of an underlying vascular malformation. With AVMs, CT may demonstrate calcification and hypodensity surrounding the lesion. The feeding arteries and draining veins are markedly enhanced after injection of contrast medium. MRI and MRA allow further clarification of the nature of the vascular supply and drainage, but standard arteriography is necessary to better demonstrate the arterial feeding system and venous drainage (Fig. 17-7).

Because AVMs have a lower risk for rebleeding than do saccular aneurysms, conservative management during the immediate posthemorrhage phase is commonly advised to prevent increased

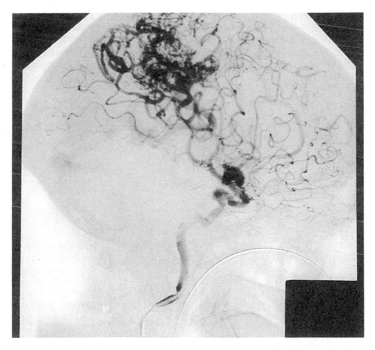

Figure 17-7.   Cerebral arteriogram: left frontoparietal AVM.

intracranial pressure (surgery is usually delayed until 1 to 2 weeks after the hemorrhage). Generally, relatively young patients with small malformations located superficially in the frontal or temporal area of the nondominant hemisphere are the best candidates for operation; very large malformations (>6 cm in diameter) involving more than one lobe or the posterior fossa and deep areas of the brain may be inoperable or unable to be resected at one sitting. Preceding embolization of feeding vessels may be required. When feasible, early excision of the entire AVM is the preferred therapy. Although newer microsurgical techniques have made safe removal of more malformations possible, many still cannot be totally excised. A commonly used scale that predicts the risk of AVM surgery is the Spetzler-Martin AVM Grading scale (Table 17-1).

Endovascular embolization also should be considered as a preparation for operation in patients with a few major arterial feeders, especially for malformations that are >3 cm and for treatment of dural AVMs. However, embolization of small feeders is associated with some risk of accidental embolization of a normal artery, which results in brain ischemia or infarct, and so this procedure should be avoided. Another possible complication associated with endovascular embolization is intracranial hemorrhage caused by rupture of an arterial feeder. Embolization alone is rarely successful for totally obliterating an AVM and is used infrequently as a sole means of treatment. Other increasingly popular treatment options for managing AVMs include various forms of radiotherapy, most notably gamma knife radiosurgery. Other forms of radiotherapy include linear accelerator (LINAC) and Bragg-peak proton beam radiosurgery.

AVMs that are located deep within the dominant hemisphere, in the brainstem, or in other highly risky areas of the brain such as the internal capsule and the thalamus are often considered to

Table 17-1.   Spetzler-Martin Arteriovenous Malformation Grading Scale

Graded Feature	Points
AVM Size	
Small, <3 cm	1
Medium, >3 cm and <6 cm	2
Large, >6 cm	3
Pattern of venous drainage	
Cortical/superficial only	0
Any draining veins into deep system	1
Eloquence of adjacent brain	
Noneloquent	0
Eloquent	1

Eloquent area: the sensorimotor, visual, and language cortex; thalamus and hypothalamus; internal capsule; brainstem; and cerebellar peduncles/deep nuclei. Noneloquent area: anterior frontal and temporal lobes, cerebellar hemisphere. Grade on a 1–5 scale = (size) + (venous drainage) + (eloquence).

be inoperable because of their inaccessibility or high risk for postoperative severe neurologic deficit and death. Even in the most experienced centers, surgical excision of an AVM with or without embolization is associated with a mortality rate of 1% to 5% and a morbidity rate of 10% to 20%.

If surgical excision is not feasible, focused radiotherapy (gamma knife or proton beam radiosurgery) alone or after embolization of the feeders or as an adjunct to embolization and resection may be considered. Radiotherapy (gamma knife) may be especially effective if the nidus is no larger than 3 to 4 cm in diameter (2 cm in the brainstem). Approximately 40% of lesions are arteriographically obliterated at 1 year after radiosurgery, 80% after 2 years, and approximately 90% after 3 years. However, intracranial hemorrhage may occur until the lesion is completely obliterated. Other complications of radiosurgery include radionecrosis of normal brain tissue and focal neurologic deficits in approximately 6% of patients (3% transient and 3% permanent). Occasionally, focal seizures occur within the first few days of treatment, usually in patients with a preexisting seizure disorder. Radiotherapy is less satisfactory for treatment of AVMs that are >3 to 4 cm in the hemispheres or >2 cm in the brainstem. (The management of unruptured AVMs is discussed further in Chapter 30).

Cavernous malformations that present with significant hemorrhage or intractable seizures typically are treated surgically if they are at an accessible site. Rarely, lesions have been treated with gamma knife radiosurgery if they were surgically inaccessible and presented with recurrent hemorrhage. **Venous malformations** are usually treated conservatively, although those that clearly are associated with intracranial hemorrhage may be considered for excision. When hemorrhage is noted in association with a venous malformation, another type of vascular malformation, most typically a cavernous malformation, is usually found to have caused the hemorrhage at the time of surgery. **Dural arteriovenous fistulae** may be treated with endovascular occlusive procedures (embolization or coils), surgical excision, or radiosurgery, depending on the size, location, and vascular characteristics.

Other Causes of Subarachnoid Hemorrhage

Other factors that may also be associated with nontraumatic SAH are (1) hypertension; (2) hematologic disorders, such as disseminated intravascular coagulation, often associated with leukemia or thrombocytopenia; (3) anticoagulant therapy; (4) cortical vein and dural sinus thrombosis; (5) primary or metastatic brain tumor; (6) cerebral vasculitis; (7) drugs, including alcohol abuse and cocaine abuse; and (8) spinal lesions. Management of these conditions is specific for each underlying pathologic process.

INTRACEREBRAL HEMORRHAGE

The onset of ICH is usually rapid, but unlike the acute, sudden onset to maximal deficit of embolism, this process typically evolves during minutes to hours without the stepwise progression of many ischemic strokes. The hemorrhage usually occurs while the patient is up and active, and it frequently presents with a severe headache and decreased level of consciousness, with nonfocal symptoms often predominating over the focal neurologic deficit. Small hemorrhages usually produce restricted focal neurologic deficit accompanied by mild or moderate nonfocal neurologic signs, and those in "silent" regions of the brain may even escape clinical detection, whereas large hemorrhages may produce early coma and signs of herniation.

Rupture of an **intracerebral hematoma** through to the cortical surface may produce associated bleeding **into the subarachnoid space**. When the hemorrhage is in the basal ganglia, thalamus, brainstem, or cerebellum, rupture into the ventricular system may occur. **ICH** occasionally also occurs **within a cerebral infarct** that results from venous thrombosis or, less commonly, arterial ischemia, together accounting for approximately 4% of cases.

Hypertension is the most frequently identified predisposing cause of nontraumatic ICH in adults. Other common causes are ruptured intracranial saccular aneurysm and vascular malformations such as AVM and cavernous malformations. Causes of ICH are reviewed in Table 8-2.

Once the diagnosis of intraparenchymal hemorrhage is established by CT or MRI of the head, one must use the clinical history, physical examination, appearance of the hematoma on CT or MRI (including location and size), and other appropriate laboratory tests to define the underlying cause of the hemorrhage, as delineated in Chapter 15. Decisions regarding diagnostic workup, medical treatment, and timing of operation should be based on both neurologic and neurosurgical criteria. General diagnostic and treatment considerations are outlined in Chapter 15. Management of patients with specifically identified underlying mechanisms for ICH is delineated in this chapter.

Primary hypertensive ICH is the most common nontraumatic brain hemorrhage and constitutes as much as 60% of all brain hemorrhages. This type of hemorrhage usually occurs with marked hypertension that produces anatomic changes, including microaneurysms and lipohyalinosis in the small intraparenchymal arteries. Less common, it occurs with moderate hypertension or even with BP in the normal range. The most common locations of hypertensive ICH are the basal ganglia and thalamus (37%; penetrating artery involved); temporal (21%), frontal (15%), or parieto-occipital (15%) lobes; cerebellum (8%); and pons (4%). In pathologic studies, these hemorrhages are described as large (>2 cm in diameter), small (1 to 2 cm in diameter), slit (<1 cm in diameter lying subcortically at the junction of white and gray matter), and petechial. Clinically, with the advent of radiologic imaging studies, the volume of the hemorrhage may be estimated from the CT scan using the ellipsoid method. The volume is estimated by measuring the width, length, and height of the hematoma, with multiplication of these measurements in centimeters and division by 2 to provide the very approximate volume in cubic centimeters. The volume of hemorrhage and the clinical status of the patient at presentation and presence and volume of intraventricular hemorrhage are important predictors of outcome, with overall volume of the hemorrhage being the most important predictor.

Management of patients with hypertensive ICH depends on the degree of hypertension; the location, surgical accessibility, and size of the hematoma; and the patientís clinical condition. Efforts should be made to (1) lower the elevated BP that set the stage for the hemorrhage and maintain BP in the appropriate range (see Chapter 15), (2) gradually reduce the mass effect (antiedema agents; see Chapter 15 and Table 11-1), and (3) prevent complications (see Chapters 11 and 15). If the patient's condition is stable and the hemorrhage is not life-threatening, a nonsurgical approach is usually recommended. In patients with lobar or cerebellar hemorrhage and associated signs of secondary deterioration related to increased intracranial pressure or brain herniation, immediate surgical treatment (evacuation of the hematoma) may be lifesaving and should be strongly considered. The results of a randomized clinical trial (International Surgical Therapy for Intracerebral Hemorrhage [STICH] Trial) of early surgery for supratentorial hemorrhage suggested that early surgery (within 24 hours of hemorrhage) was not clearly beneficial for supratentorial ICHs in general and for the lobar hemorrhage subgroup in specific. However, surgery was beneficial for the subgroup with hemorrhage ≤1 cm below the cortical surface. Emergency intervention in the setting of clinical deterioration may begin with maximal medical decompression with mannitol (1 g per kg), intubation, and hyperventilation, although the effectiveness of mannitol has not been fully investigated. High-dose steroids sometimes are used in this context, but available data do not suggest that they are effective in ICH. BP must be controlled, usually with a beta-adrenergic blocker, calcium channel blocker, or angiotensin-converting enzyme inhibitor. In patients with spontaneous ICH and a history of hypertension, a commonly recommended goal for BP reduction and maintenance is mean arterial pressure <130. Generally accepted contraindications to operation are massive hemorrhage with loss of brainstem function (such as fixed, dilated pupils and decerebrate posturing) and no response to medical therapy (see Chapter 15).

Nonhypertensive causes of ICH include ruptured vascular malformations and aneurysms; complications of anticoagulant, fibrinolytic, or antiplatelet therapy; hematologic diseases (thrombocytopenia, bleeding diathesis, hemophilia); head trauma; cerebral amyloid angiopathy; primary or metastatic brain tumors; drugs, including cocaine, alcohol, phenylpropanolamine, and heroin; CNS infection; and arteritis affecting the cerebral arteries and veins.

Ruptured vascular malformations (especially AVMs and cavernous malformations) cause approximately 5% of all ICHs (<1% of all strokes). Approximately 60% of intracranial hemorrhages associated with AVMs are intracerebral in location, whereas SAH occurs in approximately 30% of cases and ventricular hemorrhage in 10%. Headache at the onset of rupture of an AVM, rebleeding, and symptomatic cerebral vasospasm are not as prominent as with a ruptured saccular aneurysm. These ICHs usually evolve slower than those from hypertension or ruptured saccular aneurysms. The possibility of an underlying vascular malformation should be considered in patients with ICH, particularly in patients who have lobar and cortical hemorrhages with associated subarachnoid bleeding of unexplained mechanism, and especially in young adults (15 to 45 years of age). Cerebral arteriography must be considered in young adults with ICH of unknown cause and in older patients without a history of hypertension. Other diagnostic and treatment issues regarding vascular malformations are reviewed in the discussion of SAH earlier in this chapter.

ICHs that are caused by **aneurysmal rupture** are commonly managed with early surgical or endovascular intervention (within 3 days) to repair the aneurysm and sometimes to evacuate hematoma, unless contraindications exist. For patients who are in poor medical condition (severe neurologic deficit with altered level of consciousness), operation is usually delayed until the patient's condition improves with conservative management.

Cerebral amyloid angiopathy (congophilic angiopathy) is characterized by the deposition of amyloid protein in media and adventitia of leptomeningeal and cortical small arteries, arterioles, and capillaries, which is not associated with systemic amyloidosis. The amyloid angiopathy predisposes to miliary aneurysm formation or double barreling and fibrinoid necrosis of the affected vessels, which are prone to rupture in response to minor trauma or sudden changes in BP. Although the presence of amyloid seems to be strongly related to advancing age (overall, cerebral amyloid angiopathy causes approximately 15% to 20% of ICHs in the elderly), the precise mechanism for its development is unknown.

The diagnosis of cerebral amyloid angiopathy is particularly relevant in normotensive patients, primarily those who are older than 65 years and have nonhypertensive ICH, particularly in a subcortical or lobar location. However, approximately 30% of patients have coexistent hypertension. Multiple, hyperdense foci of blood on noncontrast CT of the head in lobar locations or multiple punctate hemorrhagic lesions on gradient echo MRI associated with periventricular leukoencephalopathy suggest the diagnosis of cerebral amyloid angiopathy. Recurrent intracerebral bleeding associated with amyloid angiopathy is common; minor head trauma, anticoagulation, and antiplatelet therapy have been reported as potential precipitants of the bleeding. The apolipoprotein E genotype may be useful in predicting which patients with lobar hemorrhage are at highest risk for recurrence. Carriers of the E2 or E4 allele had a higher risk for hemorrhage recurrence (28% over 2 years), compared with those with the most common E3/E3 genotype (10% over 2 years). A definitive diagnosis of cerebral amyloid angiopathy is made by biopsy of the involved brain and leptomeninges, although this is uncommonly indicated.

Because cerebral amyloid angiopathy is a widespread vascular disease that is prone to recurrence and because intraoperative hemostasis is difficult, surgical removal of lobar hemorrhage generally is not undertaken, except in situations of progressive or life-threatening hematomas in patients who are otherwise in relatively good condition. Conservative management consists of close clinical monitoring for signs and symptoms of increased intracranial pressure, maintenance of fluid and electrolyte balance, airway management, treatment of systemic cardiovascular

disorders, prevention of secondary complications, and administration of prophylactic anticonvulsants because most hemorrhages involve the cerebral cortex. Anticoagulants and
antiplatelet agents should be avoided.

ICHs that occur as a **complication of anticoagulant or fibrinolytic therapy** usually evolve more slowly than those that are
caused by hypertension. ICH that is related to the use of tissue
plasminogen activator for myocardial or cerebral infarction
tends to occur within 24 hours of infusion of these drugs. In this
situation, if possible, appropriate measures (such as protamine
for heparin and fresh frozen plasma with or without parenteral
vitamin K [1 to 2 mg intravenously] for warfarin agents) should
be taken to reverse coagulation defects.

ICH that is caused by **thrombocytopenia** is commonly treated
with platelet transfusions; for patients who have cerebrovascular
disease with a **bleeding diathesis** resulting from low prothrombin, replacement with plasma protein fraction and the administration of vitamin K are recommended. ICH that results from
hemophilia (hereditary abnormalities in factor VIII) should be
treated with early and aggressive replacement of factor VIII, in
the form of cryoprecipitate or commercial factor VIII concentrates.

Head trauma may produce intraparenchymal hemorrhage,
often in the form of cortical contusions at the site of impact of a
blow to the head (coup injury) or opposite the site of impact (con-
trecoup injury). Contusion may be associated with petechial
hemorrhage or a large area of hemorrhage with more severe
injuries, which typically are located along the hemispheric cortical surfaces, the inferior surface of the corpus callosum, the cerebral peduncles and in the rostral brainstem. In contrast to
epidural and subdural hemorrhagic components of traumatic
head injury, intraparenchymal hemorrhages are seldom treated
surgically unless they are associated with hydrocephalus or
evolving mass effect from blood. Efforts are instituted to correct
cerebral edema (see Chapter 11 text and Table 11-1) and any
associated hypocoagulable state. The recent Medical Research
Council Corticosteroid Randomisation After Significant Head
Injury (MRC CRASH) trial demonstrated a harmful effect of
early intravenous administration of corticosteroids (methylprednisolone) on 2-week mortality in patients with head injury and a
Glasgow Coma Score of 14 or less within 8 hours of injury.

Bleeding into **brain tumors** is relatively rare and may result
from primary brain tumors (for example, glioblastoma, pituitary
adenoma, medulloblastoma) or metastases (bronchogenic carcinoma, malignant melanoma, renal cell carcinoma, and choriocarcinoma). Secondary hemorrhage into a previously asymptomatic brain tumor should be suspected in patients with a history
of malignant disease or patients who present with papilledema.
Characteristic CT or MRI findings are multiple hemorrhages; ring-
like, high-density areas of blood surrounding a low-density center;
disproportionate edema and mass effect surrounding the acute
hemorrhage; and postcontrast enhancement of nodules at the
periphery of the acute hematoma or ring enhancement pattern.
Management is based predominantly on neuro-oncologic principles
and depends on the precise nature of the underlying tumor, which
is usually defined by biopsy of a systemic primary or brain lesion.

ICH that results from **cerebral arteritis** is usually characterized by preceding chronic headache; progressive intellectual
deterioration and altered consciousness; and, often, seizures,
recurrent episodes of cerebral infarction, fever, malaise, arthralgias, myalgias, weight loss, and anemia (see Chapter 16). The
diagnosis is suggested by elevated erythrocyte sedimentation
rate (typical of systemic vasculitides but uncommon in isolated
CNS angiitis) or cerebrospinal fluid findings, including elevated
protein and lymphocytic pleocytosis (occasionally found in isolated CNS angiitis). Cerebral arteriography occasionally shows
a characteristic beading pattern in multiple intracranial arteries with multiple branch occlusions; in such cases, evacuation of
the clot should be considered. The diagnosis can be confirmed
with brain biopsy before initiating immunosuppressive treatment (see Chapter 16).

INTRAVENTRICULAR HEMORRHAGE

Primary intraventricular hemorrhage is relatively rare and
usually results from vascular malformation or neoplasm of the
choroid plexus. More common, intraventricular hemorrhage
occurs as an extension of ICH or SAH. Clinically, primary hemorrhage into the ventricles produces a sudden loss of consciousness
without focal neurologic deficit (coma with periodic, generalized
tonic seizures may occur in some patients with extensive intraventricular hemorrhage). Most patients with intraventricular
hemorrhage are treated medically. However, if indications for
surgical treatment (as discussed in Chapter 15 for parenchymal
hematoma) exist, immediate evacuation of the clot should be
considered. Ventricular drainage is generally of limited value;
however, ventriculostomy can be lifesaving for patients who
have neurologic deterioration caused by acute hydrocephalus, as
shown by CT.

Cerebral Venous Thrombosis

Intracranial venous thrombosis may arise from infectious or noninfectious processes. Since the introduction of antibiotics, the frequency of venous thrombosis has decreased considerably, apparently from the prevention of thrombosis related to local head infections. In recent years, most cases of intracranial venous thrombosis have been aseptic in nature, and most of these are considered idiopathic. Other causes of aseptic intracranial venous thrombosis are polycythemia vera, leukemia, dehydration, cancer, phospholipid antibody syndromes and other primary hypercoagulable states, sickle cell disease, pregnancy, Behçet's disease and other inflammatory disorders, Crohn's disease, ulcerative colitis, dural arteriovenous fistulae, and other hyperviscosity syndromes. Sinus thrombosis has also been reported after jugular vein catheter placement and jugular thrombosis.

The clinical presentation of cerebral venous thrombosis varies, depending on the site of the lesion, its rate of progression and extension of thrombosis, and the nature of the underlying disease. Typically, the initial symptom is severe headache, which may precede other signs and symptoms by hours or days. Vomiting and focal seizures also tend to occur early in the course along with weakness and sensory disturbances that are usually progressive and may be unilateral or bilateral. Consciousness is usually altered, and language disturbances occur in approximately one fourth of patients. There is a tendency for venous infarcts to become hemorrhagic.

The diagnosis is based on the combination of clinical findings with radiographic documentation of venous occlusion. The patient's pelvis and legs are examined carefully to rule out coexistent peripheral thrombosis. The definitive diagnostic procedure has long been cerebral arteriography, but in recent years, computed tomography (CT) and magnetic resonance imaging (MRI) have proved helpful through visualization of hemorrhagic infarcts and thrombosed veins or venous sinuses. Magnetic resonance angiography (MRA) has become the standard imaging for cerebral venous thrombosis, providing excellent visualization of the venous sinuses, and is valuable for the early diagnosis of venous thrombosis (Fig. 18-1). Arteriography may still be performed in patients with a high clinical suspicion but negative or equivocal MRA.

The mortality rate is approximately 20% (hemorrhagic infarction caused by cerebral venous thrombosis is associated with the worst prognosis), but functional outcome among survivors is usually favorable, with less chance of persistent focal neurologic deficit than that for patients with arterial cerebral infarction (Fig. 18-1). Clinical presentation and underlying causes for venous infarcts vary to some extent with the location of the lesion.

Lateral sinus thrombosis commonly occurs in children and adolescents who have otitis media and may be asymptomatic, but those with propagation of thrombus into the superior sagittal

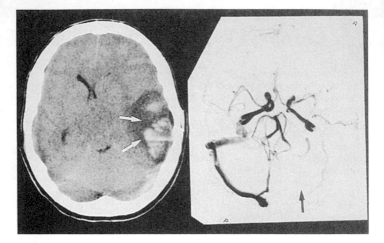

Figure 18-1.   Left. CT scan of head without contrast: area of
hemorrhagic venous infarction (arrows). Right. Magnetic resonance
angiography: asymmetry of transverse sinuses, consistent with
left transverse sinus occlusion (arrow).

sinus may experience progressive cerebral edema. If the thrombosis extends into the jugular vein, a jugular foramen syndrome
may occur (involving cranial nerves IX, X, and XI).

   Superior sagittal sinus thrombosis is the most common site of
sinus occlusion. Presenting symptoms are variable. Some lesions
may be asymptomatic, but significant thrombosis in the posterior
segments may lead to increased intracranial pressure (ICP),
papilledema, headaches, and decreased level of consciousness.

   Inferior petrosal sinus or **superior petrosal sinus thrombosis** may be associated with infections of the middle ear. The former may lead to diplopia caused by involvement of the abducens
nerve; the latter may cause facial pain from trigeminal ganglion
irritation.

   Cavernous sinus thrombosis is usually caused by paranasal
sinus infections, facial furuncles, or ear infections and characteristically produces severe headache; ipsilateral proptosis; visual
loss; chemosis; and palsies of the third, fourth, or sixth cranial
nerve or the first division of the fifth cranial nerve. Ocular signs
often become bilateral after a short period, and neck rigidity and
hemiparesis may occur. An accompanying palsy of the second and
third divisions of the fifth cranial nerve usually indicates superior petrosal sinus involvement. Thrombosis of the **jugular vein**,
lateral sinus, or torcula may produce signs of increased ICP without ventricular dilation.

   **Venous cerebral thrombosis with bland or hemorrhagic
infarction** should be suspected when focal neurologic symptoms,
especially hemiparesis accompanied by severe headache or
seizures, develop in the course of meningitis, otitis media,
or disseminated malignancy (especially lymphoma, leukemia, or
meningeal metastasis); during the postpartum period (pelvic or

other deep venous thrombosis is often present); or postoperatively. Thrombosis of cerebral veins can also occur in association with cachexia, dehydration, cardiac failure (especially congenital heart disease), inflammatory disorders such as Behçet's disease, or changes in blood coagulability (for example, primary or secondary polycythemia, use of oral contraceptives, antithrombin III deficiency, disseminated intravascular coagulation, Crohn's disease, ulcerative colitis, leukemia, polycythemia vera, hemolytic anemia, sickle cell disease, antiphospholipid antibody syndrome). Structural abnormalities such as a dural arteriovenous fistulae or tumor compressing a dural sinus can also provoke a sinus thrombosis. Some aseptic thromboses of multiple cerebral veins and sinuses are idiopathic and also involve extracranial veins simultaneously or in succession (thrombophlebitis migrans).

Treatment of intracranial venous occlusions, including those with minor hemorrhagic infarction, generally includes bed rest (the patient's head should be kept elevated at 15 to 30 degrees to improve venous drainage and lessen ICP) and hydration (with half-normal or normal saline to maintain normal fluid status). Heparin anticoagulation is standard therapy in most patients with cerebral venous thrombosis. The usual approach is to initiate anticoagulation, even if hemorrhagic transformation is noted on CT scan. Heparin should be initiated with a bolus and then ongoing intravenous infusion to attain an **activated partial thromboplastin time** two times control. Warfarin initiation is typically delayed for approximately 5 to 7 days and then is continued for at least 3 months (longer for specific hypercoagulable states). Antiplatelet agents (such as aspirin) are usually given thereafter.

In patients with severe papilledema, repeated lumbar punctures are performed, but optic nerve fenestration may be needed. Oral acetazolamide may also reduce ICP. If repeat lumbar punctures and oral acetazolamide are not successful in reducing ICP, then lumboperitoneal shunt may be needed. Prophylactic anticonvulsants are not indicated in patients with cerebral venous thrombosis. Hypotension or hypertension also should be corrected. Hypotension is particularly important because some element of dehydration may play a role in some patients with cerebral venous thrombosis. In patients with worsening cerebral edema and clinical deterioration, aggressive measures to reduce ICP should be instituted (see Chapter 11 text and Table 11-1).

When patients deteriorate in the setting of a venous thrombosis, one key concern is that the thrombosis may be propagating. Thrombolytic therapy of arteriographically proven aseptic cerebral venous thrombosis with intravenous or transjugular infusion of urokinase is considered in patients with a marked clinical deterioration in the setting of a worsening thrombosis. Anticoagulant therapy is then initiated.

Treatment of lateral sinus thrombosis that is caused by otitis media or mastoiditis usually includes removal of the infected bone, administration of antibiotics, and surgical drainage of abscesses. The jugular vein may be ligated if necessary. Antibiotics (with or without anticoagulants) should be administered to patients with septic superior sagittal sinus thrombosis or cavernous sinus thrombosis, and craniotomy with evacuation of subdural or epidural abscess should be performed when these conditions are present.

Patients in whom intracranial venous occlusion develops while they are taking oral contraceptives, antifibrinolytic agents, androgen drugs, or L-asparaginase should be advised to discontinue use of these drugs. If the disease is complicated by seizures, phenytoin, fosphenytoin, or phenobarbital should be given in loading doses as described in Chapter 13.

Other Cerebrovascular Syndromes

HYPERTENSIVE ENCEPHALOPATHY

Acute or sustained elevation of blood pressure (BP) may result in failure of cerebral autoregulatory mechanisms, with vasodilation, hyperperfusion, and exudation of fluid. Increased intracranial pressure (ICP), capillary compression, and decreased intraparenchymal blood flow may result in **hypertensive encephalopathy**.

Affected patients have malignant or uncontrolled hypertension from any of various causes, including chronic renal disease, pheochromocytoma, antihypertensive withdrawal syndrome, sympathomimetic drugs, acute toxemia of pregnancy, Cushing's syndrome, aortic dissection, and polyarteritis nodosa. The diagnostic term should be reserved for the few patients who, in addition to extreme increases in BP (diastolic pressure usually >120 mm Hg), have severe hypertensive retinopathy (papilledema, retinal hemorrhages, or exudates, with or without optic nerve infarction) or severe retinal arteriolar spasm and altered consciousness.

The syndrome usually develops during a period of several minutes to several hours and is usually characterized by diffuse, moderate to severe headache; nausea; vomiting; and various visual symptoms such as visual blurring or dimming, scintillating scotoma, or cortical blindness, with or without vivid visual hallucinations. Generalized or focal seizures or altered consciousness or behavior (anxiety, agitation, disorientation, drowsiness, confusion, or coma) are common. On examination, generalized hyperreflexia is a common early feature. Focal neurologic findings (which may be postictal) are infrequent and may reflect an underlying intracerebral hemorrhage or infarction. Computed tomography (CT) may reveal evidence of cerebral edema or ischemia (widespread low attenuation primarily involving white matter). Magnetic resonance imaging (MRI) usually demonstrates white matter edema and increased T2-weighted signal bilaterally involving the occipital lobes, the parieto-occipital junction areas, or the superior frontal lobes.

Hypertensive encephalopathy may be complicated by acute congestive heart failure, pulmonary edema, acute anuria, or microangiopathic hemolytic anemia. Prompt reduction in BP is essential and is achieved with labetalol hydrochloride (10 to 20 mg intravenously for 1 to 2 minutes, repeated or doubled every 10 to 20 minutes until desired BP is achieved or until a cumulative dose of 300 mg is reached; or 2 mg per minute by intravenous [IV] infusion), diazoxide (1 to 2 mg per kg by IV bolus, repeated every 10 minutes, not to exceed 150 mg; or 15 to 30 mg per minute by IV infusion), or sodium nitroprusside (starting with 0.3 to 0.5 µg/kg/minute intravenously, titrated to the desired effect, with the usual dose 1 to 3 µg/kg/minute).

The initial aim of antihypertensive therapy should be to reduce the patient's mean arterial BP by approximately 20%

within a few hours. Further control of BP is achieved during the next 24 hours, with a goal of reducing the diastolic pressure toward but not less than 90 mm Hg. Reduction in BP reverses the pathophysiologic processes that are responsible for the clinical symptoms.

VASCULAR DEMENTIA

Vascular or arteriosclerotic dementia constitutes approximately 10% of all cases of dementia and often contributes to dementia in Alzheimer's disease (so-called mixed dementia). It is caused by multiple bilateral cerebral infarcts, especially involving regions such as the medial temporal lobes, the medial frontal lobes, the corpus callosum, and the nondominant parietal lobe. A history of one or more strokes preceding the dementia is common, and the first symptoms of dementia commonly appear within 1 year of focal neurologic symptoms or signs. Typical clinical features of the dementia include abrupt onset and a fluctuating course with a stepwise or slowly progressive loss of function (see Chapter 2). Other common neurologic signs include hemiparesis, hemianopia, and pseudobulbar palsy. Associated atherosclerosis, hypertension, diabetes mellitus, and other risk factors for stroke are usually present. The diagnosis should be made on the basis of the historical evaluation (see Chapter 2), examination (see Chapter 5), and diagnostic imaging findings. CT findings include multiple areas of low attenuation in the subcortical white matter or multiple other areas of infarction. MRI demonstrates areas of increased T2 signal diffusely in subcortical regions, although these may be detected in the absence of dementia. Recent clinical and pathologic information suggests that vascular (multi-infarct) dementia and Alzheimer's disease may overlap much more than previously thought.

Although effective **specific treatment** of vascular dementia is still lacking, it may be possible to influence the development or progression of this disease by controlling cerebrovascular risk factors, particularly hypertension, sources of emboli, and other risk factors for atherosclerosis (see Chapters 24 to 27). Palliative **symptomatic treatment** may be useful for abulia or inattention (methylphenidate or dextroamphetamine sulfate, 10 to 60 mg, divided into two or three doses daily), depression (imipramine, amitriptyline, or desipramine, 75 to 300 mg, once a day at bedtime), pseudobulbar affect (tricyclic antidepressants), and agitated confusion (lorazepam, 0.5 to 2.0 mg, orally or intramuscularly at bedtime; haloperidol, 1 to 6 mg, orally, divided into two or three doses). One must be careful to avoid overtreatment of hypertension, which may lead to side effects such as orthostatic hypotension. Preliminary clinical data on the use of ginkgo biloba, a plant extract, for the treatment of vascular dementia are somewhat encouraging, although this agent has been associated with some increased risk for intracerebral hemorrhage. Acetylcholinesterase inhibitors such as donepezil, galantamine, and rivastigmine have not been demonstrated to be of clear benefit for the cognitive impairment of vascular dementia but are commonly used for this purpose given the difficulties in differentiating with certainty between Alzheimer's disease and vascular dementia.

Vascular dementia should be differentiated from other disorders that lead to intellectual dysfunction, such as **Alzheimer's disease** (insidious onset, slowly progressive course without focal peripheral neurologic signs or systemic illness at onset, associated with diffuse atrophy of the cortex, especially involving the frontal and temporal lobes, with characteristic neurofibrillary degeneration and senile plaques; as noted above, however, this disorder frequently overlaps with vascular or multi-infarct dementia); **brain tumor or subdural hematoma** (focal neurologic signs often accompanied by symptoms of increased ICP, history of neoplasm or trauma); **Huntington's disease** (family history, chorea); **normal-pressure hydrocephalus** (gait disturbance and incontinence); **inflammatory disease (vasculitis**—evidence of arteritis elsewhere, relatively young age of patient, history of infections that could affect the cerebral vessels, for example, syphilis or tuberculosis); **infectious diseases** (human immunodeficiency virus [HIV] infection, syphilis, meningitis); **nutritional deficiencies** (Wernicke-Korsakoff syndrome, Marchiafava-Bignami disease, pellagra, vitamin B_{12} deficiency); **other syndromes** associated with systemic disorders, such as progressive multifocal leukoencephalopathy (systemic illness such as lymphoma or HIV infection, with diffuse, rapidly progressive multifocal neurologic symptoms, sometimes associated with signs of increased ICP and seizures); **chronic drug intoxication** (alcohol, sedatives); **endocrine-metabolic disorders** (myxedema, Cushing's disease, chronic hepatic or renal encephalopathies); **posttraumatic disease** (history of head trauma); and the **pseudodementia of depression** (see Chapter 2).

BINSWANGER'S ENCEPHALOPATHY

Binswanger's encephalopathy is a rare disorder that has been associated with diffuse hemispheric demyelination that results from chronic ischemia in central white matter caused by chronic hypertensive cerebrovascular disease and arteriolar sclerosis. Clinically, this encephalopathy is characterized by progressive dementia and pseudobulbar palsy associated with periventricular low-attenuation areas on CT. There is no specific treatment for Binswanger's encephalopathy, but symptomatic therapy (as discussed above for vascular dementia) and treatment of occult hydrocephalus are recommended in appropriate situations.

Vascular Disease of the Spinal Cord

Spinovascular disease is rare compared with cerebrovascular disease. It includes spinal cord infarction, hemorrhage, transient ischemic attack, and venous disease. The clinical symptoms of spinovascular disease usually begin abruptly and vary in severity and rate of onset, depending on the affected vessel, the level of the lesion (most commonly, lower thoracic cord and conus medullaris), and underlying disease. Spinovascular diseases should be differentiated from **spinal cord compression** (primary or metastatic tumors, epidural or subdural hematoma, acute extradural abscess, spinal tuberculosis, disk prolapse, spinal trauma, and spondylosis), **transverse myelitis** (often occurs with local pain followed by paraparesis or paraplegia, numbness, and urinary retention in association with cerebrospinal fluid (CSF) lymphocytic pleocytosis and increased protein), **Guillain-Barré syndrome** (progressive weakness during a period of several days or a few weeks, occurring diffusely or beginning in the legs and spreading proximally, involving first the trunk, then arms, neck, respiration, and cranial muscles), **syringomyelia** (typical segmental dysfunction with bilateral and, occasionally, unilateral loss of cutaneous sensation and dissociated sensory loss but sparing the sense of touch, position, and vibration), **subacute combined degeneration** (often present with gait disorder and lower motor neuron signs with loss of position and vibration, with no motor or sensory level, related to vitamin B_{12} deficiency and pernicious anemia), and **Friedreich's ataxia** (a genetic disorder that gradually results in ataxia of the limbs and trunk with areflexia and dysarthria; Babinski signs; and, occasionally, pes cavus, optic atrophy, nystagmus, cardiomyopathy, and scoliosis). The diagnosis is suggested by the patient's history and is confirmed by magnetic resonance imaging (MRI). Myelography, CSF analysis, spinal arteriography, and computed tomography (CT) are not required in most cases. CSF analysis may still be useful in evaluating for the presence of an inflammatory disorder. Selective spinal arteriography is indicated when arteriovenous malformation (AVM) is either suggested but not seen on MRI or is suggested on the MRI. Special coagulation studies should also be performed in young patients with no other apparent cause. Transesophageal echocardiography or CT with contrast may be used to evaluate for thoracic segment aortic dissections, and abdominal CT may be useful for abdominal aortic abnormalities.

The general principles outlined for treatment of cerebrovascular disease (see Chapters 11 to 17) may be applied to cases in which analogies to vascular diseases of the spinal cord can be made, with additional attention to bladder and skin care and physical therapy. For subdural and epidural spinal hemorrhage, immediate operation is often necessary. Although intramedullary hemorrhages from AVMs may be removed, followed by successful resection of the malformation, hematomyelia that results from trauma with no imaging evidence of an associated compressive lesion is usually treated conservatively.

SPINAL CORD INFARCTION

The common causes of spinal cord infarction are (1) aortic disease (dissecting aneurysm, severe atherosclerosis, thrombosis) or surgical procedures such as aortic aneurysm repair, femoral artery catheterization, and coronary artery bypass grafting; (2) small vessel disease (polyarteritis nodosa, systemic lupus erythematosus, neurosyphilis, secondary endarteritis resulting from tuberculosis or borreliosis, Behçet syndrome, giant cell arteritis, or isolated central nervous system angiitis); (3) spinal or segmental artery compression or occlusion caused by embolic material, including disc fragments (fibrocartilaginous emboli); cardiac source of emboli; extradural abscess, hemorrhage, or tumor; aortic arteriography; or sickle cell disease; (4) hypotension caused by myocardial infarction, cardiac arrest, or aortic rupture; (5) vertebral artery disorders including vertebral artery dissection, atherosclerosis causing stenosis, and vertebral arteriography; (6) hypercoagulable states; and (7) spinal cord AVM.

An ischemic lesion of the spinal cord usually involves the territory of the **anterior spinal artery** (the ventral two thirds of the spinal cord [Fig. 20-1]) and produces radicular or ascending leg pain at onset; rapidly progressive paraplegia or quadriplegia (flaccid legs, which soon become spastic); areflexia (evolving after days or weeks to hyperreflexia with extensor plantar responses); sensory loss to pain and temperature to the level of the lesion; urinary and fecal incontinence; and, later, focal atrophy and wasting (with cervical or lumbar infarction). Light touch, position, and vibration sense are preserved because the dorsal columns are not affected. Infarction in the territory of the posterior spinal artery (dorsal columns and the posterior horns) is less common and involves infarction in the posterior one third of the spinal cord. This may produce loss of joint position and vibration sense below the lesion and deep tendon reflexes at the level of the lesion.

For patients with spinal cord infarction associated with suspected aortic dissection, emergency aortic operation may be indicated after medical and neurologic stabilization. Initial pharmacologic treatment often involves nitroprusside or a beta-adrenergic blocker (see Chapter 11). When the dissection involves the ascending aorta, prompt operation is usually advised. When the dissection originates beyond the origin of the left subclavian artery, pharmacologic therapy can be continued if symptoms are controlled, but surgical resection should be considered. Occasionally, dissection of the ascending thoracic aorta may also compromise cerebral blood flow because of occlusion or stenosis at the origins of the carotid, brachiocephalic, or subclavian artery.

Specific treatments are not available for spinal cord infarction; supportive care is instituted. In patients with probable atherosclerotic disease, atherosclerosis risk factors should be treated aggressively. If a patient is seen within 8 to 12 hours after symptom onset, then high-dose intravenous (IV) methylprednisolone is

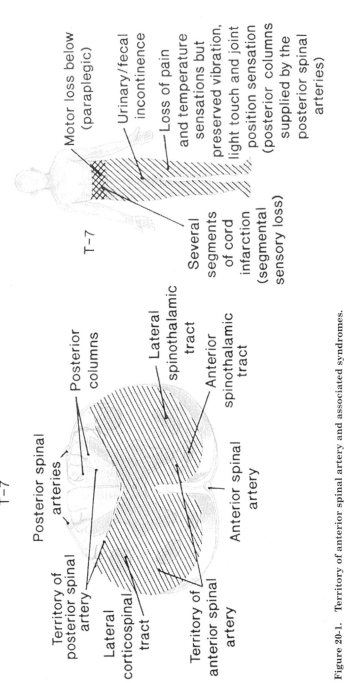

Figure 20-1. Territory of anterior spinal artery and associated syndromes.

a consideration, as is commonly used after spinal cord trauma. This involves a 30-mg per kg IV bolus, followed by an infusion of 5.4 mg/kg/hour for 24 hours if the steroids are initiated within 3 hours of symptom onset or for 48 hours if the steroids are initiated 3 to 8 hours after symptom onset. Other treatments are dependent on the specific etiology identified for the infarct and may include antiplatelet agents, anticoagulants, immunosuppressive agents, or surgical procedures.

SPINAL CORD HEMORRHAGE

Spinal cord hemorrhage is also rare compared with the frequency of brain hemorrhage. Almost all nontraumatic hemorrhages into the spinal cord are the result of AVMs, cavernous malformations, metastatic tumor, bleeding disorders, and the use of anticoagulants. The invariably sudden onset of symptoms (back or leg pain, paraparesis or quadriparesis, paraplegia or quadriplegia, sensory loss) associated with blood and xanthochromia in the CSF are the common clinical features of hematomyelia. MRI or myelography may demonstrate the swollen cord; in addition, MRI may demonstrate the hemorrhage in the cord.

Bleeding into the epidural or subdural spinal space produces rapidly evolving compressive myelopathy (sudden or gradual onset with severe back pain and a rapidly progressive paraplegia). Most common, anticoagulant use is causative, although liver disease is occasionally associated. Spinal subarachnoid hemorrhage is uncommon and most typically is caused by an AVM. Bleeding disorders, use of anticoagulants, and spinal artery aneurysms are less common causes. Clinical features include sudden onset of back or leg pain, followed by neck stiffness, but often without headache unless the blood spreads into the cranial subarachnoid space. Symptoms of myelopathy or radiculopathy may occur, helping to localize the process to a spinal cord level.

TRANSIENT SPINAL ISCHEMIC ATTACK

Transient spinal ischemic attack is a rare condition that results from emboli coming from the heart, aorta, or radicular arteries or is caused by an AVM or aortic coarctation. Hemodynamic transient spinal ischemic attacks may be caused by a stenotic arterial lesion, aortic coarctation, or spinal AVM (spinal claudication of Dejerine or aortic "steal" syndrome), usually presenting with transient paraparesis, difficulty walking, and the appearance of Babinski signs induced by exercise because blood is shunted away from the spinal cord, which causes transient ischemia.

VENOUS DISEASE OF THE SPINAL CORD

Venous disease of the spinal cord may be caused by coagulopathy with venous thrombosis, venous compression caused by an epidural mass, and spinal vascular malformations. Venous disease of the spinal cord includes hemorrhagic and nonhemorrhagic spinal infarctions, which are very rare. Venous hemorrhagic infarctions are characterized by sudden onset of symptoms (back, leg, or abdominal pain; flaccid paraparesis or paraplegia; ascending loss of sensation; disturbances of bowel and bladder function) that progress within 1 to 2 days. Nonhemorrhagic venous infarction may produce the same symptoms but more gradually; the clinical onset may be as long as 1 year, and back pain typically does not occur. There is usually evidence of venous thrombosis elsewhere. The **Foix-Alajouanine syndrome** is characterized by spinal cord necrosis involving the corticospinal tract (anterior horn cells are spared) and evidence of enlarged, tortuous, and thrombosed veins, often found in association with a vascular malformation.

Cerebrovascular Disease in Children and Young Adults

Stroke is uncommon in children who are younger than 15 years. The annual incidence is approximately 2.5 cases per 100,000 children. Ischemic strokes in young adults (aged 15 to 40 years) constitute about 5% of all cases. Although the frequency of stroke in children and young adults is far less than that in individuals who are older than 50 years, the causes are more diverse.

The frequency of specific causes of ischemic stroke in patients who are younger than 40 years depends on age. **Cerebral infarction in children** (aged 1 to 15 years) most commonly results from cardiac diseases, head and neck trauma with dissection, migraine, hematologic disease, and other large vessel occlusive diseases (Table 21-1). In contrast to arterial thrombosis in adults, arterial thrombosis in children more commonly involves the intracranial internal carotid arterial system. Infarction is more commonly subcortical in children and particularly involves the striatum and internal capsule.

CLINICAL PRESENTATION

Because cerebrovascular ischemia in children is uncommonly caused by atherosclerotic occlusive disease, transient ischemic attack (TIA) before cerebral infarction is relatively uncommon. The clinical features of cerebral ischemia are similar to those noted in adults, but seizures are more common. Aphasias usually have some expressive component even when the lesion is posterior. A less common clinical presentation that is unique to children includes recurrent or alternating hemiplegia with or without associated headache, which may be caused by hemiplegic migraine, or, less common, by bilateral carotid artery thrombosis. The clinical features of craniocervical thrombosis or cerebral embolism vary according to the area involved; the anatomic and pathophysiologic principles are analogous to those described for adults in Chapters 1 to 7.

CAUSE

The differential diagnosis of stroke in children and young adults is outlined in Table 21-1. Many of these disorders are reviewed in the setting of cerebral infarction and intracranial hemorrhage in adults (see Chapters 12 to 17). Causes of **cerebral ischemia** that occur much more commonly in children include **congenital heart disease**, head and neck **trauma** that leads to extracranial carotid or vertebral **dissection**, and distal thrombo-emboli or hemodynamic events. **Hematologic disorders** such as **sickle cell disease** are an important cause of infarction in children and lead to cerebrovascular disorders in 6% to 25% of patients (see Chapter 16, Hematologic Disease), and hematologic disorders can cause both ischemic and hemorrhagic stroke. Both ischemic and hemorrhagic events tend to occur during a painful

Table 21-1.   Differential diagnosis of stroke in children and young adults

Ischemia

Cardiac disease
  Congenital heart disease
  Rheumatic valve disease
  Mitral valve prolapse
  Patent foramen ovale
  Bacterial or marantic endocarditis
  Atrial myxoma
  Pulmonary arteriovenous fistula
  Rhabdomyoma
  Cardiac or umbilical vein catheterization
  Cardiomyopathies
  Arrhythmias
  Cardiac, thoracic surgery
Large vessel disease
  Premature atherosclerosis
  Dissection
    Traumatic
    Spontaneous
  Inherited metabolic diseases
    Homocystinuria
    Fabry's disease
    Pseudoxanthoma elasticum
    Sulfate oxidase deficiency
    MELAS syndrome
  Fibromuscular dysplasia
  Infection
    Bacterial
    Fungal
    Tuberculosis
    Syphilis
    Lyme disease
  Vasculitis
    Collagen vascular disease
      Systemic lupus erythematosus, rheumatoid arthritis, Sjögren's syndrome, polyarteritis nodosa
    Takayasu's disease
    Wegener's disease
    Cryoglobulinemia
    Behçet's disease
    Sarcoidosis
    Churg-Strauss syndrome
    Inflammatory bowel disease
    Isolated CNS angiitis
  Moyamoya disease
  Radiation
  Toxic
    Illicit drugs: cocaine, heroin, phencyclidine
    Therapeutic drugs: L-asparaginase, cytosine arabinoside
Small vessel disease
  Vasculopathy

Table 21-1. *Continued*

  Infectious
  Noninfectious
  Microangiopathy of brain, ear, and retina
Hematologic disease
  Sickle cell disease
  Leukemia
  Hypercoagulable states
    Antiphospholipid antibody syndromes
    Protein C or protein S deficiency
    Antithrombin III deficiency
    Increased factor VIII
    Resistance to activated protein C
  Disseminated intravascular coagulation
  Thrombocytosis
  Polycythemia vera
  Thrombotic thrombocytopenic purpura
Venous occlusion
  Dehydration
  Parameningeal infection (sinusitis, mastoiditis)
  Meningitis
  Neoplasm
  Polycythemia
  Leukemia
  Inflammatory bowel disease

Hemorrhage

AVM

Saccular aneurysm

Neoplasm
  Primary CNS neoplasm
  Metastatic neoplasm
  Leukemia

Hematologic
  Sickle cell disease
  Hemophilia
  Neoplasm
    Leukemia
  Thrombocytopenia
Moyamoya disease

Drug use (especially amphetamines, cocaine, phenylpropanolamine)

AVM = arteriovenous malformation; CNS = central nervous system; MELAS = mitochondrial myopathy, encephalopathy, lactic acidosis, and stroke-like episodes.

crisis and usually are seen in patients with more severe disease that includes frequent crises and decreased hematocrit value. Another cause of stroke that occurs more commonly in children than in adults is **moyamoya disease**.

The differential diagnosis in young adults mimics closely that noted in children. Important causes include **cardiogenic embolism, hematologic diseases, large vessel occlusive disease,**

and small vessel disorders. In most series, the most common causes of ischemic stroke in young adults are premature atherosclerosis, cardiogenic embolism, and use of oral contraceptives. Although **migraine** and use of **oral contraceptives** are commonly noted as potential causes of stroke in young adults, it is important to evaluate for other causes of stroke. Other risk factors for arterial occlusive disease typically are present in patients with ischemic events that are caused by oral contraceptives.

In most young adult patients with **premature atherosclerosis**, prominent risk factors are present, such as familial hypercholesterolemia, severe hypertension, and insulin-dependent diabetes. In addition, early cigarette smoking has been reported frequently in this subgroup. Less commonly, patients will have premature large vessel occlusive disease as a result of Fabry's disease or homocystinuria.

Stroke related to use of **illicit drugs** is also an important consideration in young adults. Ischemia or hemorrhage may result from use or abuse of prescription drugs or illicit drugs, including amphetamines, phenylpropanolamine, heroin, cocaine, phencyclidine, and lysergic acid diethylamide. Potential mechanisms include direct vascular effects such as vasospasm, vasoconstriction, vasculopathy without inflammation, inflammatory arteritis, prothrombotic state, and cardiac disorders such as cardiac arrhythmia and endocarditis. Intracranial hemorrhage occurs most commonly with use of cocaine, phenylpropanolamine, amphetamines, and heroin; cerebral infarction is often noted with use of heroin and cocaine.

Hypertensive encephalopathy or brain hemorrhage during a **hypertensive crisis** may result when a person receives monoamine oxidase inhibitor antidepressants and then consumes tyramine-rich products such as wine or cheese. Young adults also commonly report a history of trauma, which makes **dissection** an important cause in many series. Although **migraine** is relatively commonly associated with ischemic stroke in young adults, the importance as a causative factor or risk factor for stroke is poorly defined. Most series indicate that 10% to 15% of strokes in this age group are caused by migraine. The concurrent use of **oral contraceptives** may increase the occurrence of stroke in patients with migraine. The associations of migraine and ischemic stroke and of oral contraceptives and ischemic stroke both are accentuated in cigarette smokers.

STROKE RELATED TO INHERITED SYNDROMES

Inherited syndromes that are associated with an increased occurrence of stroke include cerebral autosomal dominant arteriopathy with subcortical infarcts and leukoencephalopathy (CADASIL), Ehlers-Danlos syndrome, pseudoxanthoma elasticum, Fabry's disease, homocystinuria, and sulfate oxidase deficiency. Although these disorders are relatively uncommon, they more typically become symptomatic in patients who are younger than 40 years.

CADASIL is a rare hereditary cerebrovascular disease that typically becomes evident in early or middle adulthood with migraine or a cerebral ischemic event. Later manifestations include recurrent subcortical ischemic strokes between 30 and 50 years of age that lead to a stepwise decline and dementia with reduced survival (mean age at death, approximately 55 years). The arteriopathy develops slowly, resulting in destruction of smooth muscle cells and thickening and fibrosis of the walls of small- and medium-sized penetrating arteries with consequent narrowing of the lumen. This impairs cerebral blood flow and produces characteristic white matter hyperintensities in T2-weighted magnetic resonance imaging on the basis of which CADASIL may be diagnosed well before the first clinically apparent stroke. Multiple lacunar infarcts, mainly in the frontal white matter and basal ganglia, lead to progressive permanent brain damage manifested as cognitive decline and finally as dementia. Although the symptoms are almost exclusively neurologic, the arteriopathy is generalized and diagnosis can be made on the basis of skin biopsy immunostaining and the identification of vascular osmophilic granules on electron microscopy. In addition, genetic testing can be performed, analyzing for the known mutations on the Notch 3 gene of chromosome 19. At present, no specific therapy for this disorder is available.

Ehlers-Danlos syndrome is an autosomal dominant disorder of unknown cause in which collagen fibers are affected and frequently leads to aneurysmal dilation or arterial dissection. Clinical features are cutaneous hyperelasticity and fragility, hypermobile joints, and occasionally carotid-cavernous fistula or aneurysmal subarachnoid hemorrhage (SAH).

Pseudoxanthoma elasticum is an autosomal recessive disorder in which degeneration and secondary calcification of the elastic tissue lead to vascular disturbances in many organs of the body, including the brain. Clinically, the disorder is characterized by yellowish papules on the neck, face, axilla, inguinal region, and periumbilical area, frequently associated with hypertension, angina pectoris, gastrointestinal bleeding, unequal radial pulses, and progressive, bilateral visual loss caused by retinitis with macular involvement. Ischemic stroke or SAH as a result of ruptured intracranial aneurysm may occur.

Fabry's disease is an X-linked recessive disorder that typically affects homozygous men in which deficiency of the enzyme alpha-galactosidase A causes accumulation of trihexyl ceramide and a resultant occlusive arteriopathy. Fabry's disease may present with dermal angiokeratomas (reddish or black) in the region of the lower abdomen and the upper thighs and is commonly associated with painful limb paresthesias and generalized hypohidrosis. Chronic renal failure, hypertension, cardiomegaly, myocardial infarction, TIAs, or cerebral infarction caused by a narrowing of blood vessel lumina may also occur. Unfortunately, no effective treatment of this disorder exists to prevent cerebrovascular complications.

Clinical features of **homocystinuria** in homozygous patients are characteristic skeletal abnormalities (tall, slender habitus; long limbs; occasional scoliosis and arachnodactyly; kyphosis; and high-arched feet) associated with mental retardation, seizures, ectopia lentis, and multiple cerebral infarctions. Deficiency of the enzyme cystathionine synthetase leads to abnormal conversion of homocysteine to methionine and increased serum homocysteine levels. Endothelial damage with premature atherosclerosis and relative hypercoagulability have been postulated as potential mechanisms.

Whether **heterozygous** patients have sufficient enzyme deficiency to cause similar vascular abnormalities is controversial. In children and young adults with cerebral ischemia of unknown cause, the patient's serum homocysteine level should be checked; if it is high, then B_{12}, B_6 (pyridoxine), and folate levels also should be evaluated. If none of the vitamin levels is low or low-normal, then an assay of fibroblast cystathione synthase activity may be performed, which requires a punch biopsy of the skin. In patients with an elevated homocysteine level, therapy with supplemental B_{12}, B_6, and folate should be considered.

Sulfate oxidase deficiency is a very rare disorder of sulfur metabolism involving increased blood sulfite and S-sulfocysteine levels; it usually manifests clinically during the neonatal period with seizures, multiple cerebral infarcts, decreased responsiveness, generalized spasms, and opisthotonos.

Mitochondrial myopathy, encephalopathy, lactic acidosis, and stroke-like episodes (**MELAS syndrome**) is an uncommon cause of strokes in children and young adults. Presenting symptoms include an abrupt onset of visual dysfunction, motor weakness, ataxia, or sensory abnormalities, often with headache and generalized cognitive decline. Seizures are also common. Imaging studies may reveal multifocal subcortical and cortical abnormalities consistent with infarction, often predominating in the posterior head regions and cerebellum. Abnormal blood test results may include increased serum lactic and pyruvic acid levels; mitochondrial DNA analysis may reveal mutations. Patients with MELAS have been treated with coenzyme Q10, riboflavin, and carnitine, but the efficacy of these agents has not been established.

OTHER CAUSES OF CEREBRAL ISCHEMIA

Moyamoya disease occurs in a bimodal distribution; children who are younger than 15 years typically present with episodes of TIA or cerebral infarction, whereas those who are older than 40 years more commonly present with intracranial hemorrhage, particularly in the basal ganglia or the thalamus. Children also tend to have more seizures and generalized cognitive impairment. The diagnosis is made on the basis of characteristic arteriographic findings, which include progressive stenosis or occlusion of the intracranial internal carotid arteries and prominent collateral formation appearing as a fine network of vessels deep in the brain. This leads to the so-called "puff-of-smoke" appearance, translated into "moyamoya" in Japanese. The cause of the changes is unknown. Small intracranial aneurysms may also be detected. Treatment options include direct extracranial artery–to–intracranial artery bypass and other indirect revascularization procedures, such as encephaloduroarteriosynangiosis, that are designed to bring blood flow from the external carotid artery into the distal internal carotid artery vasculature.

HEMORRHAGIC STROKE

The relative frequency of **hemorrhagic stroke** is higher in children and young adults than in patients who are older than 40 years, and some series have reported that the ratio of hemorrhagic stroke to ischemic stroke is 1:1 to 1.5:1 in the younger age groups. Although **arteriovenous malformations (AVMs)** are a more frequent cause of hemorrhage in younger patients than they are in older patients, **intracranial aneurysms** are still the most common cause of intracranial hemorrhage. In young children, **vein of Galen malformations** (in which the vein of Galen is enlarged, which forms a venous aneurysm or varix) may also cause hemorrhage, although hydrocephalus and congestive heart failure are more common in infants.

Intracranial saccular aneurysms that occur in children may be associated with a genetic disorder such as polycystic kidney disease, Marfan's syndrome, pseudoxanthoma elasticum, coarctation of the aorta, or Ehlers-Danlos syndrome.

In patients who are older than 15 years, AVMs and saccular aneurysms continue to be important causes of intracranial hemorrhage; however, other important causes include drug use, hematologic disorders, and hypertension. Venous occlusive disease is also in the differential diagnosis for hemorrhagic infarction in children and young adults.

LABORATORY EVALUATION

The evaluation and the treatment of ischemic and hemorrhagic disorders in children and young adults are similar to those described earlier (see Chapters 11 to 17). However, on the basis of the differential considerations presented in this chapter, additional studies that evaluate for causes that are more specific to children and young adults are necessary, with more emphasis on cardiac disorders, hematologic disorders such as hypercoagulable states, infectious and inflammatory causes, and metabolic disorders.

In addition to noninvasive studies to evaluate the extracranial and intracranial arterial system and cardiac imaging studies, detailed hematologic studies should be considered because hematologic disorders play a greater role in stroke occurrence in children and young adults than they do in older groups. Potential types of evaluation may include the sickle cell preparation; hemoglobin and serum protein electrophoresis; determination of antithrombin III level, partial thromboplastin time, fibrinogen level, and protein C and protein S levels; evaluation for resistance to activated protein C; homocysteine level; determination of antiphospholipid (anticardiolipin) antibodies; and lupus anticoagulant testing. If there is a family history of early-onset stroke or if radiographic or clinical findings suggest the presence of such a disorder, then evaluation for hereditary metabolic disorders should be performed.

TREATMENT

The general principles that are outlined for treatment of cerebrovascular disease in adults (see Chapters 11 to 17) may be applied to most cerebrovascular diseases in children and young adults. Some entities that are described in this chapter are exceedingly rare in patients who are older than 40 years, and they require treatment of the specific cause, if known.

Treatment issues for intracerebral hemorrhage (see Chapter 17) are also similar to those in adults. Ruptured intracranial aneurysms and AVMs in children are usually treated surgically. The preferred procedure for ruptured AVMs is excision, but when that is not possible, radiosurgery, embolization, or a combination of both should be considered. For unruptured AVMs, rates of future rupture are relatively low—approximately 2% per year—but are persistent over time. Because affected patients otherwise have very long life expectancies, radiosurgery (which may take 2 to 3 years to obliterate the AVM from the cerebral circulation) becomes more of a consideration for possible first-line therapy, especially for a small AVM in a location that is difficult to access surgically. The management of unruptured intracranial aneurysms is analogous to that described in Chapter 28.

PROGNOSIS

The prognosis for children with ischemic and hemorrhagic stroke is better than that for adults with a comparable lesion. Speech recovery occurs in nearly all children who are affected by cerebral infarction before the age of 5 years. Children who present with hemiplegia and seizures before age 2 years have a worse prognosis, and most have persistent behavioral changes, intellectual deficits, hemiplegia, and epilepsy.

Cerebrovascular Disease in Pregnant Patients

Although stroke is the third leading cause of death in the general population in the United States, it is uncommon among women of childbearing age. Nevertheless, cerebrovascular disease is ranked as the fifth most common cause of maternal mortality. Pregnancy has long been recognized as a factor that increases the risk for cerebrovascular disease in young women, although the magnitude of the increase in risk has been exaggerated by referral-based studies. Many of the same mechanisms that produce stroke in older age groups are responsible for strokes in pregnant women, but the distribution of mechanisms is different. Furthermore, some mechanisms are unique to pregnancy, particularly in the area of ischemic cerebrovascular disease. Evaluation and treatment of pregnant patients with cerebrovascular symptoms require an awareness of the differences in underlying pathophysiology between pregnant and non-pregnant patients. The physician must understand the potential adverse effects of diagnostic procedures and medications on the fetus as well as on the patient.

HEMORRHAGIC DISORDERS

Hemorrhagic cerebrovascular disorders cause 5% to 10% of all maternal deaths that occur during pregnancy. Most common, non-traumatic intracranial hemorrhage in pregnancy occurs within the subarachnoid space (subarachnoid hemorrhage [SAH]), within the ventricular system (intraventricular hemorrhage), or as a combination of these. Hemorrhage into each of these areas may be produced by various pathophysiologic mechanisms, most commonly (1) rupture of an intracranial aneurysm, which usually produces SAH, occasionally in association with intracerebral hemorrhage (ICH) or intraventricular hemorrhage; (2) bleeding from an arteriovenous malformation (AVM), which frequently produces SAH, ICH, or both; and (3) rupture of an intraparenchymal vessel, which results in ICH, often with some extension of the bleeding into the subarachnoid space or ventricular system.

Intracranial Aneurysm

On the basis of data collected from various referral practices during the past 40 years, the incidence of aneurysmal rupture during pregnancy has been estimated at approximately 1 in 10,000 pregnancies, approximately two to three times that of non-pregnant women of the same age group. However, data from the Rochester, Minnesota, population from 1955 to 1979 more recently revealed no instances of intracranial hemorrhage among 26,099 pregnancies, an observation suggesting that previous rates may have been overestimated. Approximately one half of the patients with ruptured aneurysms during pregnancy have had previous successful pregnancies with no difficulty. As in the general population, there is some tendency toward increasing risk with increased maternal age. During pregnancy, the risk for rupture increases with each trimester. Although one might expect the Valsalva maneuver of childbirth to increase the risk for aneurysmal rupture, very few initial ruptures have been reported during labor and delivery. However, rebleeding frequently occurs during labor and the first few weeks postpartum (Table 22-1).

Early investigation and treatment of intracranial aneurysm are important in pregnant patients, particularly when the aneurysm has produced intracranial hemorrhage. Radiographic and surgical procedures should not be delayed or avoided, although special shielding during radiography is required to protect the fetus. The clinical decisions that are involved in managing these patients vary with the type, size, and location of the aneurysm; the condition of the patient; and whether the aneurysm is symptomatic (see Chapters 14, 15, and 17).

If the intracranial aneurysm is obliterated successfully (surgically clipped, trapped, or documented to be obliterated after coil placement) from the circulation before the 35th week of gestation, the rest of pregnancy and the delivery can proceed normally. If the ruptured aneurysm cannot be obliterated completely (incompletely clipped, arterial ligation, not obliterated after coil placement, wrapped, or packed) or if an operation is not performed, vaginal delivery is generally recommended only if the rupture occurred during the first two trimesters of pregnancy. If the SAH occurred during the third trimester, delivery should be performed by cesarean section at 38 weeks of gestation. Little can be done to avoid the increased postpartum risk for rebleeding in this situation.

Intracranial Arteriovenous Malformation

AVMs cause approximately the same number of intracranial hemorrhages during pregnancy as do aneurysms. Although previous data revealed a high incidence of intracranial hemorrhage

Table 22-1.   Features of intracranial aneurysm and AVM during pregnancy

Feature	Aneurysm	AVM
Age (yr)	25–35	15–25
Peak hemorrhage risk (wk)	30–40 (third trimester)	16–20 (second trimester)
Parity	Multipara	Primipara
Risk for recurrent hemorrhage		
Same pregnancy	+ +	+ + +
Delivery	+ +	+ + +
Postpartum	+ + +	+
Subsequent pregnancies	+	+ + +

AVM = arteriovenous malformation.
From Wiebers DO. Subarachnoid hemorrhage in pregnancy. *Semin Neurol.* 1988;8:226–229, with permission of Thieme Medical Publishers.

among patients with AVM, recent data have been conflicting and have shown a minimally increased risk for pregnant patients. AVMs tend to occur in younger pregnant women (aged 15 to 25 years), and aneurysms in pregnant women aged 25 to 35 years. In contrast to aneurysms, AVMs tend to rupture during the second trimester (peak, 16 to 20 weeks of gestation), and they are more likely to hemorrhage again in the same pregnancy and in subsequent pregnancies. Rebleeding during delivery may be more common with AVMs than it is with aneurysms. However, the increased risk for AVM hemorrhage during specific trimesters and during delivery was not noted in one study (see Horton et al. [1990] in Suggested Reading for Part IV). Pregnant patients with AVMs tend to have a lower parity than those with aneurysms (Table 22-1). A patient with intracranial hemorrhage caused by a ruptured AVM is six times less likely to have had a previous normal pregnancy than a pregnant patient with aneurysmal SAH. Overall, the fetal prognosis is worse when there is known maternal intracranial AVM compared with the prognosis with intracranial aneurysm.

The mechanism for the somewhat increased risk for rupture of AVMs during pregnancy is unknown. Many investigators have suggested that the periods of greatest risk of rupture (16 to 20 weeks of gestation and at the time of labor and delivery) correlate with the greatest increases in cardiac output. Shunting through intracranial AVMs presumably increases during pregnancy. No direct measurements are available, but analogies have been made to visible cutaneous spider nevi and vascular tumors of the skin and gums. These tumors increase in size as pregnancy progresses (particularly during times of increased cardiac output) and decrease in size or disappear after delivery. Increased shunting is thought by some physicians to predispose to rupture and to focal ischemic events from the AVM. The latter condition has been noted only rarely during pregnancy.

Some pregnant patients with AVMs also present with periodic throbbing headache that appears in the same location with each episode and is indistinguishable from classic migraine. Others present with progressive neurologic deficits or seizures without evidence of associated cerebral hemorrhage or infarction. However, during pregnancy, initial presentation with SAH is approximately five to 10 times more likely than is any other type of presentation.

As noted with intracranial aneurysms, early investigation and treatment of intracranial AVMs are important in pregnant patients, particularly in the setting of intracranial hemorrhage. Radiographic and surgical procedures should not be delayed or avoided, although special shielding during radiography is required to protect the fetus. The clinical decisions that are involved in managing these patients vary with the type of vascular malformation and whether it is symptomatic (see Chapters 14, 15, and 17).

If the AVM can be totally excised before the 35th week of gestation, the rest of pregnancy and the delivery can proceed normally. If the lesion is not operable or only partially resectable and has bled during the pregnancy, elective cesarean section at 38 weeks of gestation is usually recommended, especially in a nulliparous patient. If the patient is multiparous with a proven adequate pelvis, some investigators have advocated vaginal delivery in which Valsalva maneuver is minimized by administering regional lumbar epidural anesthesia or by having the patient learn breathing techniques to be used during delivery to obviate the cardiovascular stresses that would otherwise occur.

Rupture of Intraparenchymal Vessels

Rupture of an artery, capillary, or vein within the brain parenchyma commonly results in ICH and sometimes subarachnoid or intraventricular bleeding. In both pregnant and nonpregnant women, certain underlying conditions may predispose to nontraumatic rupture of the intraparenchymal vessel. **Hypertension** is the most frequently identified predisposing cause of ICH in nonpregnant women and has been implicated in some cases of ICH in pregnant women, particularly in the setting of eclampsia. In both situations, the basal ganglia area seems to be the most common site of hemorrhage, although there are very few well-documented cases in pregnant patients.

Other conditions that have been associated with nontraumatic intracerebral bleeding in pregnancy are (1) **hematologic disorders** such as disseminated intravascular coagulation, often associated with placental abruption, leukemia, thrombocytopenia, or carcinoma; (2) **anticoagulant therapy**; (3) **cortical vein and dural sinus thrombosis**; and (4) **metastatic choriocarcinoma**. Patients with angiopathies such as systemic lupus erythematosus (SLE) might also be expected to have intracranial hemorrhage because this disorder is often exacerbated by pregnancy, but a relationship has not yet been documented.

If the pregnant patient with intraparenchymal hemorrhage survives to the time of delivery and an underlying structural lesion has been found and repaired, labor and delivery can proceed normally. The remainder of survivors should undergo either elective cesarean section at 38 weeks of gestation or vaginal delivery with epidural lumbar anesthesia, depending on the individual circumstance.

ISCHEMIC CEREBROVASCULAR DISEASE

Pregnancy appears to increase the risk for focal ischemic cerebrovascular events. However, population-based data from Rochester, Minnesota, indicated only one cerebral infarction among 26,099 pregnancies during a period of 25 years (5.1 per 100,000 patient-years of observation), a finding that suggests that previous estimates of risk (five to 15 times the expected risk) were probably exaggerated. Until recently, cerebral venous thrombosis was thought to be the cause of most focal cerebral ischemic lesions in pregnancy. However, during the past 20 years, available data in the Western literature suggest that arterial occlusions cause approximately 60% to 80% of these lesions. Arterial occlusions tend to occur during the second and third trimesters of pregnancy and during the puerperium; venous occlusions tend to occur 1 to 4 weeks after childbirth.

When the various possible causes of ischemic cerebrovascular events in pregnancy are considered, it is useful to categorize the various pathophysiologic mechanisms according to which part of the vascular system is most prominently involved: cardiac disease, large or small vessel arterial disease, hematologic disorders, venous occlusions, and other uncommon disorders.

Cardiac Disease

In pregnancy, cardiac disease may produce symptoms of focal cerebral ischemia through various mechanisms. Cardiac ischemic sources cause a higher percentage of focal ischemic neurologic deficits in pregnant patients than they do in the rest of the adult population. This is at least partially a result of the lower prevalence of advanced atherosclerosis in the younger age group. In addition, pregnancy may aggravate preexisting maternal heart disease (such as rheumatic fever, subacute bacterial endocarditis) or may cause maternal heart disease (such as peripartum cardiomyopathy).

Valve-Related Emboli

Cerebral embolization occurs in approximately 20% of patients with infective endocarditis and may be the presenting symptom. During pregnancy, *Streptococcus viridans* is the most common infective agent, particularly with preexisting rheumatic heart disease. Among cases of **subacute bacterial endocarditis** during pregnancy, 8% are enterococcal, which is particularly common after delivery, abortion, or insertion of an intrauterine device. Staphylococcal subacute bacterial endocarditis is more common among narcotic addicts and is associated with an increased risk for cerebral abscess formation and a higher fatality rate. Four distinct clinical and pathologic syndromes occur: (1) focal cerebral infarction resulting from embolic occlusion of large arteries (the most common), (2) multiple small areas of cerebral infarction producing diffuse encephalopathy, (3) meningitis from small infected emboli lodging in meningeal arteries, and (4) mycotic aneurysm formation with subsequent intracranial hemorrhage caused by septic embolization and vessel wall rupture.

There is some evidence that **rheumatic fever** is more likely to recur during pregnancy, and this occasionally causes serious maternal cardiac decompensation and death. Cerebral embolization in rheumatic heart disease may occur either during the acute illness, when inflammatory vegetations on the heart valve may detach and embolize, or, more commonly, during the chronic phase of the disease, when valvular deformity, atrial enlargement, and abnormal cardiac rhythm develop. Atrial fibrillation, congestive heart failure, atrial enlargement, and associated mitral insufficiency also increase the risk for cerebral embolization.

Mitral valve prolapse occurs in approximately 5% of otherwise healthy young women. During the past decade, cerebral ischemic events that were unrelated to other recognized risk factors have been noted in patients with this condition. However, an increased risk for cerebral embolization during pregnancy in patients with mitral valve prolapse has not yet been documented. Some have advocated close observation for the appearance of arrhythmias as well as the use of antibiotic prophylaxis and aspirin, particularly when associated mitral regurgitation is present. These recommendations, however, are not based on strong scientific evidence.

Intracardiac Thrombi

In the childbearing years, the cardiac arrhythmia that most frequently is associated with embolic brain infarction is **atrial fibrillation**, which predisposes to blood stagnation and the formation of intracardiac thrombi. During pregnancy, the risk for systemic embolism from the arrhythmia has been estimated at 10% to 23%, including a 2% to 10% risk for symptomatic brain embolism.

Also known as **peripartum cardiomyopathy**, **cardiomyopathy of pregnancy** is a syndrome that resembles other congestive cardiomyopathies and occurs during late pregnancy or the puerperium in the absence of any of the well-recognized causes of heart disease. There is still no unanimity of opinion about whether this syndrome is a specific entity caused by pregnancy or whether pregnancy unmasks preexisting latent myocardial disease. Like other congestive cardiomyopathies, this condition predisposes to blood stagnation with consequent mural thrombi, which may embolize to the cerebrum, especially from the left ventricle. Multiparous black women who are older than 30 years are at the highest risk for development of this condition. In most patients, the heart returns to normal soon after delivery, but chronic congestive heart failure develops in some women.

Acute myocardial infarction (MI) occurs in approximately one in 10,000 pregnancies, and the overall maternal mortality rate is approximately 30%. When the infarction occurs during the last month of pregnancy, the maternal mortality rate is considerably higher (approximately 50%). The frequency of cerebral embolization with acute MI during pregnancy is unknown.

The foramen ovale is anatomically patent in 15% of the population and retains the functional capacity of patency in an additional 15%. In these situations, venous emboli can enter the cerebral circulation (**paradoxical embolism**), especially after pulmonary embolization with associated increases in pulmonary arterial and right atrial pressures. The risk for paradoxical embolism increases with pregnancy because of the increased risk for thrombophlebitis in the pelvis and lower extremities, especially during early puerperium after cesarean section, forceps rotation, or manual removal of the uterus.

Large or Small Vessel Arterial Disease

Atherosclerosis

In the general population, **atherosclerosis** is the most common identifiable disease process that produces cerebral ischemia. Among women of childbearing age and even more so among pregnant women, atherosclerosis plays a smaller role in the pathogenesis of cerebral ischemic events. The number of well-studied cases is too small to allow definitive percentages, but roughly 10% of all cerebral infarctions during pregnancy are related to atherosclerosis. Young women with long-standing hypertension, diabetes mellitus, hyperlipidemia, cigarette abuse, and radiation therapy to the neck may be predisposed to the development of atherosclerosis (accelerated atherosclerosis).

In pregnancy, **hypotensive episodes** may result from acute blood loss, vasovagal-induced syncope, or epidural or spinal anesthesia. Such episodes may produce transient or permanent cerebral ischemic lesions with or without underlying atherosclerosis. The terminal branches (watershed areas) of the anterior, middle, and posterior cerebral arteries are most frequently involved. Severe intrapartum hypotension also may result in Sheehan's syndrome (pituitary necrosis) as a result of infarction in the distribution of the inferior hypophyseal artery.

Arteritis

A pregnant patient is as susceptible to pyogenic central nervous system (CNS) infections as any other person but is not unusually predisposed to them. **Leptomeningitis** that is produced by *Meningococcus* is the most common, but the frequency of cerebrovascular complications in pregnant patients with this condition is unknown. **Tuberculous meningitis** in pregnant women is rare in Western countries, but it occurs frequently in less industrialized nations. **Tertiary syphilis**, once a common cause of ischemic stroke in young patients, is now rare.

The presumably noninfectious inflammatory angiopathies include those that affect primarily the arterioles and the capillaries (**SLE**), those that affect primarily small- or medium-sized arteries (**polyarteritis nodosa, isolated CNS angiitis**), and those that affect primarily medium-sized to large arteries (**temporal arteritis, Takayasu's disease**). SLE and Takayasu's disease tend to occur in women of childbearing age.

Exacerbations of **SLE** often occur during pregnancy, and the risk for abortion and stillbirth is significantly increased. Because the cerebral vessel arteriopathy primarily affects small vessels diffusely, the CNS findings are usually those of a diffuse encephalopathy with delirium, seizures, acute cyanosis, and increased intracranial pressure. Focal or multifocal cerebral and brainstem infarcts occur, but they rarely produce recognizable arterial syndromes.

Takayasu's disease (pulseless disease) is a chronic inflammatory arteriopathy of unknown origin that results in narrowing of major-vessel ostia involving the aortic arch and its branches. Clinically, the ischemic symptoms include Takayasu's retinopathy and thromboembolic or hemodynamic focal or multifocal cerebral ischemia. There may be reduction or absence of subclavian, carotid, brachial, and radial pulses with bruits over affected or collateral vessels; secondary hypertension; aortic regurgitation; and aortic aneurysm. The course of the disease during pregnancy is variable. Approximately half of the patients will notice some increase in symptoms during pregnancy, possibly explained by the increased blood volume and cardiac output during pregnancy in conjunction with the variability of venous return caused by impingement of the enlarging uterus on the inferior vena cava. Vaginal delivery is generally preferred in these patients unless cesarean section is indicated for obstetric reasons (regional anesthesia should be used with caution because of the danger of hypotension).

Hypertension

No data are available regarding the occurrence of hypertensive lacunar infarction in pregnancy. In contrast, **hypertensive encephalopathy** frequently has been described in association with eclampsia in the second half of pregnancy. Affected patients have accelerated severe hypertension with severe hypertensive retinopathy or retinal arteriolar spasm and alteration of consciousness. Seizures and cortical blindness are often present, but focal neurologic findings are infrequent and may reflect an underlying ICH or infarction.

Intracranial Venous Occlusion

Intracranial venous thrombosis has long been recognized as a cause of cerebral infarction in pregnancy and the puerperium. Such thromboses may arise from infectious or noninfectious processes and should be diagnosed and treated as discussed in Chapter 18. The vast majority of venous thromboses occur 3 days to 4 weeks after childbirth, and 80% occur in the second or third postpartum week. Venous occlusion probably causes between 20% and 40% of cerebral infarctions during pregnancy. The overall average mortality rate of pregnant patients with cerebral venous thromboses is approximately 25%. For patients who survive, the outlook is usually good, and they have less chance of persistent focal neurologic deficit than do patients with cerebral infarction from arterial lesions.

Hematologic Disorders

In a normal pregnancy, increases in plasma fibrinogen and clotting factors VII, IX, and XI, along with decreased blood coagulation factor inactivation, produce a mild hypercoagulable state, especially during the third trimester. Similar effects have been noted with the use of birth control pills. In addition, other abnormalities in blood cell constituents and plasma proteins may result in a hypercoagulable state, with increased blood viscosity and stasis, which predispose the patient to cerebral ischemia.

The most commonly described of these disorders in pregnancy is **sickle cell disease**. The structure of red blood cells that contain hemoglobin SS or SC is altered when these cells are exposed to low oxygen tension, which increases blood viscosity and predisposes to diffuse small vessel wall ischemia from occlusion of nutrient arteries. Sickle cell crisis is relatively common in pregnancy in the setting of SS and SC disease. Rarely, pregnant patients with sickle cell trait have suffered brain infarction or sudden death.

Thrombotic thrombocytopenic purpura (TTP) is a rare syndrome that likely is a multicentric vasculitis. It occurs approximately three times as often in pregnant and puerperal women as in other women of the same age group. The hematologic and cerebrovascular manifestations are the result of secondary mechanical damage to erythrocytes. The damage causes increased use of platelets to form diffuse microthrombi, which in turn occlude terminal arterioles in the brain and produce multiple small infarcts and a fluctuating encephalopathy. Many pregnant women with TTP are admitted to the hospital during the final weeks of pregnancy, at which time petechiae, ecchymoses, and purpuric patches may be present. The management of TTP is described in more detail in Chapter 16.

Other Uncommon Conditions Associated with Pregnancy

Particles from amniotic fluid embolize to the brain and other parts of the body. These emboli tend to occur most frequently in multiparous women who are older than 30 years and who have uterine, cervical, or vaginal tears as portals for amniotic fluid to enter the systemic circulation. The clinical picture that has been described includes convulsions, sudden dyspnea, cyanosis, disseminated intravascular coagulation, shock, and death. Antemortem diagnosis is made by finding fetal epithelial cells just above the buffy coat layer of settled blood (which may be withdrawn from the right atrium while a central venous pressure catheter is placed).

Air emboli during pregnancy and the puerperium have been associated with abortion, complicated vaginal delivery, cesarean section, vaginal air insufflation, and puerperal knee–chest exercises. The symptoms are similar to those of amniotic fluid emboli. Cardiac examination may reveal a gurgling, churning heart sound that results from frothy blood.

Fat emboli have rarely been reported in pregnancy, but they occur in the setting of sickle cell crisis, in association with amniotic fluid embolization, and, independently, in obese women.

Rarely, **metastatic choriocarcinoma** may present with cerebral infarction or hemorrhagic cerebral infarction as a result of vessel occlusion by embolic chorioepithelioma cells. Once these cells lodge in blood vessels, they tend to lead to destruction and rupture of the walls of the artery. Early diagnosis is facilitated by measurement of human chorionic gonadotropin levels in the serum.

Although some authors have associated **spontaneous carotid artery dissection** with use of oral contraceptives, only one case has been described in association with pregnancy. In that case, a cerebral infarction occurred 6 days after a cesarean section that had been done after 14 hours of strenuous, unsuccessful labor.

**Evaluation and Management of Ischemic
Cerebrovascular Disease in Pregnancy**

Focal ischemic cerebrovascular disease may arise from any one of the described pathologic processes through hemodynamic and thromboembolic mechanisms. Whenever possible, management should be based on a precise definition of the underlying pathophysiologic mechanism and its appropriate treatment (as outlined above and in Chapters 16 and 17).

In the general population, patients with recent onset or an increase in the frequency of transient ischemic attack (TIA) and minor cerebral infarction are at high risk for cerebral infarction. The evaluation and treatment of patients with TIA and minor cerebral infarction are summarized in Chapter 12. There are some special issues to be considered in pregnant women.

For patients who are pregnant and have a disorder that is managed best with anticoagulation, heparin may be used more safely than warfarin. Warfarin carries considerable fetal risks, particularly in the first trimester, and in general is not recommended for use during pregnancy. For patients who are not candidates for operation, treatment with intravenously administered heparin is suggested during the first 1 to 2 weeks after the most recent TIA. Subcutaneous heparin can be self-administered for 2 to 6 weeks thereafter. Arteriography generally is not performed in pregnant patients with vertebrobasilar TIA because of the availability of noninvasive studies such as magnetic resonance angiography and transcranial Doppler ultrasonography. In these patients, medical treatment is instituted on the basis of the results of the evaluations (see Chapter 12).

In general, warfarin is avoided during pregnancy, particularly during the first trimester, because of the increased risk for teratogenic complications and fetal wastage with this therapy. Most of the evidence for this approach is based on sporadic case reports. The teratogenic complications have included one or more of the following:

1. Skeletal abnormalities such as stippling of bone epiphyses, nasal hypoplasia (saddle nose), hypertelorism, frontal bossing, short neck, short stature, and high arched palate
2. Psychomotor retardation
3. Optic atrophy or cataracts
4. Agenesis of the corpus callosum and cerebellar atrophy
5. Fetal hemorrhage

Heparin is not without risks during pregnancy, but with a molecular weight of approximately 20,000, heparin does not cross the placental barrier to a significant degree, compared with warfarin, which has a molecular weight of approximately 1,000 and crosses the placental barrier. When anticoagulation is needed during pregnancy, either unfractionated heparin, used subcutaneously every 12 hours and adjusted to keep activated partial thromboplastin time at the appropriate level, or low molecular weight heparin, adjusted by the anti–factor Xa heparin level 4 hours after injection, may be used. Warfarin may then be instituted postpartum.

There have been a few isolated reports of congenital anomalies in infants who were born to mothers who were taking aspirin. However, a prospective study by Heinonen et al. (1977), under the auspices of the National Institute of Neurological and Communicative Disorders and Stroke (see Suggested Reading for Part IV), of >50,000 pregnancies indicated that use of aspirin did not cause any congenital malformations. No definitive data are available regarding the use of ticlopidine or dipyridamole in pregnancy.

Management of patients with major ischemic stroke and progressing infarction is based on the principles outlined in this chapter and in Chapters 11, 13, and 16. For pregnant women with progressing infarction, mannitol should be avoided because of its relative lack of usefulness to the mother and because of the significant risk for fetal dehydration.

Cerebrovascular Disease Genetics

Several cerebrovascular disorders tend to run in families or are either entirely congenital in nature or largely genetically determined. These include disorders that may cause ischemic stroke, hemorrhagic stroke, and structural cerebrovascular entities.

SUBARACHNOID HEMORRHAGE/INTRACRANIAL ANEURYSM

The evaluation and management of subarachnoid hemorrhage (SAH) and intracranial saccular aneurysm were addressed in Chapters 14 and 17. Population-based studies have suggested that there is an increased occurrence of a first- or second-degree relative having had an SAH, with 20% noted in one study. In **first-degree relatives**, nearly 10% have a history of SAH, or intracranial aneurysm, far higher than would be expected in the general population.

From a **screening** perspective, among first-degree relatives of patients who had intracranial aneurysm and were 30 years or older and in families in which at least two members of the family had an intracranial aneurysm, 9% had an aneurysm confirmed. Magnetic resonance angiography (MRA) screening in first-degree relatives of those who had ruptured intracranial aneurysm and no known family history of intracranial aneurysm indicated that only 3% of first-degree relatives who were between the ages of 20 and 70 and screened with MRA had an aneurysm detected. The highest risk was noted in the siblings as opposed to their children. Risk factors for a slightly higher risk for aneurysm detection included female gender, older age, family history of polycystic kidney disease, history of hyperlipidemia, history of hypertension, and presence of hyperglycemia.

Among familial cases, the mean age of SAH is younger, and in later generations, SAH occurs at a younger age. The overall outcome may also be poorer in familial cases. Heritable disorders that are associated with intracranial aneurysm include autosomal dominant polycystic kidney disease, neurofibromatosis type 1, pseudoxanthoma elasticum, tuberous sclerosis, Marfan's syndrome, Ehlers-Danlos syndrome type IV, and hereditary hemorrhagic telangiectasia.

CEREBRAL INFARCTION

Cerebral Autosomal Dominant Arteriopathy with Subcortical Infarcts and Leukoencephalopathy

Cerebral autosomal dominant arteriopathy with subcortical infarcts and leukoencephalopathy (CADASIL) is a rare hereditary stroke disease that is caused by a mutation in Notch 3. The disorder typically begins in early or middle adulthood, with patients presenting with migraine, cerebral infarction, psychiatric disorders, or cognitive impairment. Recurrent subcortical cerebral infarctions may lead to a stepwise decline and dementia and results in reduced survival. The arteriopathy develops slowly, resulting in destruction of smooth muscle cells and thickening and fibrosis of the walls of small- and medium-sized penetrating arteries with consequent narrowing of the lumen. This impairs cerebral blood flow and produces characteristic white matter hyperintensities in T2-weighted magnetic resonance imaging (MRI) on the basis of which CADASIL may be diagnosed well before the first clinically apparent stroke. Multiple lacunar infarcts, mainly in the frontal white matter and basal ganglia, lead to progressive permanent brain damage manifested as cognitive decline and finally as dementia. Although the symptoms are almost exclusively neurologic, the arteriopathy is generalized and pathologic diagnosis is possible via skin biopsy in which osmophilic granules can be detected on electron microscopy (accumulation of pathognomonic basophilic, periodic acid-Schiff–positive, and, in electron microscopy, osmophilic material between degenerating smooth muscle cells in dermal arteries). The findings are highly specific, but the sensitivity is somewhat less than 100%. In addition to the suggestive family history and clinical features, the diagnosis can be suggested on the basis of MRI. The blood can be tested for the Notch 3 mutation. Once the diagnosis is made, the homocysteine level should be checked because there is some suggestion that these patients may be at higher risk for hyperhomocysteinemia. There are no proven therapies that will alter the course of CADASIL or reduce the risk for recurrent cerebral infarction. Treatment for CADASIL includes use of antiplatelet agents, although the efficacy is not clear. The effectiveness of aggressive atherosclerosis risk factor control is uncertain but typically is implemented. Because MRI scanning may suggest tiny hemorrhages frequently in CADASIL cases, more aggressive antiplatelet agents and anticoagulation are not usually recommended. Use of medications for dementia, such as the acetylcholinesterase inhibitors as used in Alzheimer's dementia, is of unclear efficacy.

MITOCHONDRIAL DISORDERS

Mitochondrial encephalopathy, lactic acidosis, and stroke-like episodes (MELAS) is maternally inherited and caused by mitochondrial DNA mutations, with a substitution of adenine or guanine at position 3243 (A3243G) causing 80% of cases. Patients present with intermittent confusion, migraine headaches, cerebral infarction before the age of 40, lactic acidosis in the blood, possible focal or generalized seizures, muscle biopsy showing ragged red fibers, and encephalopathy. Imaging may demonstrate ischemic stroke–like lesions, particularly affecting the occipital lobes and basal ganglia. No specific treatments are clearly efficacious. Patients sometimes are treated with coenzyme Q10, vitamin C, carnitine, and riboflavin, but the effect of any of these is uncertain.

FABRY DISEASE

Fabry disease is an X-linked disorder that is caused by a mutation in the alpha-galactosidase A gene. Neurologic presentations include burning pain in a "glove and stocking" distribution caused by a small-fiber peripheral neuropathy, and others may present with cerebral infarctions, most commonly affecting small arteries but also sometimes affecting the larger arteries. Some of the strokes may be caused by hypertension-induced small artery occlusive disease. The ischemic strokes are caused mainly by thrombosis in the setting of small artery occlusive disease. The findings of skin angiokeratomas (typically found between the umbilicus and the knees), progressive renal disease, and a specific type of corneal dystrophy known as whorl keratopathy also suggest the diagnosis.

The diagnosis can be made by a skin biopsy showing the membrane-bound electron-dense bodies in the fibroblasts and endothelial cells and also by evaluating the level of alpha-galactosidase activity in the plasma or peripheral leukocytes. The diagnosis is more difficult in women because these levels may well be normal. Enzyme replacement therapy has not been completed for cerebral ischemia prevention. Likewise, the effectiveness of any other medical therapy such as antiplatelet therapy is not certain. Cardiac abnormalities may also lead to brain embolism. The disorder is caused by deficient lysosomal galactosidase A activity. The deposits then accumulate in the endothelium and smooth muscle, including the arteries, the cornea, and throughout the nervous system.

HOMOCYSTINURIA

Homocystinuria is an autosomal recessive disorder of amino acid metabolism that most typically is caused by a defect in the gene that leads to the production of the enzyme cystathionine beta-synthase. It may also be caused by deficiencies in the production of 5,10-methylene tetrahydrofolate reductase, or homocysteine methyltransferase. The autosomal recessive disease leads to elevation of homocystine in the plasma and urine. The endothelial accumulation of homocysteine leads to premature atherosclerosis and also increased platelet adhesion. Both arterial and venous thrombosis may occur. In addition to thrombosis and premature atherosclerosis, clinical features include eye abnormalities such as optic atrophy, ectopic lens, or glaucoma; marfanoid appearance; high arched palate; mental retardation; seizures; osteoporosis; and scoliosis. Patients are treated with high-dose pyridoxine, folic acid, and vitamin B_{12}. A diet that is low in methionine and high in cystine should also be considered.

SICKLE CELL DISEASE

Sickle cell disease is an inherited disorder that occurs in 1 in 600 births in African Americans. Although much less common, it can affect people of other ethnicities. The disorder commonly leads to cerebral infarction, which occurred in 8% of children by the age of 14 in one large cohort study. In another, the occurrence of first stroke was 11% at age 20 years and 24% at age 45. Red cells that contain hemoglobin SS and are exposed to low oxygen tension alter their structure, leading to increased blood viscosity and the potential for multiple small artery occlusions. Larger arteries can also become affected through adverse changes in the small arteries that supply the arterial wall. The strokes can be either ischemic or hemorrhagic, with ischemic strokes being most common in children and intracerebral hemorrhages (ICHs) and SAHs occurring preferentially in adults. The carotid system is most commonly affected in children. Other cerebrovascular manifestations may include cortical vein and venous sinus thromboses. From a pathologic standpoint, the arterial damage leads to intimal hyperplasia with clot formation leading to ischemia. On occasion, bilateral internal carotid arterial stenoses may cause an arteriographic appearance that mimics Moyamoya disease.

The sickle cell crisis may be precipitated by hypoxia, physical exertion, stress, or acute infection. Transcranial Doppler (TCD) studies may be used to define children who are at highest risk for experiencing a cerebral infarction. Those with TCD velocities >200 cm per second are at the highest stroke risk. In the Stroke Prevention in Sickle Cell Disease (STOP) trial, children were randomly assigned to either intermittent transfusions or standard care. The goal was to keep hemoglobin S level <30% and was highly effective in reducing the risk for first stroke. In adults, chronic intermittent transfusions are often considered, but a complete evaluation is necessary to determine whether there is any other cause of the infarction. In addition to transfusion, aggressive hydration, oxygenation, and pain control are implemented.

INTRACEREBRAL HEMORRHAGE

Amyloid Angiopathy

Cerebral amyloid angiopathy and its potential for causing intracranial hemorrhage is reviewed in Chapter 17. Amyloid angiopathy can be familial, in heredity cerebral hemorrhage with amyloidosis of the Dutch type. This autosomal dominant disorder leads to amyloid deposition in the small intracranial arteries. Patients present with recurrent lobar ICHs or with vascular dementia. There is another autosomal dominant disorder, hereditary cerebral hemorrhage with amyloidosis of the Icelandic type, which is caused by a different gene mutation but with similar clinical findings.

Cerebral Malformations

Cavernous Malformations

Intracranial cavernous malformations are commonly noted on MRI and typically are angiographically occult legions. They may occur in families, most commonly associated with chromosome 7 and chromosome 3. The natural history of intracranial cavernous malformations is described in Chapter 30.

Hereditary Hemorrhagic Telangiectasia

Hereditary hemorrhagic telangiectasia (HHT), also known as Osler-Weber Rendu syndrome, is an autosomal dominant disorder that involves abnormalities of chromosome 9 or 12. Arteriovenous malformations (AVMs) commonly occur in these families intracranially and in the lung, liver, and kidney. ICH and cerebral infarction that is caused by paradoxic embolus through the pulmonary AVM both can occur. Other manifestations of the brain AVMs may include seizures and focal neurologic deficits. As is described earlier, AVMs may be treated with surgical excision, endovascular therapy, or radiosurgery.

Epistaxis, gastrointestinal bleeding, shortness of breath or hemoptysis caused by the pulmonary AVMs, and skin and mucus membrane telangiectasias all may be noted. In one study of 321 patients who had HHT and were seen at a single institution, 3.7% had a history of cerebral malformations, with 2.1% presenting with intracranial hemorrhage. In addition to AVMs, cavernous malformations and venous malformations may be seen. It is suggested that the risk for having a hemorrhage from AVMs in the setting of HHT is lower than from nonfamilial AVMs. A history of cerebral infarction or transient ischemic attack is more common than hemorrhagic disease.

SUGGESTED READING FOR PART IV

Adams HP Jr. Calcium antagonists in the management of patients with aneurysmal subarachnoid hemorrhage: a review. *Angiology.* 1990;41:1010–1016.

Adams RJ, McKie VC, Hsu L, et al. Prevention of a first stroke by transfusions in children with sickle cell anemia and abnormal results on transcranial Doppler ultrasonography. *N Engl J Med.* 1998;339:5–11.

Antiplatelet Trialists' Collaboration. Secondary prevention of vascular disease by prolonged antiplatelet treatment. *BMJ (Clin Res Ed).* 1988;296:320–331.

Asplund K. Hemodilution in acute stroke. *Cerebrovasc Dis.* 1991;1[Suppl 1]:129–138.

Atrial Fibrillation Investigators. Risk factors for stroke and efficacy of antithrombotic therapy in atrial fibrillation: analysis of pooled data from five randomized controlled trials. *Arch Intern Med.* 1994;154:1449–1457.

Auger RG, Wiebers DO. Management of unruptured intracranial aneurysms: a decision analysis. *J Stroke Cerebrovascular Dis.* 1991;1:174–181.

Auger RG, Wiebers DO. Management of unruptured intracranial arteriovenous malformations: a decision analysis. *Neurosurgery.* 1992;30:561–569.

Barnett HJ. Stroke prevention by surgery for symptomatic disease in carotid territory. *Neurol Clin.* 1992;10:281–292.

Barnwell SL, Higashida RT, Halbach VV, et al. Direct endovascular thrombolytic therapy for dural sinus thrombosis. *Neurosurgery.* 1991;28:135–142.

Ben-Yehuda D, Rose M, Michaeli Y, et al. Permanent neurological complications in patients with thrombotic thrombocytopenic purpura. *Am J Hematol.* 1988;29:74–78.

Bick RL. Disseminated intravascular coagulation: objective criteria for diagnosis and management. *Med Clin North Am.* 1994;78:511–543.

Biller J. Medical management of acute cerebral ischemia. *Neurol Clin.* 1992;10:63–85.

Biller J, Mathews KD, Love BB, eds. *Stroke in Children and Young Adults.* Boston: Butterworth-Heinemann; 1994.

The Boston Area Anticoagulation Trial for Atrial Fibrillation Investigators. The effect of low-dose warfarin on the risk of stroke in patients with nonrheumatic atrial fibrillation. *N Engl J Med.* 1990;323:1505–1511.

Bracken MB, Shepard MJ, Holford TR, et al. Administration of methylprednisolone for 24 or 48 hours or tirilazad mesylate for 48 hours in the treatment of acute spinal cord injury. Results of the Third National Acute Spinal Cord Injury Randomized Controlled Trial. National Acute Spinal Cord Injury Study. *JAMA.* 1997;277:1597–1604.

Broderick J, Talbot GT, Prenger E, et al. Stroke in children within a major metropolitan area: the surprising importance of intracerebral hemorrhage. *J Child Neurol.* 1993;8:250–255.

Brott TG, Brown RD Jr, Meyer FB, et al. Carotid revascularization for prevention of stroke: carotid endarterectomy and carotid artery stenting. *Mayo Clin Proc.* 2004;79:1197–1208.

Brown RD Jr, Evans BA, Wiebers DO, et al. Transient ischemic attack and minor ischemic stroke: an algorithm for evaluation and treatment. *Mayo Clin Proc.* 1994;69:1027–1039.

Brown RD Jr, Flemming KD, Meyer FB, et al. Natural history, evaluation, and management of intracranial vascular malformations. *Mayo Clin Proc.* 2005;80:269–281.

Buchbinder R, Detsky AS. Management of suspected giant cell arteritis: a decision analysis. *J Rheumatol.* 1992;19:1220–1228.

Butler RN, Ahronheim J, Fillitt H, et al. Vascular dementia: an updated approach to patient management. A roundtable discussion: part 3. *Geriatrics.* 1994;49:39–40, 43–46.

CAPRIE. A randomized, blinded trial of clopidogrel versus aspirin in patients at risk of ischaemic events (CAPRIE). *Lancet.* 1996;348:1329–1338.

Chakravarty K, Elgabani SH, Scott DG, et al. A district audit on the management of polymyalgia rheumatica and giant cell arteritis. *Br J Rheumatol.* 1994;33:152–156.

Chimowitz MI, Lynn MJ, Howlett-Smith H, et al. Comparison of Warfarin and aspirin for symptomatic intracranial arterial stenosis. *N Engl J Med.* 2005;352:1305–1316.

Chobanian A, Bakris G, Black H, et al. The Seventh Report of the Joint National Committee on Prevention, Detection, Evaluation, and Treatment of High Blood Pressure: The JNC 7 Report. *JAMA.* 2003;289:2560–2572.

Collins R, Baigent C, Sandercock P, et al. Antiplatelet therapy for thromboprophylaxis: the need for careful consideration of the evidence from randomised trials. Antiplatelet Trialists' Collaboration. *BMJ.* 1994;309:1215–1217.

Connolly SJ, Laupacis A, Gent M, et al. Canadian Atrial Fibrillation Anticoagulation (CAFA) Study. *J Am Coll Cardiol.* 1991;18:349–355.

Coull BM, Levine SR, Brey RL. The role of antiphospholipid antibodies in stroke. *Neurol Clin.* 1992;10:125–143.

Croce MA, Dent DL, Menke PG, et al. Acute subdural hematoma: nonsurgical management of selected patients. *J Trauma.* 1994;36:820–826.

Crowell RM, Ojemann RG, Ogilvy CS. Spontaneous brain hemorrhage: surgical considerations. In: Barnett HMJ, Stein BM, Mohr JP, Yatsu FM, eds. *Stroke: pathophysiology, diagnosis, and management.* 2nd ed. New York: Churchill Livingstone; 1992:1169–1187.

Davis WD, Hart RG. Cardiogenic stroke in the elderly. *Clin Geriatr Med.* 1991;7:429–442.

Desmond DW, Moroney JT, Lynch T, et al. The natural history of CADASIL: a pooled analysis of previously published cases. *Stroke.* 1999;30:1230–1233.

Diener HC, Bogousslavsky J, Brass LM, et al., on behalf of the MATCH investigators. Aspirin and clopidogrel compared with clopidogrel alone after recent ischaemic stroke or transient ischaemic attack in high-risk patients (MATCH): randomised, double-blind, placebo-controlled trial. *Lancet.* 2004;364:331–337.

Diener HC, Cunha L, Forbes C, et al. European Stroke Prevention Study 2: dipyridamole and acetylsalicylic acid in the secondary prevention of stroke. *J Neurol Sci.* 1996; 143:1–13.

Dodick DW, Meissner I, Meyer FB, et al. Evaluation and management of asymptomatic carotid artery stenosis. *Mayo Clin Proc.* 2004;79:937–944.

Donnan GA. Investigation of patients with stroke and transient ischaemic attacks. *Lancet.* 1992;339:473–477.

The Dutch TIA Trial Study Group. A comparison of two doses of aspirin (30 mg vs. 283 mg a day) in patients after a transient ischemic attack or minor ischemic stroke. *N Engl J Med.* 1991;325:1261–1266.

EAFT (European Atrial Fibrillation Trial) Study Group. Secondary prevention in non-rheumatic atrial fibrillation after transient ischaemic attack or minor stroke. *Lancet.* 1993;342:1255–1262.

The EC/IC Bypass Study Group. Failure of extracranial-intracranial arterial bypass to reduce the risk of ischemic stroke: results of an international randomized trial. *N Engl J Med.* 1985;313:1191–1200.

Eden OB, Lilleyman JS. Guidelines for management of idiopathic thrombocytopenic purpura. *Arch Dis Child.* 1992;67:1056–1058.

Einhaupl KM, Villringer A, Meister W, et al. Heparin treatment in sinus venous thrombosis. *Lancet.* 1991;338:597–600.

Erbguth F, Brenner P, Schuierer G, et al. Diagnosis and treatment of deep cerebral vein thrombosis. *Neurosurg Rev.* 1991;14:145–148.

Ernst E, Pittler MH. Ginkgo biloba for dementia. A systematic review of double-blind, placebo-controlled trials. *Clin Drug Invest.* 1999;17:301–308.

European Carotid Surgery Trialists' Collaborative Group. MRC European Carotid Surgery Trial: interim results for symptomatic patients with severe (70–99%) or with mild (0–29%) carotid stenosis. *Lancet.* 1991;337:1235–1243.

Executive Committee for the Asymptomatic Carotid Atherosclerosis Study. Endarterectomy for asymptomatic carotid artery stenosis. *JAMA.* 1995;273:1421–1428.

Farrell B, Godwin J, Richards S, et al. The United Kingdom transient ischemic attack (UK-TIA) aspirin trial: final results. *J Neurol Neurosurg Psychiatry.* 1991;54:1044–1054.

Feldmann E, Tornabene J. Diagnosis and treatment of cerebral amyloid angiopathy. *Clin Geriatr Med.* 1991;7:617–630.

Flemming KD, Brown RD Jr. Secondary prevention strategies in ischemic stroke: identification and optimal management of modifiable risk factors. *Mayo Clin Proc.* 2004;79:1330–1340.

Flemming KD, Brown RD Jr, Petty GW, et al. Evaluation and management of transient ischemic attack and minor cerebral infarction. *Mayo Clin Proc.* 2004;79:1071–1086.

Fletcher AE, Bulpitt CJ. How far should blood pressure be lowered? *N Engl J Med.* 1992;326:251–254.

Fulgham JR, Ingall TJ, Stead LG, et al. Management of acute ischemic stroke. *Mayo Clin Proc.* 2004;79:1459–1469.

Gent M, Blakely JA, Easton JD, et al. The Canadian American Ticlopidine Study (CATS) in thromboembolic stroke. *Lancet.* 1989;1:1215–1220.

Gorelick PB, Richardson D, Kelly M, et al. Aspirin and ticlopidine for prevention of recurrent stroke in black patients. *JAMA.* 2003;289:2947–2957.

Grubb R, Derdeyn C, Fritsch S, et al. Importance of hemo-dynamic factors in the prognosis of symptomatic carotid occlusion. *JAMA*. 1998;280:1055–1060.

Hacke W, Kaste M, Fleschi C, et al. Intravenous thrombolysis with recombinant tissue plasminogen activator for acute hemispheric stroke: the European Cooperative Acute Stroke Study (ECASS). *JAMA*. 1995;274:1017–1025.

Haley EC Jr, Brott TG, Sheppard GL, et al. Pilot randomized trial of tissue plasminogen activator in acute ischemic stroke: the TPA Bridging Study Group. *Stroke*. 1993;24:1000–1004.

Haley EC Jr, Kassell NF, Torner JC. The International Cooperative Study on the Timing of Aneurysm Surgery: the North American experience. *Stroke*. 1992;23:205–214.

Haley EC Jr, Kassell NF, Torner JC, et al. A randomized trial of two doses of nicardipine in aneurysmal subarachnoid hemorrhage: a report of the Cooperative Aneurysm Study. *J Neurosurg*. 1994;80:788–796.

Hart RG, Kanter MC. Hematologic disorders and ischemic stroke: a selective review. *Stroke*. 1990;21:1111–1121.

Hass WK, Easton JD, Adams HP Jr, et al. A randomized trial comparing ticlopidine hydrochloride with aspirin for the prevention of stroke in high-risk patients: Ticlopidine Aspirin Stroke Study Group. *N Engl J Med*. 1989;321:501–507.

Haynes RB, Taylor DW, Sackett DL, et al. Prevention of functional impairment by endarterectomy for symptomatic high-grade carotid stenosis. North American Symptomatic Carotid Endarterectomy Trial Collaborators. *JAMA*. 1994;271:1256–1259.

Heinonen OP, Slone D, Shapiro S. *Birth Defects and Drugs in Pregnancy*. Littleton, MA: Publishing Sciences Group; 1977.

Hobson RW II, Weiss DG, Fields WS, et al. Efficacy of carotid endarterectomy for asymptomatic carotid stenosis. The Veterans Affairs Cooperative Study Group. *N Engl J Med*. 1993;328:221–227.

Horton JC, Chambers WA, Lyons SL, et al. Pregnancy and the risk of hemorrhage from cerebral arteriovenous malformations. *Neurosurgery*. 1990;27:867–871.

Jonas S. Anticoagulant therapy in cerebrovascular disease: review and meta-analysis. *Stroke*. 1988;19:1043–1048.

Kaku DA, Lowenstein DH. Emergence of recreational drug abuse as a major risk factor for stroke in young adults. *Ann Intern Med*. 1990;113:821–827.

Komsuoglu SS, Komsuoglu B, Ozmenoglu M, et al. Oral nifedipine in the treatment of hypertensive crises in patients with hypertensive encephalopathy. *Int J Cardiol*. 1992;34:277–282.

Manno EM, Atkinson JL, Fulgham JR, et al. Emerging medical and surgical management strategies in the evaluation and treatment of intracerebral hemorrhage. *Mayo Clin Proc*. 2005;80:420–433.

Martin N, Khanna R, Rodts G. The intensive care management of patients with subarachnoid hemorrhage. In: Andrews BT, ed. *Neurosurgical intensive care*. New York: McGraw-Hill; 1993;291–310.

Mascio RD, Marchioli R, Tognoni G. From pharmacological promises to controlled clinical trials to meta-analysis and back: the case of nimodipine in cerebrovascular disorders. *Clin Trials Metaanal.* 1994;29:57–79.

Mayer SA, Brun NC, Begtrup K, et al. Recombinant activated Factor VII for acute intracerebral hemorrhage. *N Engl J Med.* 2005;352:777–785.

Mayo Asymptomatic Carotid Endarterectomy Study Group. Results of a randomized controlled trial of carotid endarterectomy for asymptomatic carotid stenosis. *Mayo Clin Proc.* 1992;67:513–518.

Mendelow AD, Gregson BA, Fernandes HM, et al. Early surgery versus initial conservative treatment in patients with spontaneous supratentorial intracerebral haematomas in the International Surgical Trial in Intracerebral Haemorrhage (STICH): a randomised trial. *Lancet.* 2005;365:387–397.

Meyer FB, ed. *Sundt's Occlusive Cerebrovascular Disease.* 2nd ed. Philadelphia: WB Saunders; 1994.

Mohr JP, Thompson JL, Lazar RM, et al.; Warfarin-Aspirin Recurrent Stroke Study Group. A comparison of warfarin and aspirin for the prevention of recurrent ischemic stroke. *N Engl J Med.* 2001;345:1444–1451.

Molyneux A, Kerr R, Stratton I, et al.; International Subarachnoid Aneurysm Trial (ISAT) Collaborative Group. International Subarachnoid Aneurysm Trial (ISAT) of neurosurgical clipping versus endovascular coiling in 2143 patients with ruptured intracranial aneurysms: a randomised trial. *Lancet.* 2002;360:1267–1274.

MRC Asymptomatic Carotid Surgery Trial (ACST) Collaborative Group. Prevention of disabling and fatal strokes by successful carotid endarterectomy in patients without recent neurological symptoms: randomised controlled trial. *Lancet.* 2004;363: 1491–1502.

National Institute of Neurological Disorders and Stroke rt-PA Stroke Study Group. Tissue plasminogen activator for acute ischemic stroke. *N Engl J Med.* 1995;333:1581–1587.

North American Symptomatic Carotid Endarterectomy Trial Collaborators. Beneficial effect of carotid endarterectomy in symptomatic patients with high-grade carotid stenosis. *N Engl J Med.* 1991;325:445–453.

O'Donnell HC, Rosand J, Knudsen KA, et al. Apolipoprotein E genotype and the risk of recurrent lobar intracerebral hemorrhage. *N Engl J Med.* 2000;342:240–245.

Petersen P, Boysen G, Godtfredsen J, et al. Placebo-controlled, randomised trial of warfarin and aspirin for prevention of thromboembolic complications in chronic atrial fibrillation: the Copenhagen AFASAK study. *Lancet.* 1989;1: 175–179.

Pickard JD, Murray GD, Illingworth R, et al. Effect of oral nimodipine on cerebral infarction and outcome after subarachnoid haemorrhage: British aneurysm nimodipine trial. *BMJ.* 1989;298:636–642.

Poungvarin N, Bhoopat W, Viriyavejakul A, et al. Effects of dexamethasone in primary supratentorial intracerebral hemorrhage. *N Engl J Med.* 1987;316:1229–1233.

PROGRESS Collaborative Group. Randomised trial of a perindopril-based blood-pressure lowering regimen among

6105 individuals with previous stroke or transient ischaemic attack. *Lancet.* 2001;358:1033–1041.

Ramsey RG. *Neuroradiology.* 3rd ed. Philadelphia: WB Saunders; 1994:174–224.

Riela AR, Roach ES. Etiology of stroke in children. *J Child Neurol.* 1993;8:201–220.

Roberts I, Yates D, Sandercock P, et al. Effect of intravenous corticosteroids on death within 14 days in 10,008 adults with clinically significant head injury (MRC CRASH trial): randomised placebo-controlled trial. *Lancet.* 2004;364:1321–1328.

Rogvi-Hansen, Boysen G. Intravenous glycerol treatment of acute stroke: a statistical review. *Cerebrovasc Dis.* 1992;2:11–13.

Rothrock JF, Hart RG. Antithrombotic therapy in cerebrovascular disease. *Ann Intern Med.* 1991;115:885–895.

Sabbadini G, Francia A, Calandriello L, et al. Cerebral autosomal dominant arteriopathy with subcortical infarcts and leucoencephalopathy (CADASIL). Clinical, neuroimaging, pathological and genetic study of a large Italian family. *Brain.* 1995;118:207–215.

The SALT Collaborative Group. Swedish Aspirin Low-Dose Trial (SALT) of 75 mg aspirin as secondary prophylaxis after cerebrovascular ischaemic events. *Lancet.* 1991;338:1345–1349.

Sherman DG, Dyken ML Jr, Fisher M, et al. Antithrombotic therapy for cerebrovascular disorders. *Chest.* 1992;102[Suppl 4]: 529S–537S.

Shuaib A. Alteration of blood pressure regulation and cerebrovascular disorders in the elderly. *Cerebrovasc Brain Metab Rev.* 1992;4:329–345.

Stam J. Thrombosis of the cerebral veins and sinuses. *N Engl J Med.* 2005;352:1791–1798.

Stein BM. Surgical decisions in vascular malformations of the brain. In: Barnett HJM, Stein BM, Mohr JP, et al., eds. *Stroke: pathophysiology, diagnosis, and management.* 2nd ed. New York: Churchill Livingstone; 1992:1093–1133.

Steinberg MH. Sickle cell anemia: pathophysiology, management, and prospects for the future. *J Clin Apheresis.* 1991;6:221–223.

Stroke Prevention in Atrial Fibrillation Investigators. Stroke Prevention in Atrial Fibrillation Study: final results. *Circulation.* 1991;84:527–539.

Tefferi A, Hoagland HC. Issues in the diagnosis and management of essential thrombocythemia. *Mayo Clin Proc.* 1994;69:651–655.

Viitanen M, Kalimo H. CADASIL: hereditary arteriopathy leading to multiple brain infarcts and dementia. *Ann N Y Acad Sci.* 2000;903:273–284.

Vinuela F, Halbach W, Dion JE, eds. *Interventional Neuroradiology: Endovascular Therapy of the Central Nervous System.* New York: Raven; 1992.

Wiebers DO. Ischemic cerebrovascular complications of pregnancy. *Arch Neurol.* 1985;42:1106–1113.

Wiebers DO. Subarachnoid hemorrhage in pregnancy. *Semin Neurol.* 1988;8:226–229.

Wiebers DO. Intracranial aneurysm. *Curr Ther Neurol Dis.* 1990;3:192–194.

Wiebers DO, Piepgras DG, Meyer FB, et al. Pathogenesis, natural history, and treatment of unruptured intracranial aneurysms. *Mayo Clin Proc.* 2004;79:1572–1583.

Wijdicks EFM, Kallmes DF, Manno EM, et al. Subarachnoid hemorrhage: neurointensive care and aneurysm repair. *Mayo Clin Proc.* 2005;80:550–559.

Yadav JS, Wholey MH, Kuntz RE, et al. Protected carotid-artery stenting versus endarterectomy in high-risk patients. *N Engl J Med.* 2004;351:1493–1501.

Primary Prevention of Cerebrovascular Disorders

As medicine moves into the 21st century with the added pressure of increasing costs and limited resources, successful reduction of the impact of stroke on the population will require shifting emphasis from treatment of end stages of generalized atherosclerosis and other underlying diseases to primary prevention of underlying diseases and stroke. This approach will require, in many cases, more sophisticated and more definitive studies to identify, verify, and better explain the relative importance of known risk factors, the interactions of various risk factors, and the existence of currently unknown or unverified risk factors.

Successful primary prevention of stroke is now becoming possible with the identification of important risk factors such as hypertension, cardiac disease, transient ischemic attack, asymptomatic carotid artery stenosis or occlusion, cigarette smoking, diabetes mellitus, and sickle cell disease, which may be modified by medical treatment or other means. Other factors that are not as strongly correlated with an increased risk for stroke but are amenable to treatment or to some kind of modification include hypercoagulable states (including increased concentration of fibrinogen), migraine, contraceptive use, drug abuse, low body and environmental temperature in the cold season, and dyslipidemia (including a high ratio of total cholesterol to high-density lipoprotein cholesterol). It should be noted that the reason some of these factors (such as dyslipidemia) have not been as strongly correlated with increased stroke risk may relate to most existing studies not examining various subtypes of ischemic stroke (such as atherosclerotic ischemic stroke), and many not even distinguishing ischemic versus hemorrhagic stroke. A family history of stroke, advanced age, sex, and race are untreatable risk factors, but they may be useful for identifying individuals at higher risk for stroke who might then be more motivated to address other risk factors. Stroke is preventable in at least 80% of cases. It can be prevented by identifying individuals who are at high risk (see Appendix D) and initiating a cost-effective approach to address the reversible risk factors. An even greater impact can be realized by instituting broader healthy lifestyle components across the population, beginning in young age groups and focused on preventing stroke risk factors before they develop.

Current American Heart Association guidelines for primary prevention of cardiovascular disease and stroke recommend risk factor screening in adults to begin at age 20 years, with blood pressure (BP), body mass index, waist circumference, and pulse (to screen for atrial fibrillation) to be recorded at least every

2 years and fasting serum lipoprotein profile (or total and high-density lipoprotein cholesterol if fasting is unavailable) and fasting blood glucose measured according to a person's risk for hyperlipidemia and diabetes, respectively (at least every 5 years if no risk factors are present and every 2 years if risk factors are present). For all adults ≥40 years of age or people with two or more risk factors (such as smoking, elevated BP, total/low-density lipoprotein cholesterol, electrocardiogram-documented left ventricular hypertrophy, or diabetes mellitus), the absolute risk for developing coronary heart disease and stroke can be ascertained (see Appendix D). Control of risk factors should be aimed at lowering the absolute risk for developing coronary heart disease and stroke to the extent possible.

Modifiable Lifestyle and Environmental Factors

Much of the desirable reduction in risk factors for stroke requires modification of environmental factors and maintenance of an appropriate lifestyle, including cessation of cigarette smoking, dietary adjustment, weight control, physical activity, cessation of drug abuse, modification of oral contraceptive use, and maintenance of adequate personal and environmental temperatures during the cold season.

CIGARETTE SMOKING

Smoking increases the risk for stroke by approximately 40% in men and 60% in women. Cigarette smoking raises the blood fibrinogen concentration, enhances platelet aggregation, and increases hematocrit level and blood viscosity. It is one of the most powerful risk factors that contribute to the development of carotid atherosclerosis and also seems to contribute significantly to the development of intracranial aneurysms. Second-hand smoke may also increase the risk for stroke. Smoking cessation substantially decreases the risk for subsequent stroke in a remarkably short time and is particularly vital for patients who present with cerebral or retinal ischemic events. The risk for stroke decreases substantially each year after cessation of cigarette smoking, and by the end of 5 years, the risk is nearly that of a person who never smoked. The physician should review with the patient who smokes the benefits of quitting and the risk of continuing. Smoking or nicotine dependence centers have become increasingly sophisticated at assessing the nature and the severity of an individual's dependence, determining which of several different strategies is most likely to succeed for a given patient's situation and providing needed support. Nicotine patches or nicotine replacement gum (initial dose depends on number of cigarettes smoked per day) or bupropion may be useful smoking cessation aids unless contraindications exist.

DIET

Diet may help to prevent stroke in two ways: It can prevent the development and the progression of stroke risk factors, such as atherosclerosis, hypertension, hyperlipidemia, ischemic heart disease, and diabetes mellitus, and it can provide beneficial food components, such as fruits and vegetables, that can independently reduce the risk for stroke. In coronary atherosclerosis, preliminary evidence suggests that to stabilize or reverse atheroma, dietary intake of fat (especially saturated fat) must be reduced to <10% of the total caloric intake and cholesterol to <5 mg per day (major sources of saturated fatty acids and cholesterol are meat, eggs, and dairy products) through a very low-fat vegetarian diet. Such results have been associated with total serum cholesterol levels of 150 mg per dl or below. The same principles may also apply to carotid and other large-vessel atherosclerosis.

However, randomized, controlled trials have not yet been reported, except with respect to coronary arthrosclerosis. There is also some evidence that eating fish or other plant-based sources of omega-3 fatty acids (flax seed, soybeans, soybean oil, walnuts) more than two times per month and using reduced-fat milk (along with other appropriate dietary modifications) may reduce the risk for stroke. Restriction of dietary salt (to approximately 6 to 7 g per day) or sodium intake (to approximately 2 to 3 g per day) helps in the prevention and management of hypertension. In hot, humid climates, the reduction in dietary sodium should be modified to accommodate for the loss of sodium in such extreme conditions. In general, patients should be discouraged from consuming salt-rich foods or adding salt to already prepared foods. Ensuring an adequate intake of potassium, calcium, and magnesium may also help to keep blood pressure (BP) under control.

In the typical American diet, approximately 40% to 45% of the dietary caloric intake is in the form of fat (most of which is saturated fat), and the cholesterol intake is approximately 400 mg per day. The standard low-fat diet (see Appendix F-1) seeks to reduce fat consumption to approximately 30% of the dietary caloric intake (saturated fat constituting <10% of calories) and cholesterol consumption to approximately 300 mg. This diet is recommended as a minimal modification for general health reasons, even for individuals without atherosclerosis. It is recommended to match energy intake with energy needs.

An even more healthful alternative for prevention of atherosclerosis in the general population and the diet that is strongly recommended for individuals with symptomatic or asymptomatic coronary or craniocervical atherosclerosis is a very low-fat diet (see Appendix F-2) because coronary atherosclerosis appears to progress with the typical American diet and standard low-fat diets. A very low-fat diet is aimed at reducing fat intake to 10% to 20% of the total calories and cholesterol intake to 5 to 10 mg per day or less.

Recent data from the Harvard School of Public Health have indicated that individuals who consumed at least five to six servings of fruits and vegetables per day were approximately 30% less likely to have an ischemic stroke over a 10-year period than those who ate fewer than three servings per day. Each daily serving was associated with a 6% reduction in risk. The most potent effects were found in orange juice and other citrus fruits and juices; green leafy vegetables; and such cruciferous vegetables as broccoli, cauliflower, brussel sprouts, and cabbage.

Calorie restriction to achieve and maintain ideal body weight is recommended to control obesity, particularly because appropriate weight reduction enhances the regulation of hypertension and type 2 diabetes mellitus. Ideal body weight determinations based on height and weight (see Appendix F-3) are appropriate for some people but should not be considered necessary for everyone. In general, a healthy adult needs approximately 30 to 35 kcal per kg of body weight. With any type of restrictive diet, it is generally recommended that patients take a multivitamin and mineral supplement to ensure adequate intake of various nutrients such as iron, vitamin B_{12}, vitamin D, magnesium, and calcium, particularly if patients are likely to avoid certain food groups.

Dietary recommendations are most effective when they are specific (see recommended reading for Section V—*Stroke-Free for Life* [Wiebers, 2002] and *When Lightening Strikes* [Feigin, 2003]—for more detailed dietary suggestions and examples). It may be helpful for a dietitian or similarly trained physician to interview individual patients to more fully characterize eating patterns and daily calorie intake and to design the most appropriate and comfortable diet. In some patients, adherence to the modified diet should be monitored under medical supervision. It is particularly helpful for patients who are making the transition to a very-low-fat, very-low-cholesterol diet to realize that numerous products that now are on the market can help individuals give up meats, egg yolks, and dairy products without giving up their flavor or texture. The number of these products is growing steadily, and many are available in regular supermarkets as well as health food stores. Some of these products, such as several readily available butter substitutes, contain ingredients (such as sitosterol esters) that reduce low-density lipoprotein and total cholesterol levels.

PHYSICAL EXERCISE

Increased relative weight (body mass index ≥ 24.9 kg per m^2) or obesity (body weight $>10\%$ above ideal weight) is associated with increased BP, cholesterol, blood glucose, uric acid, and relative risk for death from cardiovascular disease. In most cases, appropriate weight reduction may be achieved by dietary modification in association with physical exercise. Medical supervision, especially in the early stages of a weight control program, is desirable. A sedentary lifestyle predisposes to obesity, hypertension, glucose intolerance, hypertriglyceridemia, and reduced high-density lipoprotein (HDL) cholesterol levels.

Regular exercise has been shown in several recent studies to reduce the risk for stroke. It improves the health of the cardiovascular system, reduces weight and BP, increases HDL levels and reduces triglycerides, prevents or helps control diabetes mellitus, reduces stress, and may counter symptoms of depression. In general, exercise can be obtained by (1) altering daily lifestyle to incorporate appropriate levels of physical exertion into an overall routine or (2) undertaking regular aerobic recreational or sporting activities (as a rule, patients with moderate to severe hypertension or coronary artery disease should avoid isometric or static exercise) at least three times a week or frequent brisk walking from 30 to 45 minutes as often as six times per week. To facilitate the aerobic aspect of the program, the individual should warm up slowly to lessen anaerobic exercise, which may lead to early fatigue.

Exercise regimens should be tailored to the individual and, as appropriate, may be based on results of a baseline treadmill electrocardiographic test. The target heart rate should be 50% to 75% of the maximal heart rate during the treadmill exercise study or the calculated maximal pulse rate for the patient's age (220 − age). In general, deconditioned patients can be asked to walk briskly for approximately 15 minutes per session (two times a day) for the first week, 20 minutes per session (two times a day) for the second week, 25 minutes per day in a single session for the third week, 30 minutes per day in a single session for the fourth week, and thereafter 40 to 60 minutes six times weekly; the pulse rate should be recorded and any symptoms or complications reported at each exercise session. Preliminary evidence indicates that this amount of regular aerobic exercise (such as running, jogging, swimming, dancing, tennis, racquetball, bicycling, cross-country skiing, hiking, mountain climbing, aerobics classes) in combination with a strict vegetarian diet and various stress reduction techniques (without medication) may reverse coronary atherosclerosis.

ORAL CONTRACEPTIVES

Oral contraceptives (especially when used by someone who smokes cigarettes or is hypertensive) can cause systemic thromboembolism and result in ischemic stroke and cerebral vein thrombosis in women of childbearing age. Replacement of high-estrogen contraceptives with low-estrogen compounds or an alternative contraceptive strategy should be considered for women with ischemic cerebrovascular disease without other identifiable cause. Special precautions should be taken by women who have other stroke risk factors, particularly hypertension and cigarette smoking.

HORMONE REPLACEMENT THERAPY

There is evidence that hormone replacement therapy (HRT), especially a combination of estrogen with progestin, increases the risk for stroke by approximately 33%, especially ischemic stroke. It also appears to increase the risk for coronary heart disease and dementia. Therefore, HRT (especially those that contain both estrogen and progestin) should only be prescribed for temporary use to treat menopausal symptoms. For perimenopausal and menopausal women who take HRT (especially a combination of estrogen with progestin), counseling should be provided about benefits and harms of HRT based on the individual risks. In most cases, HRT should be stopped if the person has had an ischemic stroke, transient ischemic attack, carotid artery stenosis, or atrial fibrillation unless the benefit outweighs the risk for the specific indication. More intensive prophylaxis should be used when HRT has not been stopped.

ALCOHOL

Accumulating evidence suggests that the relationship between alcohol and stroke depends on the type of stroke as well as the amount and consistency of alcohol consumed. A recent meta-analysis showed that, compared with abstainers, individuals who consumed >60 g of alcohol per day had an increased risk for both hemorrhagic (odds ratio [OR] 2.18) and ischemic (OR 1.69) stroke. Consumption of <12 g of alcohol per day was associated with a decreased relative risk for ischemic (OR 0.80) and total (OR 0.83) stroke and consumption of 12 to 24 g per day with a decreased risk for ischemic stroke (OR 0.72). Chronic heavy alcohol consumption and binge drinking may exert their harmful effects through changes in BP, platelet aggregability, blood coagulation, triglyceride levels, and cardiac status (paroxysmal atrial fibrillation and cardiomyopathy). Mild to moderate alcohol consumption may exert its beneficial effects through lipid and coagulation mechanisms.

DRUG ABUSE

Alcohol, heroin, amphetamines, cocaine, phencyclidine, and other recreational drugs may produce cerebral infarction or hemorrhage associated with vasculitis, vasospasm, noninflammatory vasculopathy, cardiac dysfunction including arrhythmias, hypercoagulability and hypocoagulability, or acute circulatory abnormalities (such as hypertensive crisis). Cessation of drug abuse and recreational drug use may prevent stroke in many young adults.

AMBIENT TEMPERATURE

Avoidance of low body and environmental temperatures in the cold season is recommended because they are associated with increased BP, fibrinogen levels, and cholesterol concentration and may increase the risk for stroke, particularly hemorrhagic subtypes, in people with cardiovascular disease and other risk factors.

Asymptomatic Carotid and Vertebral Stenosis

ASYMPTOMATIC CAROTID STENOSIS

The treatment of patients with asymptomatic carotid disease (bruit, stenosis, or occlusion) continues to be somewhat controversial, although recent data have clarified some aspects. It is generally accepted that all patients with asymptomatic carotid bruits should be evaluated with a complete neurologic examination, including ophthalmoscopy and one or more of the noninvasive carotid artery techniques, including carotid duplex ultrasonography and oculopneumoplethysmography. If abnormalities suggest relatively high-grade lesions (stenosis of >60%) or there is evidence of cholesterol or fibrin platelet retinal emboli, then aggressive atherosclerosis risk factor modification and antiplatelet therapy generally are used with or without carotid endarterectomy (CEA) or carotid angioplasty with stent placement (CAS), which may benefit some of these patients. Although the effectiveness of antiplatelet agents for reducing stroke in these patients has not been proved, these agents may also be beneficial for reducing the risk for myocardial infarction. Antiplatelet therapy also generally is recommended for patients who have lesser degrees of carotid stenosis (non–pressure-significant lesions) and have other direct evidence for or risk factors associated with generalized atherosclerosis. In the setting of asymptomatic carotid occlusive disease, aspirin typically is selected as the antiplatelet agent. There is no specific indication in these patients for clopidogrel or aspirin in combination with sustained-release dipyridamole, unless they require one of these treatments for a nonneurologic indication.

Data from the Asymptomatic Carotid Atherosclerosis Study (ACAS) and the Medical Research Council Asymptomatic Carotid Surgery Trial (ACST) indicate that selected patients with reduction in the diameter of the carotid artery of >60% may benefit from CEA in addition to use of aspirin and management of risk factors. It is important to realize that there are different measurements of carotid artery stenosis; for example, 70% stenosis recorded using the criteria used in the North American Symptomatic Carotid Endarterectomy Trial (NASCET) equals approximately 80% European Carotid Stenosis Trial (ECST) stenosis (Fig. 25-1). In ACAS, participating surgical investigators performed CEA with a combined perioperative morbidity and mortality rate of <3%. The risk during 5 years for the primary outcome (any stroke or death within 30 days postoperatively or any **ipsilateral stroke** or death from stroke thereafter) was 5.1% (approximately 1% per year) for patients who were treated surgically and 11.0% (approximately 2% per year) for those who were treated without operation. The relative risk reduction was 53%, with a 66% reduction in men (statistically significant) and 17% in women (not statistically significant). The perioperative morbidity and mortality were higher in women,

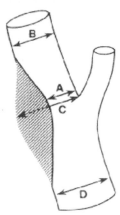

ECST method: $\dfrac{C-A}{C} \times 100\%$ stenosis

NASCET method: $\dfrac{B-A}{B} \times 100\%$ stenosis

CC method: $\dfrac{D-A}{D} \times 100\%$ stenosis

Figure 25-1.   Different measurements of carotid artery stenosis.

contributing to the lack of clear benefit in women. Evaluation of secondary end points revealed that the differences between the operation and nonoperation groups with respect to **total stroke and ipsilateral major stroke and death** were not statistically significant, although there was a trend in favor of operation.

The ACST was a large, prospective, randomized trial that compared CEA with conservative management among 3120 asymptomatic patients with >60% stenosis as demonstrated on ultrasonography. During a maximum of 5 years of follow-up, the 5-year stroke risk was 6.4% in those who were treated with CEA compared with 11.8% in those who were treated medically. Fatal or disabling stroke was also reduced by CEA, with the 5-year risk of 3.5% in the CEA cohort and 6.1% in those who were treated medically (p = 0.004). In the subgroup analyses, as opposed to the ACAS outcome, a statistically significant benefit was noted in both men and women. However, the benefit was not noted in those who were older than 75 years.

These data suggest that CEA, performed in centers with low (<3%) perioperative morbidity and mortality, should be considered for high-grade asymptomatic carotid stenosis in selected patients with a life expectancy of at least 5 years. In patients with significant medical problems that may preclude general anesthesia, surgical management is contraindicated and management with antiplatelet agents is more appropriate. Additional features that make operation more compelling are progressing stenosis despite risk factor management, very-high-grade lesions, and relatively localized rather than diffuse atherosclerotic disease (see Appendix E-6).

Patients who have a high-grade carotid stenosis and are at increased risk for CEA may also be considered for CAS. In the Stenting and Angioplasty with Protection in Patients at High Risk for Endarterectomy (SAPPHIRE) trial, 334 patients with a condition that could increase the risk of CEA, with either a 50% symptomatic stenosis or 80% asymptomatic stenosis, were randomly assigned to either CEA or CAS. More than 70% of patients had an asymptomatic stenosis. The primary end point was the occurrence of a major cardiovascular event within 1 year of treatment: death, stroke, or myocardial infarction within 30 days of intervention or death or ipsilateral stroke between 31 days and 1 year. Overall, among those who underwent CAS, 12.2% had a primary end point, compared with 20.1% of those who underwent CEA. In those with an asymptomatic stenosis, the occurrence of a primary end point was 9.9% in the CAS group, compared with 21.5% in those who underwent CEA. There was no comparison group of patients who were treated conservatively. The CEA risk in these asymptomatic patients was far higher than in any previous clinical trial. Whether the outcome of these asymptomatic patients who are at higher risk of a procedure is improved with CEA or CAS compared with those who are treated with aggressive risk factor control and antiplatelet therapy is uncertain. Given the substantial occurrence of adverse outcomes in both treatment groups, one must be very careful in selecting patients for a procedure, particularly if they are considered to be at increased risk of CEA or CAS because of some underlying condition.

ASYMPTOMATIC VERTEBRAL STENOSIS

In the presence of stenosis or occlusion of the proximal vertebral arteries, the cervical anastomotic network usually provides efficient alternative blood flow. The natural history of vertebrobasilar ischemia that results from asymptomatic vertebral artery occlusive disease is relatively benign, and corrective surgical or endovascular procedure in the proximal or distal portions of the artery is relatively risky; thus, medical management that includes aggressive atherosclerosis risk factor control and antiplatelet therapy is the treatment of choice. Alternative treatment approaches, such as anticoagulants, endovascular procedures, and open operation, are considerations in patients with symptomatic vertebrobasilar stenosis, as outlined in Chapters 12, 13, and 16.

Hypertension

Hypertension (systolic or diastolic) is an important risk factor for ischemic and hemorrhagic stroke in male and female individuals at all ages. **Stage 2 hypertension** (blood pressure [BP] ≥160/100 mm Hg) increases the risk for stroke to approximately four times that of normotensive individuals (BP <140/90 mm Hg). **Stage 1 hypertension** (BP 140 to 159/90 to 99 mm Hg) increases the risk for stroke to approximately two times that of normotensive individuals. Atherosclerosis occurs with increased frequency and severity in patients with chronic hypertension. However, the more specific nonatherosclerotic cerebrovascular abnormality in patients with sustained hypertension consists of lipohyalinosis and fibrinoid necrosis with microaneurysm formation in penetrating arterioles. Such lesions may lead to lacunar infarction or intracerebral hemorrhage. It is important to recognize that several modifiable lifestyle components can affect BP favorably, including diet (low sodium, low fat, low cholesterol, low calorie, high fruits and vegetables), weight/body mass index (obesity is a risk factor), exercise (particularly aerobic exercise), limited alcohol intake (2 oz or less per day), and stress reduction. These components should be a staple of hypertension treatment even if medication is required.

Hypertension is also a highly prevalent abnormality. As many as 50 million Americans have elevated BP (systolic BP [SBP] ≥140 mm Hg or diastolic BP [SBP] ≥90 mm Hg) or are taking antihypertensive drugs. Reducing BP to a normal range produces a corresponding decline in the occurrence of stroke. Although most ischemic strokes occur in individuals with prehypertension or stage 1 hypertension, the incidence of both ischemic or hemorrhagic stroke is reduced substantially by treatment of hypertension. A currently used classification (Seventh Report of the Joint National Committee on Detection, Evaluation and Treatment of High Blood Pressure, 2003) categorizes BP levels into four groups: normal level, SBP <120 and DBP <90 mm Hg; prehypertension (not a disease category), SBP 120 to 139 mm Hg or DBP 80 to 89 mm Hg; stage 1 hypertension, SBP 140 to 159 mm Hg or DBP 90 to 99 mm Hg; and stage 2 hypertension, SBP ≥160 mm Hg or DBP ≥100 mm Hg. The key messages of this report are as follows: (1) In those who are older than 50 years, SBP of >140 mm Hg is a more important cardiovascular disease (CVD) risk factor than DBP; (2) beginning at 115/75 mm Hg, CVD risk doubles for each increment of 20/10 mm Hg; (3) those who are normotensive at 55 years of age will have a 90% lifetime risk for developing hypertension; (4) prehypertensive individuals (SBP 120 to 139 mm Hg or DBP 80 to 89 mm Hg) require health-promoting lifestyle modifications to prevent the progressive rise in BP and CVD; (5) for uncomplicated hypertension, thiazide diuretic should be used in drug treatment for most, either alone or combined with drugs from other classes (angiotensin-converting enzyme inhibitors [ACE-I], angiotensin-receptor blockers, beta-blockers, calcium channel blockers); (6) regardless of therapy or care, hypertension will be controlled only if patients are motivated to stay on their treatment plan. Positive experiences, trust in the clinician, and empathy improve patient motivation and satisfaction. In more than two thirds of individuals, hypertension cannot be controlled on one drug and will require two or more antihypertensive agents selected from different drug classes; therefore, a combination therapy of two or three drugs (one of which usually will be a thiazide diuretic) is commonly needed to achieve optimal BP levels. The committee recommends considering initiation of combination therapy in some patients with stage 2 hypertension ($\geq$160/100 mm Hg). There is evidence that lowering BP to optimal goal levels seems to be more important than specific drug selection. For most people, a reasonable goal of treatment to lower BP involves stabilization of SBP at or below 120 to 140 mm Hg and DBP at or below 80 to 90 mm Hg. However, on the basis of more recent linear associations between BP levels and the risk for stroke, many experts recommend lowering and maintaining BP at levels of 120/80 mm Hg or below.

In selecting drugs and providing long-term drug therapy, the physician should try to prescribe the fewest number of drugs in the smallest effective amount and lowest frequency. In this respect, monotherapy (especially for initial treatment) is desirable, but if monotherapy proves ineffective even after the dose is increased to or near maximal levels (usually after 1 to 3 months), then combination therapy may help (if a diuretic is not chosen as the first drug, then it may be useful as a second-step agent). Initial pharmacologic therapy of patients with primary hypertension without target-organ changes or with cardiovascular disorders usually includes beta-adrenergic blocking drugs, angiotensin-converting enzyme inhibitors (ACE-I), calcium antagonists, or diuretics. The initial therapy of patients with bilateral renal arterial disease, stenosis in an artery to a solitary kidney, or renal insufficiency may be loop diuretics. For these patients, two or more antihypertensive medications should be considered to achieve goal BP (<140/90 mm Hg or <130/80 mm Hg). In other clinical situations, centrally acting alpha$_2$ agonists, peripheral-acting adrenergic antagonists, or direct vasodilators may be used as initial agents.

In clinical trials, antihypertensive therapy has been associated with reductions in stroke incidence averaging 35% to 40%; myocardial infarction, 20% to 25%; and heart failure, >50%. No specific agent has proven to be clearly superior to all others for stroke protection, and there is evidence that initiating and maintaining BP reduction for stroke prevention is a more important issue than choice of initial agent.

Beta-adrenergic blockers are common first-line agents that are well tolerated and available in many forms. They are especially indicated in young patients with "hyperkinetic" circulations, but they are relatively or absolutely contraindicated in patients with congestive heart failure, asthma, chronic bronchitis, bronchospasm, bradycardia (sinus rate <60 beats per minute), heart block, sick sinus syndrome, insulin-dependent diabetes mellitus, administration of monoamine oxidase inhibitors (mainly used in psychiatry for the treatment of depressive disorders and in neurology for the treatment of Parkinson's disease), and dyslipidemia. (In patients with hyperlipidemia, labetalol or cardioselective beta$_s$-blockers such as atenolol, metoprolol, and acebutolol may be used.) The most common side effects of beta-adrenergic blockers are heart failure, bronchospasm, Raynaud's phenomenon (episodic vasoconstriction of arteries and arterioles of the fingers, toes, and sometimes the face brought on by cold or emotional stimuli), depression, fatigue, and hypotension.

ACE-I (benazepril, captopril, cilazapril, enalapril, fosinopril, lisinopril, perindopril, quinapril, ramipril, and spirapril) are relatively contraindicated in patients with renal failure (reduction of dose is required) and may cause hyperkalemia in patients with renal impairment or in those who are receiving potassium-sparing agents. Side effects (chronic cough, urticarial rash, loss of taste, angioedema, proteinuria, fever, leukopenia, pancytopenia, and acute renal failure in bilateral renal artery stenosis) are uncommon. Captopril is especially indicated for the treatment of resistant hypertension and hypertension associated with renal artery stenosis.

Angiotensin II antagonists (AIIAs; candesartan, eprosartan, irbesartan, losartan, olmesartan, telmisartan, valsartan) are contraindicated in patients with hypersensitivity to any component of the drugs as well as in pregnancy and lactation. Possible side effects include changes in renal function (in hypertensive patients with severe renal impairment or renal artery stenosis, periodic monitoring of serum potassium and creatinine levels should be considered). Special caution is indicated in patients who have hemodynamically relevant aortic or mitral valve stenosis or obstructive hypertrophic cardiomyopathy and in patients with intravascular volume depletion (correction of hypovolemia should precede initiation of the treatment with AIIAs). AIIAs are especially indicated in patients who are intolerant to ACE-Is (as a result of, for example, cough and renal dysfunction observed in approximately 20% of patients who receive ACE-I), can be used in patients with renal failure (caution is required in severe impaired renal function: creatinine clearance <30 mL/min/1.73 m^2 body surface area), and usually do not require initial dose adjustment in elderly patients.

Some **calcium channel blockers** are available in extended-release forms, allowing once-daily therapy (diltiazem, verapamil, amlodipine, felodipine, and nifedipine), whereas others generally are taken twice daily (isradipine) or thrice daily (nicardipine and nifedipine). Among these drugs, dihydropyridines (amlodipine, felodipine, isradipine, nicardipine, and nifedipine) may cause dizziness, headache, flushing, peripheral edema, and tachycardia, whereas the side effects of others (diltiazem and verapamil) are symptomatic reduction in heart rate and heart block.

Distal potassium-losing diuretics (hydrochlorothiazide, chlorthalidone, and metolazone), **loop diuretics** (furosemide, bumetanide, and ethacrynic acid), and **distal potassium-sparing diuretics** (spironolactone, amiloride, and triamterene) are particularly effective in elderly patients. Among these diuretics, thiazides (hydrochlorothiazide, chlorthalidone, and metolazone) have the longest duration of action and so are preferable over the others, but they also may cause hypokalemia, hyperglycemia, and hyperuricemia, which restrict the use of high doses in some patients. Distal potassium-losing diuretics are contraindicated in patients with diabetes mellitus, hyperuricemia, and primary aldosteronism; adverse effects include potassium depletion, hyperglycemia, hyperuricemia, dermatitis, and purpura. Contraindications for loop diuretics are hyperuricemia and primary aldosteronism; they also may produce potassium depletion, hyperuricemia, nausea, vomiting, and diarrhea. Distal potassium-sparing diuretics should be avoided in patients with renal failure. Among the side effects of spironolactone are hyperkalemia, diarrhea, gynecomastia, and menstrual irregularities; amiloride and triamterene may produce hyperkalemia, nausea, vomiting, leg cramps, nephrolithiasis, and gastrointestinal disturbances.

Less commonly used antihypertensive drugs include **centrally acting alpha$_2$-agonists** (clonidine, guanabenz, methyldopa, guanfacine, and clonidine patch), **peripheral-acting adrenergic antagonists** (guanadrel, guanethidine, rauwolfia serpentina, and reserpine), and **direct vasodilators** (hydralazine and minoxidil). None of the **centrally acting** alpha$_2$-**agonists** should be withdrawn abruptly because of possible rebound hypertension, and they should be avoided in patients who may not comply with treatment. Among these agents, only methyldopa is contraindicated in patients with pheochromocytoma or active hepatic disease (intravenous infusion) and during administration of monoamine oxidase inhibitors; however, all of these agents may cause postural hypotension. In addition, clonidine and guanabenz may produce drowsiness, insomnia, or lupus-like syndrome. Side effects of methyldopa include sedation, fatigue, diarrhea, impaired ejaculation, fever, chronic hepatitis, acute ulcerative colitis, gynecomastia, and lactation. Adverse reactions of guanfacine include dry mouth, sedation, asthenia, dizziness, constipation, and impotence.

Peripheral-acting adrenergic antagonists may cause serious orthostatic and exercise-induced hypotension and are contraindicated in patients with pheochromocytoma and during administration of monoamine oxidase inhibitors. Also, rauwolfia alkaloids should be avoided in patients with peptic ulcer or depression, and guanethidine and guanadrel should not be used for patients with severe coronary artery disease or cerebrovascular insufficiency.

Direct vasodilators should be taken with diuretics and beta-adrenergic blockers because of their side effects of fluid retention and reflex tachycardia. Hydralazine may cause headache, anorexia, vomiting, diarrhea, and lupus-like syndrome, and minoxidil may produce hair growth on the face and body, coarsening of facial features, and pericardial effusion.

Treatment of malignant hypertension (very severe hypertension but without severe symptoms or progressive target-organ complications and severe perioperative hypertension) must be provided within 24 hours and usually includes intravenous or intramuscular administration of rapidly acting antihypertensive drugs such as direct vasodilators, adrenergic inhibitors, calcium or ganglionic blockers, or sympatholytic agents.

Dyslipidemia

To illustrate the heterogeneity that exists among various dyslipidemias, some of the different primary (inherited) and secondary disorders associated with each lipoprotein phenotype are outlined in Table 27-1. Major apolipoproteins associated with chylomicrons and very-low-density lipoproteins (VLDL) are B, C, and E; with low-density lipoproteins (LDL), B; and with high-density lipoproteins (HDL), A-I and A-II.

Causes of secondary hyperlipidemia must be sought and treated. **Secondary hypercholesterolemia** may be associated with hypothyroidism, nephrotic syndrome, obstructive liver disease, acute intermittent porphyria, pregnancy, anorexia nervosa, and certain drugs (such as thiazide diuretics, retinoids, glucocorticoids, cyclosporine, progestins, and androgens). **Secondary hypertriglyceridemia** may result from diabetes mellitus, obesity, alcohol intake, excess intake of refined sugars, chronic renal failure, myocardial infarction, infections (bacterial, viral), systemic lupus erythematosus, dysglobulinemia, glycogen storage disease (type I), lipodystrophy, nephrotic syndrome, bulimia, autoimmune disorders, pregnancy, and certain drugs (such as beta-adrenergic blockers, retinoids, and estrogens). The most common causes of **secondary combined hyperlipidemia** include hypothyroidism; nephrotic syndrome; chronic renal failure; liver disease; Werner's syndrome; acromegaly; and certain drugs, such as thiazide diuretics, glucocorticoids, and retinoids.

Blood lipid abnormalities (particularly elevated levels of LDL cholesterol; low levels of HDL, HDL_2, and HDL cholesterol; and high levels of fasting triglycerides), which contribute to craniocervical atherosclerosis, are important risk factors for ischemic stroke (more in Western societies than in Asian populations). There is also limited evidence of an inverse association between serum cholesterol values and the risk for intracerebral hemorrhage or subarachnoid hemorrhage. Correction of these and other lipid abnormalities that lead to atherosclerosis is expected to be beneficial primarily for the prevention of atherosclerotic ischemic stroke.

Therapy for lipid disorders must be individualized and includes dietary changes (the basic and preferred initial step for most patients), maintenance of ideal body weight, aerobic exercise, and pharmacologic agents. A decade or two ago, most cardiologists and other clinicians accepted a total cholesterol value of <200 or even 240 mg/dl as a reasonable target for patients with or without symptomatic atherosclerosis. In recent years, the primary goal of blood lipid management has been to get the LDL cholesterol level <160 mg per dl if one or no risk factor is present; LDL cholesterol <130 mg per dl if two or more risk factors are present and 10-year absolute risk for cardiovascular disease and stroke is <20%; or LDL cholesterol <100 mg per dl if two or more risk factors are present and 10-year absolute risk for cardiovascular disease and stroke is ≥20% or if the patient

Table 27-1. Classification of primary and secondary blood lipid disorders

Group (Fredrickson Phenotype)	Lipoprotein in Excess	Primary Dyslipidemias			Secondary Dyslipidemias		
		Typical Lipid Range			Typical Lipid Range		
		Total Cholesterol (mg/dl)	Total Triglyceride (mg/dl)	Most Common Causes	Total Cholesterol (mg/dl)	Total Triglyceride (mg/dl)	Most Common Causes
I	Chylomicrons	300–500	5000–6000	LPL or apoprotein C-II deficiency	300–400	3000–6000	Systemic lupus erythematosus
IIA	LDL	350–400	<250	Familial (heterozygote) hypercholesterolemia, familial defective apoprotein B, familial combined hyperlipidemia	300–400	100	Obesity, hypothyroidism, nephrotic syndrome, hepatoma
		250–325		Polygenic hypercholesterolemia			
		400–800	<250	Familial (homozygote) hypercholesterolemia			

IIB	LDL	240–350	300–1000	Familial combined hyperlipidemia Polygenic hypercholesterolemia or familial hypercholesterolemia plus familial hypertriglyceridemia	300–400	250–500	Cushing's syndrome, dysglobulinemia, acute intermittent porphyria, anorexia nervosa, Werner's syndrome
III	β-VLDL	300–450	300–1000	Familial dysbetalipoproteinemia	300–500	300–800	Dysglobulinemia
IV	VLDL	200–240	300–700	Familial combined hyperlipidemia, familial hypertriglyceridemia	200–250	300–700	Obesity, diabetes mellitus, estrogen therapy, acromegaly
V (mild)	Chylomicrons VLDL	200–300	500–1000	Familial combined hyperlipidemia plus LPL deficiency			Cushing's syndrome, acute viral hepatitis, dysglobulinemia, alcoholic hyperlipidemia, third-trimester pregnancy

(Continued)

Table 27-1. *Continued*

Group (Fredrickson Phenotype)	Lipoprotein in Excess	Primary Dyslipidemias			Secondary Dyslipidemias		
		Typical Lipid Range		Most Common Causes	Typical Lipid Range		Most Common Causes
		Total Cholesterol (mg/dl)	Total Triglyceride (mg/dl)		Total Cholesterol (mg/dl)	Total Triglyceride (mg/dl)	
V (severe)	Chylomicrons VLDL	300–1000	2000–6000	LPL deficiency Apoprotein C-II deficiency	600–800	2000–6000	Poorly controlled diabetes mellitus, estrogen therapy, alcoholic hyperlipidemia

LDL = low-density lipoprotein; LPL = lipoprotein lipase; VLDL = very-low-density lipoprotein.

has diabetes. Secondary goals (if LDL cholesterol is at goal range) are as follows: If triglycerides are >200 mg per dl, then use non-HDL cholesterol as a secondary goal; non-HDL cholesterol <190 mg per dl for one or no risk factor; non-HDL cholesterol <160 mg per dl for two or more risk factors and 10-year CVD risk ≤20%; non-HDL cholesterol <130 mg per dl for individuals with diabetes or for two or more risk factors and 10-year CVD risk >20%. Other recommended targets for therapy are triglycerides <150 mg per dl and HDL cholesterol >40 mg per dl in men and >50 mg per dl in women. Even more recently, the National Cholesterol Education Program Adult Treatment Panel revised its recommendations to advocate target LDL cholesterol levels of 70 mg per dl or less in very-high-risk patients such as those with known coronary artery disease, diabetes mellitus, the metabolic syndrome, or a recent cardiac event. This is in keeping with recent evidence that coronary atherosclerosis may continue to progress at total cholesterol levels of 200 mg per dl and that coronary atherosclerotic lesions may be stabilized or regressed by maintaining a total cholesterol level of 150 mg per dl or less and a daily cholesterol intake of <5 mg (see Appendix F).

Therefore, for general health purposes in individuals who do not have symptomatic or asymptomatic coronary or craniocervical atherosclerosis, it is recommended that, at a minimum, patients follow a low-fat diet aimed at lowering total fat and saturated fat in the diet to 30% and 10% of total calories, respectively, and restricting total cholesterol intake to <300 mg per day (see Appendix F-1). An even more healthful approach to prevention of atherosclerosis is to adopt the stricter, very-low-fat diet, an approach that is strongly recommended for patients with known symptomatic or asymptomatic coronary or craniocervical atherosclerosis (see Appendix F-2). This diet is aimed at restricting total fat intake to 10% to 20% of total calories and cholesterol intake to 5 to 10 mg per day or less.

The approach for increasing a low HDL cholesterol value includes smoking cessation, weight loss, dietary measures, and exercise. There is evidence that regular aerobic exercise done for 20 to 30 minutes three to five times per week may increase HDL cholesterol levels and improve the blood lipid profile.

Patients with isolated increases in VLDL levels usually respond well to weight reduction, avoidance of large amounts of fructose and sucrose, and restriction of ethanol. Increasing the intake of omega-9 monounsaturated fatty acids such as oleic acid (olive oils, rapeseed oil) and omega-3 fatty acids (fish oils) also may help to lower triglyceride and LDL cholesterol levels in these patients. Patients with increases in both VLDL and LDL levels should be advised to restrict the intake of cholesterol and saturated fats and to increase the intake of fiber and complex carbohydrates (beans, oat bran, and other forms of soluble fiber).

Patients with elevated LDL cholesterol levels (≥100 mg per dl) should receive appropriate dietary counseling. Patients with isolated increases in LDL levels (especially patients with familial hypercholesterolemia) often have a less dramatic response to weight loss and dietary changes. If the LDL goal is not reached after 6 months of dietary therapy, lipid-lowering drug therapy should be considered.

In recent years, several clinical trials involving HMG-CoA reductase inhibitors (statins) in patients with coronary artery disease and/or various cardiovascular risk factors with elevated or even average levels of LDL cholesterol have demonstrated substantial relative risk reductions of stroke varying from 19% to 35%. There is also some evidence that statins have important neuroprotective properties that likely attenuate the effects of ischemia on the brain vasculature and parenchyma. These benefits have led many to conclude that statins should be used routinely for secondary stroke prevention, particularly in the setting of ischemic atherosclerotic disease, and in circumstances in which LDL cholesterol levels <100 mg per dl cannot be achieved with lifestyle changes.

Other Host Factors

TRANSIENT ISCHEMIC ATTACK

Because transient ischemic attack (TIA) predisposes to stroke, its prevention (modification of lifestyle as outlined in Chapter 24 and therapy for hypertension, atherosclerosis, cardiac disease, or other cerebrovascular risk factors) and treatment (surgical, medical, or lifestyle modification) reduces the risk for subsequent cerebrovascular events. Patients must be aware that it is important to get immediate medical consultation whenever the **warning signs** of acute ischemic cerebrovascular disease occur (see Appendix E-1 and Chapter 12). Warning signs include sudden weakness or numbness of the face, arm, and leg, especially on one side of the body; sudden darkening or loss of vision, particularly in one eye; loss of speech or trouble talking or understanding speech; and sudden unexplained dizziness, unsteadiness, double vision, or sudden fall, especially along with any of the other symptoms.

The evaluation and treatment of TIA are outlined in Chapters 12 and 16.

CARDIAC DISEASE

Because cardiac diseases (particularly congestive heart failure, coronary artery disease, valvular disease, arrhythmias, and left ventricular hypertrophy seen by electrocardiography) predispose to stroke, prevention and specialized treatment of these cardiovascular contributors can be anticipated to reduce the occurrence of stroke. (The specific treatment of patients with cardiac disorders that are already causing TIA or stroke is outlined in Chapter 16.) Regarding primary prevention, smoking cessation, dietary adjustment and weight control, physical exercise, and control of hypertension and blood lipid abnormalities (in particular, reducing elevated levels of total and low-density lipoprotein cholesterol and increasing the high-density lipoprotein cholesterol fraction) may be beneficial. Aspirin, 75 to 325 mg daily, may reduce the risk for ischemic heart disease (prophylactic use of aspirin is not advisable in individuals with poorly controlled hypertension because of possible increased risk for hemorrhagic stroke). Individual decisions are required regarding therapy for specific cardiac diseases.

To prevent stroke and improve outcomes in patients with recent myocardial infarction (especially if the infarct is large; if it involves the anterior/septal ventricular wall; or if it is associated with atrial fibrillation, congestive heart failure, thrombi, or cerebral or retinal ischemic events), thrombolytic therapy followed by anticoagulant therapy is often recommended. Therapy with heparin or low-molecular-weight heparin, and may be followed by oral anticoagulant therapy (warfarin) alone (International Normalized Ratio [INR], 2.0 to 3.0). The most efficacious duration of therapy is not known. Recent data indicate that after acute myocardial infarction, patients who were treated with high-intensity oral anticoagulants

(INR 3.0 to 4.0) or aspirin with medium-intensity oral anticoagulants (INR 2.0 to 2.5), compared with those who received aspirin alone, had reductions in recurrent myocardial infarction, stroke, and death (see van Es et al. [2002] in Suggested Reading for Part V). Prior studies in one European country indicated the cost-effectiveness of oral anticoagulant therapy (see Asplund et al. [1993] in Suggested Reading for Part V). Oral anticoagulant therapy is generally followed by daily antiplatelet therapy (most commonly aspirin 75 to 325 mg).

Among **cardiac arrhythmias**, atrial fibrillation is the most powerful risk factor for embolic brain infarction. Therefore, every attempt should be made to restore sinus rhythm in appropriate cases, preferably with electric or pharmacologic cardioversion, especially if atrial fibrillation is of recent onset (<48 hours). Many issues must be considered before cardioversion is performed, such as the potential for maintaining sinus rhythm after the procedure, the benefit of cardioversion, and risk for adverse complications, including risk for systemic embolic events. The best candidates for long-term successful cardioversion are patients who have short-term atrial fibrillation with no significant atrial enlargement and with minimal coronary artery disease. Conversion of atrial fibrillation to a normal rhythm is associated with risk for embolization, which often occurs within 48 hours after conversion. Therefore, anticoagulant therapy with heparin should usually precede cardioversion, especially in patients with associated mitral valve disease, cardiac enlargement, congestive heart failure, or previous embolization. People without previous heart disease and embolization may be exempted from such heparin therapy if transesophageal echocardiogram shows no thrombus in the heart. If acute cardioversion has failed, it is usually recommended to repeat cardioversion after 3 to 4 weeks of anticoagulation with warfarin. If sinus rhythm is not restored, long-term stroke prevention through anticoagulation with warfarin or aspirin or other antiplatelet drugs should be considered. The antithrombotic therapy should be combined with long-term pharmacologic maintenance of sinus rhythm.

The decision should be made on the basis of data available from clinical trials, although some questions persist in regard to safety of anticoagulation in patients who are older than 75 years and in regard to the efficacy of aspirin in some subgroups. Lone atrial fibrillation indicates patients without any associated clinical risk factors such as previous stroke or TIA, diabetes mellitus, hypertension, congestive heart failure, coronary artery disease, or valvular disease such as mitral valve disease or prosthetic valves. Patients younger than 60 years without clinical risk factors have a low risk for stroke and require no treatment or treatment with aspirin. In patients aged 60 to 75 years, those with lone atrial fibrillation may be treated with aspirin; for patients older than 75 years, anticoagulation should be used (warfarin; INR 2.0 to 3.0), unless contraindications exist, with close monitoring of INR. In patients with atrial fibrillation and any risk factors, chronic anticoagulation with warfarin (INR 2.0 to 3.0) should be used, although, again, warfarin must be used cautiously in patients who are older than 75 years (the recommended target INR in these patients is approximately 2.0).

In pregnant patients, subcutaneously administered heparin is often given throughout pregnancy, or, alternatively, warfarin is administered only during the second and third trimesters up until gestation week 37, at which time heparin again should be given (see Chapter 22).

Cardiac surgery of many types also is associated with an increased risk for cerebral ischemia. Improvements in the pump oxygenator and surgical techniques have helped to reduce the occurrence of multifocal ischemic syndromes. Anticoagulant therapy may reduce the frequency of postoperative embolization, particularly in patients with prosthetic mitral valves. The protective value of alternative or supplemental treatment with antiplatelet agents and neuroprotective drugs has also been suggested.

In patients with **rheumatic fever**, treatment with salicylates, corticosteroids, and antibiotics (benzathine penicillin G, intramuscularly or orally, or erythromycin orally) should be instituted. Antibiotic prophylaxis (usually with a monthly intramuscular injection of 1.2 million U of benzathine penicillin G or oral penicillin, 200,000 units, twice daily) generally is advocated for children with one or more episodes of acute rheumatic fever and should be given through the school years until the patient is 18 years of age. For individuals with onset of rheumatic fever after the age of 18, antibiotic prophylaxis is suggested for a minimum of 5 years after the episode. Antibiotic prophylaxis is also generally recommended for patients with a history of rheumatic heart disease, especially pregnant patients and for procedures associated with bacteremia, to prevent **infective endocarditis.** The risk for infective endocarditis is also increased in women who are taking oral contraceptive pills.

In patients with **aortic stenosis or regurgitation** or in patients with **mitral stenosis or regurgitation**, an appropriate surgical procedure (aortic balloon valvuloplasty or valve replacement) should be considered. The most efficacious treatment to prevent stroke in patients with **mitral valve prolapse** associated with ischemic cerebral or retinal events is controversial. Asymptomatic mitral valve prolapse occurs in approximately 5% of the population, with a marked preponderance in women. Thus, it is difficult to define the causative relationship of mitral valve prolapse with stroke of unknown cause. In general, in patients with no other cause despite a comprehensive evaluation for a cerebral ischemic event that may be embolic in nature, mitral valve prolapse may be managed with at least short-term warfarin anticoagulation followed by antiplatelet therapy. Patients with more severe mitral regurgitation may require valve replacement.

For prevention of ischemic stroke in patients with **prosthetic heart valves**, warfarin anticoagulation typically is used, and dipyridamole may be added for patients who have ongoing thromboembolic events while receiving warfarin. A combination of warfarin and aspirin typically is not recommended because it prolongs bleeding time and increases hemorrhage risk, although the combination sometimes is necessary for patients with recurrent symptoms, despite an increase in INR and additional treatment with dipyridamole.

Although the benefit of antibiotic prophylaxis against **infective endocarditis** has not been clearly proved, most cardiologists recommend prophylaxis for patients with significant valvular disease, particularly patients with prosthetic valves. To prevent ischemic stroke in patients with **cardiomyopathy**, treatment that includes bed rest, digitalis, diuretics, and sodium restriction is recommended. Anticoagulants should be used if any embolic complications have occurred, if definite mural thrombi are seen on echocardiography, or if the ejection fraction decreases to <30%.

DIABETES MELLITUS

Typically, patients have more than one risk factor for cardiac disease. Clustering of risk factors is usually manifested as hypertension, truncal (central) obesity, dyslipidemia, and insulin resistance. Several factors have an impact on insulin resistance, including weight, a sedentary lifestyle, hyperglycemia, and multiple medications.

There are two major types of diabetes. In type 1 diabetes (insulin-dependent diabetes mellitus), onset typically occurs before the person is 30 years of age, and the diabetes may be associated with ketoacidosis, which often occurs in lean individuals with a dependence on exogenous insulin. In type 2 diabetes (non-insulin-dependent diabetes mellitus), individuals typically are older, most are obese, and ketoacidosis usually does not develop in the absence of exogenous insulin. Diagnosis is usually made on the basis of a fasting glucose level (≥140 mg per dl) and typical clinical symptoms such as polyuria, polyphagia, and polydipsia, often with weight loss. Hypoglycemic therapy (if not urgent) is usually started with diet and exercise. Second-step treatment usually includes oral hypoglycemic agents (sulfonylureas and/or metformin with ancillary use of acarbose and thiazolidinediones), and third-step therapy is insulin. Goals in diabetes management are normal fasting plasma glucose (<110 mg per dl) and near normal HbA1c (<7%).

Vascular complications include accelerated atherosclerosis in large vessels and microangiopathy, most commonly involving retinal and renal vasculature. Diabetes mellitus is a risk factor for stroke and, in particular, for ischemic stroke (cerebral infarction). Because diabetes is often associated with other risk factors for atherosclerosis, such as hypertension and dyslipidemia, patients with diabetes must be followed closely for co-occurring processes and treated aggressively (for example, blood pressure should be lowered to <120/80 mm Hg and LDL cholesterol to <100 mg/dL). Treatment of the diabetes to bring the glucose level into a normal range may also decrease the occurrence of stroke.

Unruptured
Intracranial Aneurysms

Unruptured intracranial aneurysms (UIAs) constitute a significant public health issue. Several large autopsy studies have reported a wide range in the overall frequency of intracranial aneurysms, varying from 0.2% to 9.9%. More recent prospective angiographic and autopsy studies indicate an overall frequency of 2% to 4%, suggesting that among the U.S. population, approximately 6 to 12 million people have or will have intracranial aneurysms.

The magnitude of the problem of UIAs is increasing as a result, at least in part, of the increasing age of the population, because these lesions generally develop with increasing age. In addition, in recent years, the widespread use of computed tomography (CT) and magnetic resonance imaging (MRI) has greatly increased the numbers of aneurysms that are discovered incidentally. The quality of these techniques has also improved, including magnetic resonance angiography (MRA) and computed tomographic angiography (CTA) studies.

Besides the fortuitous discovery of UIAs on CT, CTA, MRI, or MRA studies that are done for unrelated reasons, UIAs may be discovered when a physician investigates subarachnoid hemorrhage (SAH) from a different source, such a separate aneurysm or an arteriovenous malformation (AVM), or investigates aneurysmal symptoms other than rupture. These symptoms include the following:

1. Cranial nerve palsies (most commonly cranial nerves II, III, IV, and VI)
2. Compression of other central nervous system structures (including the brainstem and the pituitary)
3. Persistent and often focal vascular headaches that are usually of relatively recent onset and new character
4. Focal ischemic symptoms from distal embolization of aneurysmal clot
5. Seizure foci resulting from impingement on supratentorial brain structures

Headache may be caused by a sudden dilation of the aneurysm or by chronic compression of pain-sensitive structures, such as the ophthalmic and maxillary divisions of the trigeminal nerve. Such headaches are usually persistent and focal, corresponding to the location of the aneurysm. They may also be associated with cranial nerve palsies. However, sudden and unusually severe headache associated with nausea or vomiting is always suspicious for a warning leak (or minor SAH) from an intracranial aneurysm. In these cases, CT or MRI studies should be obtained, and if negative and no signs of mass effect exist, then lumbar puncture should be performed.

When decisions about management of UIAs need to be made, it is very important to recognize that ruptured intracranial aneurysms and UIAs constitute distinctly different clinical entities and need to be considered and treated as such. Previously ruptured intracranial aneurysms have a much greater likelihood of subsequent growth and rupture than do those that are previously unruptured. Furthermore, recent studies have confirmed that the natural history and behavior of UIAs cannot be extrapolated by looking at characteristics of patients with aneurysms that are discovered after rupture. Much confusion regarding this issue has related to not recognizing the major differences between the following two questions: (1) What is the probability of a ruptured aneurysm being a certain size? (2) What is the probability of future rupture of a given-sized aneurysm discovered before rupture? The second of these questions is relevant to the clinical treatment of patients with UIAs. The key issue is that little is learned about the natural history of referring to characteristics of patients with ruptured aneurysms. This statement applies not only to aneurysm size but also to location. Available information suggests that most aneurysms that will rupture do so at the time they form or soon after and that the critical size for rupture is lower for aneurysms that rupture early.

Among patients with UIAs, there should be a distinction between patients without a history of SAH (group 1) and those with a history of SAH from a different source, most commonly another aneurysm that was successfully repaired (group 2).

Epidemiologic information from multiple vantage points suggests that most intracranial aneurysms that develop never rupture. It therefore is desirable to identify which unruptured aneurysms are at greatest risk for subsequent rupture when deciding which ones to repair. Optimal medical care of patients with UIAs also involves predicting which patients will have the greatest likelihood of success and the lowest complication rates from repairing UIAs and reconciling these data with the natural history data involving UIAs and with the patients' informed perspective regarding their desire to have the aneurysm treated.

Following a comprehensive publication of Phase I results of the International Study of Unruptured Intracranial Aneurysms (ISUIA) (NEJM, 1998), an expert panel convened by the American Heart Association concluded that "in consideration of the apparent low risk of hemorrhage from incidental small (<10 mm) aneurysms in patients without previous SAH, treatment rather than observation cannot be generally advocated." Other authors came to similar conclusions on the basis of cost-utility analysis and evidence-based medial approaches.

More recent ISUIA information from Phases I and II (Lancet, 2003) includes a large prospective natural history cohort and extensive outcomes information regarding open surgery and endovascular repair of UIAs. This newest ISUIA data generally support the earlier recommendations about patient management but allows a more individualized, detailed, and sophisticated assessment of the risks of natural history versus the risks of surgical and/or endovascular repair based upon more than aneurysm size. Nonetheless, for group 1 patients with aneurysms <7 mm in diameter, it is very unlikely that the natural history of these lesions can be improved, particularly in older patients and in those with aneurysms in the anterior circulation. On the basis of current data, it is not possible to establish that a family history of UIA or SAH increases risk in this group. It is important to note that available natural history studies, including ISUIA, include very few symptomatic patients with small UIAs, particularly those with acute or changing symptoms and virtually no patients with observed aneurysmal growth; these rare circumstances may constitute exceptions to the broader principle. For most other patients with UIA, more substantial rupture rates apply according to aneurysmal size and location, but this does not necessarily suggest that repair is advisable or desirable. It is very important to compare size-, site-, and group-specific natural history rates with size-, site-, and age-specific morbidity and mortality associated with UIA repair (Table 29-1; Figures 29-1 to 29-3). Higher natural history risk is often but not invariably associated with higher treatment morbidity and mortality.

A critical element in decision making is the age of the patient, primarily because age has a major effect on operative morbidity and mortality but relatively little effect on natural history. This effect of age is most notable in patients who are approximately 50 years and older for open surgery and approximately 70 years and older for endovascular repair.

In general, the UIA rupture risk is lowest for asymptomatic group 1 patients with UIAs <7 mm in diameter in the anterior circulation. Surgical morbidity and mortality generally are most favorable for asymptomatic patients who are younger than 50 years and have UIAs in the anterior circulation that are <24 mm in diameter and no history of ischemic cerebrovascular disease. Endovascular morbidity and mortality may be less age dependent, and this appears to favor endovascular procedures,

Table 29-1.   Five-year cumulative rupture rates according to UIA size, location, and patient group, among patients in the unoperated cohort ($N = 1692$)[a]

Aneurysm Location	No. of Patients	Aneurysm Size				
		<7 mm		7–12 mm	13–24 mm	≥25 mm
		Group 1[b]	Group 2[c]			
Cavernous	210	0.0	0.0	0.0	3.0	6.4
AC/MC/IC	1037	0.0	1.5	2.6	14.5	40.0
Post-P comm	445	2.5	3.4	14.5	18.4	50.0

AC = anterior communicating or anterior cerebral artery; Cavernous = cavernous carotid artery; IC = internal carotid artery (not cavernous carotid artery); MC = middle cerebral artery; Post-P comm = vertebrobasilar, posterior cerebral arterial system, or the posterior communicating artery; UIA = unruptured intracranial aneurysm.
[a]Values are percentages unless indicated otherwise.
[b]Patients had no history of subarachnoid hemorrhage (SAH).
[c]Patients had a history of SAH from a separate aneurysm.
Reprinted from *Lancet*. 2003;362:103–110, with permission from Elsevier.

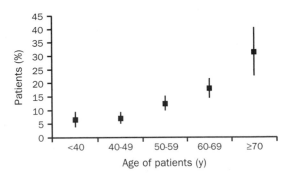

Figure 29-1.   Poor surgical outcomes (death, Rankin score of 3 to 5, or impaired cognitive status) at 1 year by patient age. Error bars represent 95% confidence intervals. Reprinted from *Lancet*. 2003;362:103–110, with permission from Elsevier.

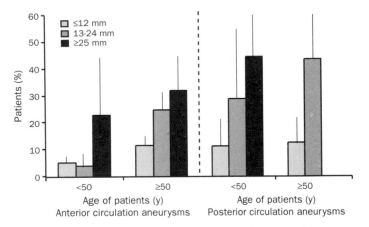

Figure 29-2.   Poor surgical outcomes (death, Rankin score of 3 to 5, or impaired cognitive status) at 1 year by patient age and aneurysm site and size. Error bars represent 95% confidence intervals. Reprinted from *Lancet*. 2003;362:103–110, with permission from Elsevier.

particularly in patients who are between the ages of 50 and 70 years. It is also important to consider the immediate versus long-term risk with regard to treatment effectiveness and durability. This issue reinforces the need for long-term follow-up in patients after open surgery and endovascular procedures to assess not only the immediate and short-term complications but also long-term effectiveness and durability.

Routine screening for UIAs with noninvasive tests such as CT/CTA or MRI/MRA in asymptomatic patients would be expected to have a very low yield in the general population,

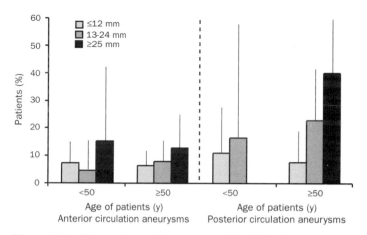

Figure 29-3. Poor endovascular outcomes (death, Rankin score of 3 to 5, or impaired cognitive status) at 1 year by patient age and aneurysm site and size. Error bars represent 95% confidence intervals. Reprinted from *Lancet.* 2003;362:103–110, with permission from Elsevier.

because although aneurysms are often prevalent at autopsy, they generally develop with increasing age. Even among patients with other predisposing medical conditions, such as autosomal dominant polycystic kidney disease, routine screening for UIAs may have a very low yield, particularly in younger individuals. Among those with autosomal dominant polycystic kidney disease, noninvasive screening is recommended typically in certain subgroups of patients, namely those with a family history of intracranial aneurysm or SAH. Also, in families without clear inherited conditions that predispose to aneurysm or SAH, if two or more family members have intracranial aneurysm or SAH, screening of the first-degree relatives with either MRA or CTA is usually considered. Although screening usually is not performed in families with only one member affected by SAH or aneurysm, some family members may request screening for reassurance; in such circumstances, noninvasive screening is usually performed with either MRA or CTA.

Among patients with both UIA and intracranial AVM, the UIA usually will be located within the feeding system of the AVM. These UIAs seem to be more prone to future growth and rupture than are UIAs in general. When intervention is contemplated, repairing the UIA before addressing the AVM is generally recommended, especially in patients with large UIAs, because sudden changes in the hemodynamics of the feeding system may predispose to aneurysmal rupture.

Regarding candidates for carotid endarterectomy (CEA) who also have UIAs, the sudden change of hemodynamics in the distal carotid artery system from correcting a pressure-significant stenosis may predispose to enlargement or rupture of a previously unruptured intracranial aneurysm. Conversely, among patients with severe carotid artery stenosis, clipping of a UIA could increase the risk for perioperative ischemic stroke with decreases in perfusion pressure during anesthesia or other factors related to increased thrombogenesis. Although available information is too sparse to allow definitive conclusions, it appears that CEA should be approached with somewhat increased caution in patients with UIAs, particularly in patients with UIAs 7 mm or larger in diameter in the ipsilateral carotid artery system and in patients with UIAs and a history of SAH from a separate aneurysm.

When repair of UIAs is considered, it is noteworthy that evidence suggests substantially lower complication rates are associated with institutions and physicians treating a larger number of these patients each year. Therefore, identifying physicians and institutions with substantial ongoing experience with these procedures is very important. For those who have UIAs and are not treated with coiling, clipping, or other intervention, UIAs generally are monitored annually with MRA or CTA for 2 to 3 years and then every 2 to 5 years thereafter if the UIAs are clinically and radiographically stable. Patients are also generally advised to avoid smoking (and passive smoke), heavy alcohol consumption, stimulant medications and drugs, and excessive straining and Valsalva maneuvers that result in major acute increases in blood pressure. Daily physical activities usually need not be altered. Although there are many other medical reasons to treat chronic hypertension, data from ISUIA and other studies indicate that chronic hypertension likely has little or no effect on aneurysmal development or future rupture of UIAs.

Unruptured Intracranial Vascular Malformations

Intracranial vascular malformations such as arteriovenous malformation (AVM), cavernous malformation (CM), capillary telangiectasia, venous malformation, and vein of Galen malformation are congenital developmental abnormalities (except most dural and extracerebral AVMs and some CMs may be acquired) and usually take many years before they become clinically apparent. The presentation and the natural history depend on the vascular malformation subtype, location, size, and other characteristics. Some of these lesions can cause serious neurologic signs and symptoms, whereas others are typically asymptomatic and are benign.

Arteriovenous malformations are congenital and are the most commonly clinically recognized form of intracranial vascular malformation. Symptoms of unruptured AVMs often appear in adolescence or later (most frequently in the third and fourth decades of life) and usually produce intracranial hemorrhage (intracerebral is most common; subarachnoid hemorrhage (SAH) and intraventricular hemorrhage are less common), recurrent unilateral headache (which may resemble migraine), focal or generalized seizures, a pulsatile noise in the head called pulsatile tinnitus, progressing neurologic deficits, or, rarely, transient focal neurologic symptoms that mimic transient ischemic attacks. Not infrequently, they are discovered fortuitously, detected on cross-sectional brain imaging that is performed for an unrelated reason. AVMs are occasionally associated with a cranial or orbital bruit. They may not be seen on computed tomography (CT) imaging without contrast, except calcification or low attenuation may be noted. Magnetic resonance imaging (MRI) is very sensitive to the detection of AVMs, with signal voids on T1 and T2 imaging and often some degree of hemosiderin. MRA provides more information regarding the nature of the feeding arteries and draining veins, but an arteriogram typically is needed to evaluate the AVM in detail and aids in defining the optimal management.

Cavernous malformations may be detected on MRI scanning, often with the cavernoma causing no neurologic signs or symptoms. When they do present with symptoms, seizures are most common, including focal or generalized seizures. Focal neurologic deficits or nonspecific headache may also occur. Symptoms are caused by small hemorrhages that occur within the lesion or at the periphery, although significant intraparenchymal hemorrhage is rare. CT with contrast enhancement may demonstrate a characteristic mulberry-shaped lesion with calcification, although MRI typically is necessary to detect these angiographically occult lesions. MRI demonstrates a mixed increased and decreased signal lesion on both T1 and T2 imaging, with surrounding hemosiderin. They may be multiple, particularly in the familial cases.

Capillary telangiectasias are anomalies of capillary-sized vessels, which characteristically are located in the brainstem or the cerebellum. They are usually asymptomatic (when associated with the syndrome of Rendu-Osler-Weber, they may be clinically recognized elsewhere in the body) and have little risk for hemorrhagic complications.

Intracranial **venous malformations** are the most common vascular malformation noted on autopsy and are usually asymptomatic. On occasion, they may cause seizures, focal neurologic symptoms, or trigeminal neuralgia. Rarely intracranial hemorrhage occurs, although in most cases, some other vascular malformation type—usually a CM—is found to be occurring along with the venous malformation and is the cause of the hemorrhage. They may be seen on CT with contrast as a enlarged draining vein and on MRI as a flow void, sometimes with the radial "caput medusa" appearance. On arteriography (venous phase), they are represented by a deep prominent vein of varying size and may be associated with the caput medusa pattern. Asymptomatic venous malformations have a benign prognosis, rarely causing hemorrhage or other neurologic symptoms

Dural arteriovenous fistulae (DAVF) or dural AVMs are vascular malformations in one of the major venous sinuses. These typically acquired lesions present with clinical symptoms dependent on the site of the lesion. Lesions in the superior sagittal sinus may cause papilledema with vision loss; those in the cavernous sinus cause diplopia, exophthalmos, and vision loss; transverse/sigmoid sinus lesions may cause pulsatile tinnitus; and cortical lesions may cause seizures or neurologic deficit. Dilated veins on a CT head scan may suggest their presence, but a CT is usually normal. MRI may show the dilated veins and feeding arteries. An arteriogram is needed to characterize these lesions best and should include selective external carotid artery injection because they often receive arterial supply from the external carotid artery.

Vein of Galen malformations usually manifest with cyanosis and respiratory distress in the neonatal period, seizures and hydrocephalus in infancy, and headache and SAH in older children and adults. Scalp or face veins may be enlarged.

NATURAL HISTORY AND MANAGEMENT OF VASCULAR MALFORMATIONS

In view of this background information, doubts continue about the optimal management of patients with unruptured vascular malformations, and dogmatic statements cannot be made on the basis of current scientific knowledge. However, certain guidelines seem reasonable. All patients who have indeterminate symptoms that might suggest an intracranial vascular malformation should undergo noninvasive tests such as CT with contrast enhancement, MRI, or MRA. Conventional arteriography should be considered for the definitive diagnosis and characterization of the lesion in patients who are appropriate candidates for treatment intervention.

The decision regarding conservative or surgical treatment (including radiosurgery and endovascular embolization) of an **AVM** must be made individually on the basis of the following factors: (1) the clinical presentation and type of malformation; (2) the location, size, and anatomy of the malformation; (3) the patient's age and overall health; (4) the patient's and the physician's thorough awareness of the potential problems associated with suggested aggressive treatment; and (5) the availability of a vascular and stereotactic neurosurgeon, neuroradiologist, and radiotherapist who are experienced in the treatment of vascular malformations.

AVMs present with hemorrhage in 60% to 70% of cases. The risk for hemorrhage when they are detected before first hemorrhage is 2% to 3% per year, a risk that does not seem to decrease over time. Given this long-term annual risk for hemorrhage, the lifetime risk for hemorrhage in those with a previously unruptured AVM is approximated by the following formula: lifetime risk in percent = 105 minus the patient's age in years. Among patients who present with hemorrhage, the risk for hemorrhage is increased early, up to 6% to 12% risk during at least the first year, but decreased to the baseline hemorrhage risk by the third year after hemorrhage. After a second hemorrhage, the risk for recurrence is at least 25% during the first year.

Several potential predictors of hemorrhage may be defined at the time of AVM diagnosis. Clinically, previous hemorrhage is a very strong predictor of future hemorrhage. Periventricular and intraventricular location and small size may be of some importance. The nature of the arterial feeders and venous drainage, delineated on MRA or arteriography, also need to be considered. In the arterial system, the presence of aneurysms on the feeding arteries, including those that are very distal on the feeding arteries called intranidal aneurysms, and perforator arterial supply both may increase the risk for hemorrhage. A single draining vein, primarily deep venous drainage, and impaired venous draining seem to be important in predicting an increased risk for hemorrhage.

In general, elective surgical resection or radiosurgery should be considered before rupture, particularly in young patients who are otherwise healthy, with AVMs whose size, venous drainage, arterial supply, and location allow relatively safe excision. If a previously untreated asymptomatic unruptured AVM ruptures, if seizures that are associated with the lesion are medically intractable, if there is evidence of progressive neurologic deficit associated with an unruptured vascular malformation, or if the patient wants the reassurance of taking the risk of treatment, then appropriate intervention should also be considered. Patients with untreatable vascular malformations should be observed with recommendations to avoid taking antiplatelet or anticoagulant drugs, and those with hypertension should be advised to control their blood pressure within the normal range. Women of childbearing age should be aware that the risk for intracranial hemorrhage of previously unruptured AVM may be somewhat higher during a pregnancy, although most women complete the pregnancy without a significant problem.

When possible, total removal of an AVM surgically with or without preceding embolization is the preferred approach to treatment, especially for patients who have had recent rupture (Fig. 30-1). Generally, relatively young patients with a small AVM in the nondominant hemisphere located superficially in the frontal or temporal area are the best candidates for operation.

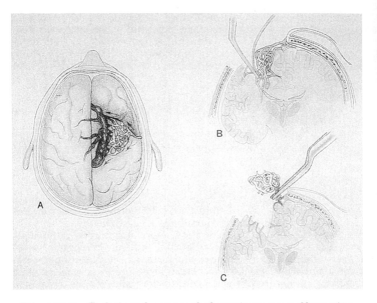

Figure 30–1. Technique for removal of arteriovenous malformation.

Very large AVMs (>6 cm in diameter) that involve more than one lobe or the posterior fossa and deep areas of the brain may be inoperable or cannot be resected at one sitting and are considered for multimodality treatment that may include surgical intervention with preceding endovascular embolization of the arterial feeders and possible radiosurgery for any residual AVM.

AVMs that are located deep within the dominant hemisphere, in the brainstem, or in other high-risk areas of the brain such as the internal capsule and the thalamus are usually considered to be at higher surgical risk because of their inaccessibility or higher risk for postoperative neurologic deficit. Even in the most experienced centers, **surgical excision** of these AVMs with or without embolization is associated with a mortality rate of 1% to 5% and a morbidity rate of 10% to 20%. In this case, **focused radiotherapy (gamma knife radiosurgery)** or **proton beam radiation** alone or after embolization of the feeders or as an adjunct to embolization and resection may be considered. Gamma knife radiotherapy may be especially effective if the nidus is no larger than 2 cm in diameter. Approximately 40% of patients have arteriographic obliteration of the lesion at 1 year after radiosurgery, 84% after 2 years, and approximately 97% after 3 years. However, intracranial bleeding may occur before obliteration of the AVM. Radiotherapy alone is less optimal for treatment of large AVMs (>3 cm in every dimension) and may result in radionecrosis of normal brain tissue with associated neurologic deficit or hydrocephalus.

Endovascular embolization, balloon or coil placement, should also be considered as a preparation for operation in patients who have a few major feeders supplying the AVM, especially for AVMs that are >2 cm in diameter, and for treatment of dural AVFs (usually excluding those involving the tentorium). Possible complications associated with endovascular procedures include intracranial hemorrhage caused by rupture of an arterial feeder and cerebral ischemia; the risk for a permanent complication is approximately 10%.

The natural history of clinically unruptured **capillary telangiectasias** is usually benign. The natural history of clinically unruptured **venous malformations** is also typically benign, and conservative management is usually indicated, unless hemorrhage, seizure disorder that is resistant to medical management, or progressive neurologic deficit occurs.

The natural history of **CMs** is dependent on presentation and lesion location. Among those who present with symptoms other than hemorrhage, the overall risk for having a clinically significant hemorrhage is <1% per year. However, if a symptomatic hemorrhage has occurred, then the risk for having another hemorrhage is approximately 5% in the next year. Location is another important issue, with deep lesions (including the brainstem, deep cerebellar, thalamus, and basal ganglia) carrying the highest risk of approximately 4% per year, compared with approximately 0.4% per year for superficial lesions. Symptomatic CMs with intractable seizure or multiple hemorrhages may lead to consideration of surgical excision. Radiosurgery typically is not used for CMs. However, that is sometimes considered for lesions causing recurrent hemorrhage and located in areas at high risk for surgical resection such as the brainstem and subcortical region. However, the efficacy of this treatment approach in arteriographically occult lesions is uncertain.

DAVF vary greatly in their natural history, based on the site and nature of the lesion. They can cause hemorrhage, and the risk is approximately 2% per year. Predictors of hemorrhage after detection include the presence of a venous varix, cortical drainage, retrograde venous drainage, and drainage into the vein of Galen. Locations that are associated with a higher risk for more serious neurologic outcome include those in the tentorium, orbital lesions, and those in the middle cranial fossa. Individuals who present with hemorrhage, seizures, or neurologic deficit are usually treated aggressively. Lesions that cause pulsatile tinnitus alone may be managed conservatively, unless the tinnitus is severe. Treatment options include surgical excision, radiosurgery, and therapeutic embolization, with surgery most often considered for cases that present with hemorrhage or other severe neurologic symptoms. In other cases, radiosurgery, sometimes followed by particulate embolization, provides the optimal management approach.

The natural course of a **vein of Galen malformation** that presents with severe cardiac failure in the first few weeks of life is invariably fatal, and therapeutic measures generally have been futile, but for older children who present with mild or none of the major complications (cardiac failure or progressive hydrocephalus) of this lesion, shunting procedures and interruption of feeding arteries may be considered.

Hematologic Disease

Sickle cell disease is an inherited disease that is characterized by the presence of an abnormal hemoglobin. Stroke (most commonly ischemic) is a major complication of **sickle cell disease**, which typically develops when a person is between the ages of 9 and 15 years but can be observed in adults as well. Cerebral infarction in sickle cell disease is associated with an occlusive vasculopathy that involves the distal intracranial segments of the cerebral arteries (usually stenosis or occlusion of the intracranial arteries of the circle of Willis, sometimes with a moyamoya disease appearance on arteriography), with documented thrombosis formation in some cases. Stroke (including silent strokes) affects approximately 40% of children with sickle cell disease. As recommended by the National Heart, Lung, and Blood Institute and the American Stroke Association, transcranial Doppler ultrasound should be used more widely in children with sickle cell disease to detect elevated blood flow velocity indicative of vessel disease and high risk for future stroke. To decrease the risk for stroke in sickle cell disease, patients should be advised to avoid excesses of unaccustomed physical exertion, hypoxia (as occurs in high altitude or with climbing), exposure to excessive heat, stress, and acute infection. A primary prevention strategy for clinical stroke using chronic blood transfusions to keep the sickle hemoglobin (Hb S) below 30% of total hemoglobin was documented recently (90% risk reduction of stroke) in the Stroke Prevention in Sickle Cell Anemia Trial. Other "anti-sickling" treatment strategies (such as hydroxyurea, "anti-endothelial" therapy, prevention of red cell dehydration) and agents such as decitabine and short-chain fatty acids are currently under investigation.

Management of **other hematologic diseases** (such as polycythemia, thrombotic thrombocytopenic purpura, dysproteinemia, thrombocythemia, leukemia) and conditions and circumstances that result in a **hypercoagulable state** (such as cancer, pregnancy, trauma, postoperative period, postpartum period, disseminated intravascular coagulation), which increases the risk for stroke, is specific to each underlying cause. (A more complete discussion of hematologic disease can be found in Chapters 16 and 17.)

SUGGESTED READING FOR PART V

Adams RJ, Brambilla DJ, Granger S, et al. STOP Study. Stroke and conversion to high risk in children screened with transcranial Doppler ultrasound during the STOP study. *Blood*. 2004;103:3689–3694.

Asplund K, Marke LA, Terent A, et al. Costs and gains in stroke prevention: European perspective. *Cerebrovasc Dis*. 1993; 3(suppl 1):34–42.

Atrial Fibrillation Investigators. Risk factors for stroke and efficacy of antithrombotic therapy in atrial fibrillation. Analysis of pooled data from five randomized controlled trials. *Arch Intern Med*. 1994;154:1449–1457.

Bailar J. Hormone-replacement therapy and cardiovascular diseases. *N Engl J Med*. 2003;349:521–522.

Baker WH, Howard VJ, Howard G, et al. Effect of contralateral occlusion on long-term efficacy of endarterectomy in the asymptomatic carotid atherosclerosis study (ACAS). ACAS Investigators. *Stroke*. 2000;31:2330–2334.

Bederson JB, Awad I, Wiebers DO, et al. Recommendations for the management of patients with unruptured intracranial aneurysms: A statement for healthcare professionals from the Stroke Council of the American Heart Association. *Circulation*. 2000;102:2300–2308; *Stroke*. 2000;31:2742–2750.

Bonita R, Duncan J, Truelsen T, et al. Passive smoking as well as active smoking increases the risk of acute stroke. Tob Control. 1999;8:156–160.

Brown RD Jr. Simple risk predictions for arteriovenous malformation hemorrhage. *Neurosurgery*. 2000;46:1024.

Brown RD Jr, Flemming KD, Meyer FB, et al. Natural history, evaluation and management of intracranial vascular malformations. *Mayo Clin Proc*. 2005;80:269–281.

Brown RD Jr, Wiebers DO, Forbes G, et al. The natural history of unruptured intracranial arteriovenous malformations. *J Neurosurg*. 1988;68:352–357.

Chobanian AV, Bakris GL, Black HR, et al. Joint National Committee on Prevention, Detection, Evaluation, and Treatment of High Blood Pressure. National Heart, Lung, and Blood Institute. National High Blood Pressure Education Program Coordinating Committee. The Seventh report of the Joint National Committee on Prevention, Detection, Evaluation, and Treatment of High Blood Pressure. *Hypertension*. 2003; 42:1206–1252; *JAMA*. 2003;289:2560–2572.

Connolly HM, Huston J III, Brown RD Jr, et al. Intracranial aneurysms in patients with coarctation of the aorta: A prospective magnetic resonance angiography study of 100 patients. *Mayo Clin Proc*. 2003;78:1491–1499.

Cushman WC, Ford CE, Cutler JA, et al. Success and predictors of blood pressure control in diverse North American settings: The antihypertensive and lipid-lowering treatment to prevent heart attack trial (ALLHAT). *J Clin Hypertens (Greenwich)*. 2002;4:393–404.

Di Bari M, Pahor M, Franse LV, et al. Dementia and disability outcomes in large hypertension trials: Lessons learned from the systolic hypertension in the elderly program (SHEP) trial. *Am J Epidemiol*. 2001;153:72–78.

Executive Committee for the Asymptomatic Carotid Atherosclerosis Study. Endarterectomy for asymptomatic carotid artery stenosis. *JAMA.* 1995;273:1421–1428.

Expert Panel on Detection, Evaluation, and Treatment of High Blood Cholesterol in Adults. Executive Summary of the Third Report of the National Cholesterol Education Program (NCEP). Expert Panel on Detection, Evaluation, and Treatment of High Blood Cholesterol in Adults. (Adult Treatment Panel III). *JAMA.* 2001;285:2486–2497.

Feigin VL. *When Lightening Strikes.* New Zealand: Harper Collins; 2003.

Feigin VL, Wiebers DO. Environmental factors and stroke: A selective review. *J Stroke Cerebrovasc Dis.* 1997;6:108–113.

Gallus AS, Baker RI, Chong BH, et al. Consensus guidelines for warfarin therapy. Recommendations from the Australasian Society of Thrombosis and Haemostasis. *Med J Aust.* 2000;172:600–605.

Gibbs GF, Huston J III, Qian Q, et al. Follow-up of intracranial aneurysms in autosomal dominant polycystic kidney disease. *Kidney Int.* 2004;65:1621–1627.

Gould KL. Reversal of coronary atherosclerosis. Clinical promise as the basis for noninvasive management of coronary artery disease. *Circulation.* 1994;90:1558–1571.

Grady D, Herrington D, Bittner V, et al. Cardiovascular disease outcomes during 6.8 years of hormone therapy: Heart and Estrogen/Progestin Replacement Study follow-up (HERS II). *JAMA.* 2002;288:49–57.

Halliday A, Mansfield A, Marro J, et al. MRC Asymptomatic Carotid Surgery Trial (ACST) Collaborative Group. Prevention of disabling and fatal strokes by successful carotid endarterectomy in patients without recent neurological symptoms: Randomised controlled trial. *Lancet.* 2004;363: 1491–1502.

Hurlen M, Abdelnoor M, Smith P, et al. Warfarin, aspirin, or both after myocardial infarction. *N Engl J Med.* 2002;347:969–974.

International Study of Unruptured Intracranial Aneurysms Investigators: Unruptured intracranial aneurysms—risk of rupture and risks of surgical intervention. *N Engl J Med.* 1998;339:1725–1733.

Kappelle LJ, Eliasziw M, Fox AJ, et al. Small, unruptured intracranial aneurysms and management of symptomatic carotid artery stenosis. North American Symptomatic Carotid Endarterectomy Trial Group. *Neurology.* 2000;55:307–309.

Kernan WN, Inzucchi SE, Viscoli CM, et al. Insulin resistance and risk for stroke. *Neurology.* 2002;59:809–815.

Krauss RM, Eckel RH, Howard B, et al. AHA Dietary Guidelines. Revision 2000: A statement for healthcare professionals from the Nutrition Committee of the American Heart Association. *Circulation.* 2000;102:2284–2299.

Lawes CM, Bennett DA, Feigin VL, et al. Blood pressure and stroke: An overview of published reviews. *Stroke.* 2004;35:1024.

Lee CD, Folsom AR, Blair SN. Physical activity and stroke risk: A meta-analysis. *Stroke.* 2003;34:2475–2481.

Lee IM, Paffenbarger RS Jr. Physical activity and stroke incidence: The Harvard Alumni Health Study. *Stroke.* 1998;29:2049–2054.

Maher CO, Piepgras DG, Brown RD Jr, et al. Cerebrovascular manifestations in 321 cases of hereditary hemorrhagic telangiectasia. *Stroke*. 2001;32:877–882.

Mast H, Young WL, Koennecke HC, et al. Risk of spontaneous haemorrhage after diagnosis of cerebral arteriovenous malformation. *Lancet*. 1997;350;1065–1068.

MRC Asymptomatic Carotid Surgery Trial (ACST) Collaborative Group. Prevention of disabling and fatal strokes by successful carotid endarterectomy in patients without recent neurological symptoms: Randomised controlled trial. *Lancet*. 2004;363:1491–1502.

Neal B, MacMahon S, Chapman N. Effects of ACE inhibitors, calcium antagonists, and other blood-pressure-lowering drugs: Results of prospectively designed overviews of randomised trials. Blood Pressure Lowering Treatment Trialists' Collaboration. *Lancet*. 2000;356:1955–1964.

Nyquist PA, Brown RD Jr, Wiebers DO, et al. Circadian and seasonal occurrence of subarachnoid hemorrhage and intracerebral hemorrhage. *Neurology*. 2001;56:190–193.

Ogilvy CS, Stieg PE, Awad I, et al. AHA Scientific Statement: Recommendations for the management of intracranial arteriovenous malformations: A statement for healthcare professionals from a special writing group of the Stroke Council. American Stroke Association. *Stroke*. 2001;32:1458–1471.

Ornish D, Brown SE, Scherwitz LW, et al. Can lifestyle changes reverse coronary heart disease? The Lifestyle Heart Trial. *Lancet*. 1990;336:129–133.

Pearson TA, Blair SN, Daniels SR, et al. AHA guidelines for primary prevention of cardiovascular disease and stroke: 2002 update. Consensus Panel guide to comprehensive risk reduction for adult patients without coronary or other atherosclerotic vascular diseases. *Circulation*. 2002;106:388–391.

Phan TG, Brown RD Jr, Wiebers DO. Asymptomatic carotid artery stenosis. In: Noseworthy JH, ed. *Neurological therapeutics, principles and practice*. London: Martin Dunitz; 2003: 420–423.

Phan TG, Huston J III, Brown RD Jr, et al. Intracranial saccular aneurysm enlargement determined using serial magnetic resonance angiography. *J Neurosurg*. 2002;97:1023–1028.

Pollock B, Gorman D, Coffey R. Patient outcomes after arteriovenous malformation radiosurgical management: Results based on a 5- to 14-year follow-up study. *Neurosurgery*. 2003;52:1291–1297.

Porter P, Willinsky R, Harper W, et al. Cerebral cavernous malformations: Natural history and prognosis after clinical deterioration with or without hemorrhage. *J Neurosurg*. 1997;87: 190–197.

Prospective studies collaboration. Cholesterol, diastolic blood pressure, and stroke: 13,000 strokes in 450,000 people in 45 prospective cohorts. *Lancet*. 1995;346:1647–1653.

Raaymakers TW. Aneurysms in relatives of patients with subarachnoid hemorrhage: Frequency and risk factors. MARS Study Group. Magnetic Resonance Angiography in Relatives of patients with Subarachnoid hemorrhage. *Neurology.* 1999;53:982–988.

Reynolds K, Lewis B, Nolen JD, et al. Alcohol consumption and risk of stroke: A meta-analysis. *JAMA.* 2003;289:579–588.

Ronkainen A, Hernesniemi J, Puranen M, et al. Familial intracranial aneurysms. *Lancet.* 1997;349:380–384.

Rothwell PM, Goldstein LB. Carotid endarterectomy for asymptomatic carotid stenosis: Asymptomatic Carotid Surgery Trial. *Stroke.* 2004;35:2425–2427.

Sacks FM, Svetkey LP, Vollmer WM, et al. Effects on blood pressure of reduced dietary sodium and the Dietary Approaches to Stop Hypertension (DASH) diet. DASH-Sodium Collaborative Research Group. *N Engl J Med.* 2001;344:3–10.

Straus SE, Majumdar SR, McAlister FA. New evidence for stroke prevention. Scientific Review. *JAMA.* 2002;288:1388–1395.

Suk SH, Sacco RL, Boden-Albala B, et al. Abdominal obesity and risk of ischemic stroke: The Northern Manhattan Stroke Study. *Stroke.* 2003;34:1586–1592.

The Homocysteine Studies Collaboration. Homocysteine and risk of ischemic heart disease and stroke. *JAMA.* 2002;288:2015–2022.

Tsang TSM, Barnes ME, Bailey KR, et al. Left atrial volume: Important risk marker of incident atrial fibrillation in 1655 older men and women. *Mayo Clin Proc.* 2001;76:467–475.

van Es RF, Jonker JJ, Verheugt FW, et al. Aspirin and coumadin after acute coronary syndromes (the ASPECT-2 study): a randomized controlled trial. *Lancet.* 2002;360:109–113.

Wald NJ, Law MR. A strategy to reduce cardiovascular disease by more than 80%. *BMJ.* 2003;326:1419.

Wang TJ, Massaro JM, Levy D, et al. A risk score for predicting stroke or death in individuals with new-onset atrial fibrillation in the community. The Framingham Heart Study. *JAMA.* 2003;290:1049–1056.

Wassertheil-Smoller S, Hendrix SL, Limacher M, et al. Effect of estrogen plus progestin on stroke in postmenopausal women: The Women's Health Initiative: A randomized trial. *JAMA.* 2003;289:2673–2684.

Wathen CN, Feig DS, Feightner JW, et al. Hormone replacement therapy for the primary prevention of chronic diseases: recommendation statement from the Canadian Task Force on Preventive Health Care. *Can Med Assoc J.* 2004;170:1535–1537.

Whelton SP, Chin A, Xin X, et al. Effect of aerobic exercise on blood pressure: A meta-analysis of randomized, controlled trials. *Ann Intern Med.* 2002;136:493–503.

Wiebers DO. *Stroke-Free For Life. The Complete Guide to Stroke Prevention and Treatment.* New York: Harper Collins/Quill Books; 2002.

Wiebers DO, Piepgras DG, Meyer FB, et al. Pathogenesis, natural history, and treatment of unruptured intracranial aneurysms. *Mayo Clin Proc.* 2004;79:1572–1583.

Wiebers DO, Whisnant JP, Huston J III, et al. International Study of Unruptured Intracranial Aneurysms Investigators. Unruptured intracranial aneurysms: Natural history, clinical outcome, and risk of surgical and endovascular treatment. *Lancet.* 2003;362:103–110.

Yadav JS, Wholey MH, Kuntz RE, et al. Protected carotid-artery stenting versus endarterectomy in high-risk patients. *N Engl J Med.* 2004;351:1493–1501.

Assessing and Discussing Prognosis and Natural History of Cerebrovascular Disorders

Carotid or Vertebral Artery Occlusive Disease

Carotid or vertebral artery disease may be asymptomatic or symptomatic. Factors that are associated with an increased risk for ischemic stroke related to carotid or vertebral artery occlusive disease include age, cigarette smoking, hypertension, ischemic heart disease, diabetes, and hyperlipidemia.

ASYMPTOMATIC CAROTID ARTERY DISEASE

Carotid bruit occurs in 4% to 5% of the population aged 45 to 80 years. However, a carotid bruit is merely a reflection of turbulence in the artery and a relatively poor predictor of underlying internal carotid stenosis in asymptomatic patients. Bruits are noted in approximately 40% of patients with 50% or more linear carotid stenosis (≥75% cross-sectional area stenosis) and 10% of those with <50% linear stenosis. Patients who have carotid bruit and have asymptomatic pressure-significant occlusive lesions of the carotid system (abnormal ocular pneumoplethysmography) are at greater risk for stroke than patients who have bruit and have normal ocular pneumoplethysmography (twofold) and the general population (sevenfold). In one study, the annual stroke rate during a period of 3 years among patients with carotid bruit was 3.4% in those with pressure-significant stenosis on ocular pneumoplethysmography, 1.5% in those with normal ocular pneumoplethysmography, and 0.5% in a normal age- and sex-matched population. Similar figures have been documented for patients with high-grade asymptomatic carotid stenoses diagnosed on carotid ultrasonography.

Various characteristics of the bruit, including location, loudness, and pitch, are relatively poor predictors of underlying stenosis. Bruits with a diastolic component in addition to the usual systolic component generally have an associated underlying high-grade stenosis. An ocular bruit is a relatively good predictor of some degree of underlying internal carotid artery siphon stenosis, although the stenosis may not be severe.

Patients with asymptomatic carotid bruits are at greater risk than the general population for all forms of atherosclerotic vascular disease. The risk for myocardial infarction (MI) is also increased (approximately 2.5 times) in patients with asymptomatic carotid bruit, and MI is the leading cause of death. However, these patients are at far less risk for ischemic stroke than are patients with symptomatic bruits or stenoses (see below). The risk for stroke in elderly individuals with asymptomatic carotid bruit is relatively small, but it increases significantly in patients of all ages when associated with hypertension.

The **degree of stenosis** in the carotid artery is a better predictor of stroke risk. In one study of asymptomatic patients, Doppler ultrasonographic evidence of >75% stenosis was associated with a 5.5% (during a mean of 28 months) annual risk for stroke. The range of stroke risk that was reported for patients with asymptomatic high-grade (≥75% cross-sectional stenosis) carotid stenosis was 2% to 5.5% during the first year, but the risk after the first year decreased, particularly if the stenosis was stable. Stroke risk depends on the percentage of stenosis, progression of stenosis between noninvasive examinations, and the presence or absence of ulceration. In the Asymptomatic Carotid Atherosclerosis Study (ACAS), stroke risk among asymptomatic patients with 60% or more carotid stenosis was 11% during a mean of approximately 5 years; these patients were treated with aspirin and correction of risk factors. Similar findings were noted in the Asymptomatic Carotid Stenosis Trial (ACST), in which the 5-year stroke risk was 11.8% in the medically treated group, in patients with at least a 60% carotid stenosis.

The presence of **ulceration** seems to increase the risk for subsequent stroke, depending on the size and the extent of the ulceration. However, these lesions are difficult to define in many cases, even with conventional arteriography. When ulcers are identified on conventional cut-film arteriography, their size can be defined by multiplying the length and the width of the ulcer in millimeters. The presence of small "A" ulcers (<10 mm^2) is not associated with an increased risk for stroke, but the presence of "B" ulcers (10 to 40 mm^2) or "C" ulcers (>40 mm^2) has been associated with stroke rates of 4.5% and 7.5% per year, respectively (in "C" ulcers, the rate of stroke may be somewhat independent of associated carotid stenosis).

Data from ACAS indicate that there may be a select group of otherwise relatively healthy patients with 60% or more carotid stenosis (diameter reduction) who have a lower risk for ipsilateral stroke and death with carotid endarterectomy (CEA) than do patients who are treated with aspirin and reduction of risk factors, when CEA is performed with $<3\%$ surgical morbidity and mortality. The risk for any stroke or death within 30 days postoperatively or any ipsilateral stroke or death after 30 days was 5.1% for surgical patients and 11.0% for those who were treated medically for 5 years. The resultant 66% relative risk reduction in men was statistically significant, but the reduction was not statistically significant in women (17%). Perioperative morbidity and mortality were higher in women and contributed to the lack of clear benefit in women. With respect to overall stroke rates and ipsilateral major stroke and death, the difference between the groups that had surgery and the groups that did not have surgery was not statistically significant, although there was a trend favoring surgery. In another large, randomized trial, ACST, CEA was compared with conservative management in patients with $>60\%$ carotid stenosis. The 5-year stroke risk was 6.4% in the CEA group, compared with 11.8% in the medically treated group. Fatal or disabling stroke was also reduced by surgery, with the 5-year risk of 3.5% in the CEA cohort and 6.1% in those who were treated medically ($p = 0.004$). Women and men both were benefited by CEA.

Patients who have severe carotid stenosis and are at increased risk for CEA may also be considered for carotid angioplasty with stent placement (CAS). In the Stenting and Angioplasty with Protection in Patients at High Risk for Endarterectomy (SAPPHIRE) trial, asymptomatic patients with at least an 80%

carotid stenosis were treated with either CEA or CAS. More than 70% of patients had an asymptomatic stenosis. The primary end point was the occurrence of a major cardiovascular event within 1 year of treatment: death, stroke, or MI within 30 days of intervention, or death or ipsilateral stroke between 31 days and 1 year. The risk for a major cardiovascular event was 12.2% in those who were treated with CAS and 20.1% of those who underwent CEA.

Some patients with an asymptomatic carotid stenosis may be found to have a contralateral carotid occlusion. In ACAS, in a post hoc analysis, the 163 patients with contralateral carotid occlusion at baseline were compared with the 1,485 with patent contralateral carotid artery. In those with contralateral occlusion, the risk for ipsilateral stroke over 5 years of follow-up for medical treatment was 3.5%, compared with 5.5% for surgical treatment. In those with a patent contralateral carotid artery, the 5-year stroke risk was 11.7% for medical treatment and 5.0% for surgical treatment. The reason for this somewhat paradoxical finding in the study post hoc analysis was not certain, but was thought to be due to a particularly benign natural history among those with a contralateral occlusion treated medically.

Anesthesia and surgery do not seem to pose substantial additional risks for stroke for patients with carotid bruits, although some have suggested that a subgroup of patients with bruit and asymptomatic, hemodynamically significant stenosis (as defined by abnormal oculopneumoplethysmography) may be at increased risk for stroke during peripheral vascular or cardiac surgery.

SYMPTOMATIC CAROTID ARTERY DISEASE

Symptomatic carotid artery disease includes symptoms that are related to transient or persistent monocular visual loss, hemispheric transient ischemic attack (TIA), and ischemic stroke. In patients with symptoms of carotid system cerebral ischemia, a localized or diffuse carotid bruit is approximately 75% predictive of ipsilateral moderate- or high-grade carotid stenosis. When both carotid arteries are assessed together, a carotid bruit is 85% predictive of moderate to severe stenosis at any extracranial carotid site. Patients who present with TIA or minor stroke related to severe carotid stenotic lesions ($\geq$70% linear stenosis) are at risk for stroke at the rate of 13% per year for 2 years after onset of symptoms. Patients who present with hemispheric TIA, recent TIA, increasing frequency of TIA, or high-grade stenosis have stroke rates that are higher than those in patients with transient monocular blindness, a remote event, a single event, or less stenosis.

The risk for stroke is lower among patients who present with amaurosis fugax than the risk in patients with hemispheric TIA. In one study, the risk for stroke in patients who presented with amaurosis fugax was one half that of patients who presented with hemispheric TIA in the setting of 70% or more ipsilateral carotid stenosis. The risk in both groups increased with increasing degrees of stenosis. Patients who are seen early after the onset of symptoms, particularly patients with multiple TIAs, are at increased risk for stroke. In another study, patients with five or more TIAs within 14 days before medical attention had a higher risk for subsequent stroke than did those with fewer than four spells. Increasing frequency or severity of ischemic cerebro-vascular events also likely indicates a high risk for stroke, although definitive data are unavailable. Patients who have had an ischemic stroke continue to be at risk for subsequent strokes at the rate of 5% to 9% per year; approximately 25% to 45% of patients have another stroke within 5 years of the original event.

Plaque characteristics may have an important effect on subsequent ischemic events. Echolucent and heterogeneous plaques are present in approximately 70% of symptomatic patients (compared with 20% to 30% of asymptomatic patients). These types of plaques generally have a high content of lipid or intraplaque hemorrhage, which may lead to plaque ulceration and a greater embolic potential. Patients with echolucent or heterogeneous plaques seem to have a neurologic event rate two to four times that of patients with echogenic plaques. Patients who present with TIA or minor stroke with high-grade carotid artery stenosis in the absence of arteriographic evidence of ulceration have a 2-year stroke rate of 17%, in contrast to a 2-year stroke rate of 30% when ulceration is present with similar degrees of stenosis.

In symptomatic patients with carotid stenosis, the combined morbidity and mortality with CEA is 2% to 6% in centers that are experienced and expert in performing the procedure. Patients who present with TIA are at somewhat lower operative risk than patients with stroke. After CEA, the risk for ipsilateral hemispheric stroke is 1% to 2% per year in patients who present with TIA and 2% to 3% per year for those with previous stroke.

VERTEBROBASILAR SYSTEM OCCLUSIVE DISEASE

Although atherosclerotic occlusive disease of the vertebral arteries is less common than it is in the carotid system, the development of disease in both is associated with the same or similar risk factors. Approximately 90% of stenoses in the vertebral system involve the origins of the vertebral arteries. Natural history data are sparse regarding patients with asymptomatic vertebral stenosis. In the small studies available, the risk of brainstem stroke is <1% to 2% per year, but it is higher if associated with basilar stenosis. The risk for any stroke or MI is much higher than that in the general population because of co-occurring anterior circulation atheromatous occlusive disease and coronary artery disease. Hemodynamic compromise of distal flow in the basilar artery also does not occur in unilateral proximal vertebral artery stenosis.

Cervical portions of the vertebral arteries are uncommonly affected by atherosclerosis. The frequency of cerebral infarction in this subgroup is unknown, although it likely is higher than that in patients with lesions at the origin. The basilar artery typically is affected by atherosclerosis in the proximal portion. Natural history data are also somewhat lacking for this entity. Symptomatic basilar artery stenosis or occlusion is associated with a high rate of recurrent stroke (approximately 10% to 20%) within 1 year. The risk in asymptomatic patients is uncertain.

Overall, both referral-based and population-based studies indicate that stroke rates after TIA or minor stroke do not differ substantially according to whether the initial symptoms were localized to the anterior or posterior circulation.

Transient Ischemic Attack

Approximately one third of patients with transient ischemic attack (TIA) (including all underlying mechanisms) have an ischemic stroke within 5 years of the first attack. In a population-based study, the risk for stroke was approximately 7% at 1 month, 10% at 6 months, and 13% at 12 months after a TIA. Approximately 50% of all strokes after TIA occur within 1 year, irrespective of the territory involved (carotid or vertebrobasilar system). The causes of death after carotid or vertebrobasilar TIA are similar (approximately 45% cardiac and 30% hemorrhagic or ischemic stroke). Survival is nearly 90% at 1 year after the first TIA and approximately 70% at 5 years, 50% at 8 years, and 40% at 10 years. After a TIA, women who are older than 70 years have a worse survival rate than do men who are older than age 70, but women who are younger than 70 years have a better survival rate than that of their male counterparts.

In a large multihospital study with a single health maintenance organization in California, the risk for stroke after TIA was 11% at 3 months, with half of strokes within the first 2 days. An increased risk for subsequent stroke was predicted by the following factors: age >60 years (odds ratio [OR] 1.8), diabetes mellitus (OR 2.0), symptom duration >10 minutes (OR 2.3), and weakness (OR 1.9) or speech impairment (OR 1.5) as a symptom of the TIA.

The overall risk for major vascular events remains high for 10 to 15 years after a TIA, with the 10-year risk for stroke of approximately 20% and the risk for myocardial infarction or death from coronary heart disease approximately 30%. Therefore, it is important to maintain preventive treatments in patients with TIA in the long term, even in seemingly "low risk" patients who have already survived free of stroke for several years.

The probability of stroke after TIA strongly correlates with the patient's age at onset (the relative risk for subsequent stroke is 1.45 for each 10 years of increasing age) and a high frequency of TIAs in a short time after the initial event (five or more TIAs within 2 weeks is associated with a subsequent ischemic stroke rate of approximately 20% in the first 3 months and 30% in the first 6 months). Amaurosis fugax alone is associated with a better prognosis (approximately half the ischemic stroke risk) compared with that of hemispheric TIA. Patients whose TIA includes only sensory symptoms of short duration (10 minutes or less) seem to be more likely to experience recurrent TIA than ischemic stroke after the index TIA. In patients with >70% extracranial carotid stenosis, the risk for stroke within 2 years after diagnosis is 12% in those who present with retinal ischemia and 28% in those with hemispheric ischemic events. Gender does not predict the risk for stroke in individual cases, but women generally have a more benign prognosis after TIA than do men. The natural history and prognosis of TIA specifically associated with carotid stenosis are discussed in Chapter 32.

Cerebral Infarction

MORTALITY

After a person has had cerebral infarction (CI) (also referred to as ischemic stroke), the 30-day **case fatality rate** is approximately 20%. **Survival** after the first cerebral infarction is approximately 70% at 1 year, 50% at 5 years, 30% at 8 years, and 25% at 10 years. The most common **causes of death early** after CI are transtentorial herniation, pneumonia, cardiac disorders, pulmonary embolus, and septicemia. Patients who present with altered sensorium and hemiplegia frequently die of herniation. Death from herniation occurs more commonly on day 1 or 2 after the onset of infarct than on any other days and considerably less frequently after day 7. Overall, nearly 40% of deaths from any cause occur within 48 hours. Other causes of death within the first month include pneumonia, cardiac disease, pulmonary embolus, and septicemia. The cause of death is dependent on the time after the initial stroke. In the first month, half of the deaths are due to the initial CI, approximately one quarter are caused by respiratory infection, and approximately one tenth are due to cardiovascular events. After the first month and during the first year after first CI, respiratory infection and cardiac causes are far more common causes of death than neurologic factors related to the first CI or recurrent CI. Overall, during the first 10 years after initial CI, cardiac disorders and pulmonary causes are the most common causes of death, followed by neurologic factors as a result of the initial CI, recurrent stroke, and malignancy.

Significant independent **predictors of death** within 5 years after CI are age (increased age is associated with a decreased survival rate), previous myocardial infarction (MI), atrial fibrillation present at the time of stroke, and congestive heart failure anytime before stroke. Survival rates in patients with symptoms that resolve within the first 3 weeks after the CI (an event that is sometimes referred to as reversible ischemic neurologic deficit) is similar to those of patients with transient ischemic attack and better than those of patients with major CI.

Long-term CI mortality differs on the basis of the **stroke mechanism.** The 5-year mortality for each cerebral infarction mechanism is as follows: large artery atherosclerosis with stenosis, 30%; cardioembolic, 80%; lacunar (small vessel disease), 35%; and stroke of unknown cause, 50%.

STROKE RECURRENCE

Recurrent CI occurs in approximately 30% of patients within 5 years, although symptoms of coronary artery disease or peripheral vascular disease also may ensue. **MI** occurs in patients who present with CI at a rate of approximately 4% to 5% per year. Significant independent predictors of recurrent stroke after CI are cardiac valve disease (including replacement) and congestive heart failure. The probability of recurrent stroke among patients with a probable cardiac source of emboli is 2% at 1 month, 5% at 1 year, and 32% at 5 years. The early risk for recurrent stroke differs on the basis of the CI subtype. The risk for recurrent stroke at 1 year on the basis of stroke mechanism is as follows: large artery atherosclerosis with stenosis, 25%; cardioembolic, 15%; lacunar (small vessel disease), 5%; and stroke of unknown cause, 15%. The difference in recurrent stroke risk on the basis of subtype is particularly important early after the initial CI, with those with large artery atherosclerosis having a 9% recurrence risk at 1 week after the first. Long term, the recurrence risk does not differ on the basis of CI subtype.

FUNCTIONAL OUTCOME

In general, approximately 60% to 70% of patients have early (1 month) functional disability after a stroke. This rate usually improves to approximately 60% in 3 months and 50% in 1 year. Although some late improvement may occur for up to 2 years after the event, most improvement occurs within 6 months. Severe neurologic deficits with no return of motor function within 1 month; marked cognitive-perceptual dysfunction, apraxia, or impairment in construction ability (especially with lesions in the dominant hemisphere or the frontal lobes); and urinary incontinence 2 weeks after a stroke are indicators of a poor functional prognosis and identify patients who are likely to need long-term care. Functional outcome differs on the basis of the cerebral infarction mechanism. In a population-based study, Rankin Disability Scale was different both at 3 months and at 1 year after the stroke. Lacunar strokes (small vessel disease) were associated with milder deficits compared with the other subtypes. At 90 days after the CI, the risk for being severely disabled or dead (Rankin status IV, V, or VI) on the basis of the stroke mechanism is as follows: large artery atherosclerosis with stenosis, 30%; cardioembolic, 55%; lacunar (small vessel disease), 5%; and stroke of unknown cause, 35%.

In addition to these prognostic indicators, previous stroke, symptomatic systemic diseases (such as cardiac or pulmonary insufficiency or frequent angina pectoris), severe mental abnormalities, lack of spouse's or family members' involvement in the rehabilitation process, and a duration of >30 days from onset of stroke to rehabilitation are other factors that may hinder recovery.

In the first days after a stroke, the patient's paralyzed muscles are usually flaccid, and the deep tendon reflexes are depressed. However, spasticity gradually develops, and deep tendon reflexes increase. Early development of spasticity in the arm generally is considered a favorable sign for a better outcome. Motor recovery tends to occur in the first 2 to 3 months, and leg improvement is usually better than arm improvement. In patients with hemiparesis, only approximately 20% have persistent severe hemiparesis at 6 months after the event, and at 1 year, 50% have perceptible weakness. Arm function improves partially or completely in 40% of patients who present with severe weakness. Complete arm paralysis at onset and minimal improvement at 4 weeks are predictive of poor outcome.

Hemineglect or sensory deficits that cause impaired proprioception usually improve. Aphasia may continue to improve for

1 year or more after onset of symptoms, and global aphasia may improve more in the second 6 months than in the first 6 months. Aphasia in left-handed patients, regardless of the hemisphere involved, tends to be milder and resolves more rapidly than that in right-handed patients with a left hemisphere lesion.

Intracerebral Hemorrhage

For individuals with intracerebral hemorrhage (ICH), the reported 30-day survival rate ranges from 40% to 70%; immediate functional prognosis with ICH is usually better than that with cerebral infarction because of differences in the amount of brain tissue damaged. The prognosis for individuals with **lobar hematomas** is usually better than that for individuals with other forms of ICHs. The overall mortality rate is approximately 15% to 30%; approximately 50% of survivors have full functional recovery. Predictors of poor outcome after lobar hemorrhage include hemorrhage of >40 ml, intraventricular extension of the hemorrhage, and degree of midline shift. The outcome of **caudate hemorrhage** is usually benign, and patients typically have full recovery without permanent neurologic deficit. Even with intraventricular extension, which is common, the prognosis is still relatively good.

For individuals with **putaminal hemorrhage**, the mortality rate is approximately 40%, although the range of clinical presentations is marked and typically depends on the volume of hemorrhage. Progressive neurologic deficit with hemiplegia and coma at admission correlate with poor functional outcome among survivors, whereas a normal level of consciousness, normal extraocular movements, and partial hemiparesis portend a better functional level among survivors. Radiologic imaging characteristics that are predictive of a poor prognosis include large hemorrhage size and intraventricular extension.

The outlook for functional status for patients with **thalamic hemorrhage** is usually poor, directly depending on the size of the lesion; hemorrhages that are >3 cm in diameter are almost always fatal. Intraventricular extension is common in thalamic hemorrhage but is not necessarily associated with a poor prognosis unless hydrocephalus occurs. Level of consciousness at presentation is also a good predictor of survival.

In **brainstem hemorrhage**, death usually occurs within a few hours, but, occasionally, patients with a small hemorrhagic lesion may survive, with functional level dependent on the site and size of hemorrhage and on the severity of symptoms at onset.

The clinical course in **cerebellar hemorrhage** is unpredictable; as the hours pass, some patients who are alert or drowsy on admission can suddenly become stuporous and then comatose as a result of progressive brainstem compression, whereas others with a similar clinical status at admission have complete functional recovery (vermis hemorrhage is associated with relatively poor survival rates). Patients who have progression have a much better prognosis with surgery if they are still arousable when taken to the operating room than do patients who are in coma. Computed tomography (CT) findings showing hydrocephalus, intraventricular hemorrhage, and hemorrhage of 3 cm or more are also associated with a poor prognosis. Overall, survivors of cerebellar hemorrhage typically have a good functional prognosis.

Primary intraventricular hemorrhage often has a benign clinical course with full recovery, but significant hemorrhage may cause death from progressive hydrocephalus.

Recurrent cerebral hemorrhage is uncommon, in part because of the high 30-day mortality rate. Nevertheless, recurrent hemorrhage represents approximately 2% to 4% of all cases of primary ICH.

Overall, **unfavorable prognostic signs** of ICH for early survival are (1) decreased level of consciousness after the ictus (especially comatose state), (2) large hematoma (>40 ml), (3) midline shift on CT or magnetic resonance imaging, (4) intraventricular blood volume of 20 ml or more, (5) advanced age (especially patients who are older than 65 years), (6) limb plegia, (7) early hyperglycemia, and (8) early fever.

Much of the natural history data refer to all cases of ICH or to cases that are not associated with underlying vascular malformation or intracranial aneurysm, the majority of which are caused by hypertensive vascular disease. However, the natural history differs if a specific cause is detected. Approximately 10% to 25% of patients with ICH from an **arteriovenous malformation (AVM)** die within 30 days, and 25% of survivors have persistent, long-term morbidity. The risk for recurrent hemorrhage is 6% to 12% during the first year after the initial bleed, 2% to 6% during the second year, and then returns to a long-term, persistent risk of 2% to 3% per year. Given this long-term annual risk for hemorrhage, the lifetime risk for hemorrhage in those with a previously unruptured AVM is approximated by the following formula: lifetime risk in percent = 105 minus the patient's age in years. Clinical and radiologic predictors of an increased risk for hemorrhage are not known with certainty. Some have reported an increased risk for hemorrhage with small lesions, whereas others have noted the character of the venous drainage system (such as a single draining vein, primarily deep drainage, or impairment in venous outflow) to be important predictors. In the arterial system, the presence of aneurysms on the feeding arteries, including those that are very distal on the feeding arteries called intra-nidal aneurysms, and perforator arterial supply both may increase the risk for hemorrhage. Patients with co-occurring **AVMs and aneurysms** have a higher risk for ICH, approximately 7% per year.

Dural arteriovenous fistulae (or **dural arteriovenous malformations**) may also cause intracranial hemorrhage, although the risk is not known with certainty. Some hemorrhages can be fatal, although the mortality rate is lower than that associated with intraparenchymal AVM.

Cavernous malformations have a lower risk for clinically significant hemorrhage, <1% per year among those who present with symptoms other than hemorrhage. Deep lesions (including the brainstem, deep cerebellar, thalamus, and basal ganglia) carry the highest risk for hemorrhage, approximately 4% per year, compared with approximately 0.4% per year for superficial lesions. After the first symptomatic hemorrhage, the risk for a recurrent hemorrhage is approximately 5% in the next year. Complete recovery occurs in most cases, although the natural history data are incomplete. Fatal hemorrhage is extremely rare. Women may be at increased risk for hemorrhage.

The risk for hemorrhage from **venous malformations** is extremely low. They may occasionally cause seizures, focal neurologic symptoms, or trigeminal neuralgia. Some investigators have reported that if a hemorrhage occurs with radiologic demonstration of a venous malformation, there likely will be a different vascular malformation subtype—typically a cavernous malformation—detected underlying the hemorrhage. Others believe that venous malformations, particularly those in the cerebellum, may cause intracranial hemorrhage, although the risk is extremely low.

Intracranial aneurysms may also cause ICH with relatively little subarachnoid hemorrhage (SAH). The overall prognosis is similar to that of aneurysmal SAH (see Chapter 36) but may be somewhat better if there is minimal subarachnoid blood.

Subarachnoid Hemorrhage

The 30-day case fatality rate in patients with subarachnoid hemorrhage (SAH) from population-based studies since 1960 has ranged from 32% to 67%. Among the more recent studies, the case fatality rate is approximately 40%. If the patient is seen at 24 hours after SAH, the mortality rate at 30 days is decreased to approximately 35%, at 48 hours to about 30%, at 1 week to about 25%, and at 2 weeks to 10%. Approximately 10% of patients die before they receive medical attention. Mortality after 30 days declines substantially, leveling off between 30 and 60 days. Significant predictors of outcome are the patient level of consciousness and clinical grade at admission. The probability of survival is better for patients with no neurologic deficit other than cranial nerve palsy (Hunt and Hess clinical grade 1 or 2) and worse for patients who present with coma, decerebrate rigidity, and moribund appearance (Hunt and Hess clinical grade 3, 4, or 5). The 30-day probability of survival is <20% for patients with clinical grades 4 and 5 and approximately 70% with grades 1 and 2. In addition, intracerebral hematoma or a history of hypertension increases the probability of death in patients with SAH.

One of the major causes of mortality after initial SAH is aneurysmal rebleeding. The rebleeding rate is approximately 2% per day during the first 10 days (total, approximately 20%). The occurrence of rebleeding is a little less than 30% at 30 days and about 1.5% per year after 30 days. In patients with clinical grade 1, 2, or 3, the probability of having isolated cranial nerve palsies or an altered level of consciousness in the first 30 days after SAH is nearly 50%.

Among survivors of SAH, approximately one third remain dependent. Even physically independent survivors are likely to experience some change in their lives, such as ongoing cognitive deficits (especially memory problems in about 50% of survivors) and problems with mood (about 40%) and speech (about 15%). Limited available data suggest that only about one third of independent survivors report no reduction in quality of life at 18 months after SAH.

Patients who have SAH of unknown origin and in whom cerebral arteriography and other laboratory studies do not show an aneurysm or other cause of the hemorrhage (such as vascular malformation or tumor) have a relatively good prognosis, with a rate of recurrent hemorrhage of approximately 2% to 10% within a follow-up period as long as 15 years.

Patients with SAH localized to the perimesencephalic region without extension into the Sylvian fissures or interhemispheric fissure (called pretruncal hemorrhage or perimesencephalic hemorrhage) have a very benign prognosis if their cerebral arteriograms are normal. The recovery period is very short, and patients are almost always able to return to work and other activities with no decrease in their quality of life. The risk for rebleed is extremely low, although some patients may have early deterioration after presentation because of hydrocephalus. Delayed cerebral ischemia is also uncommon.

In general, SAH that is caused by an arteriovenous malformation (AVM) is associated with a much lower 30-day case fatality rate (10% to 20%) than that caused by saccular aneurysm. Vasospasm and delayed ischemic neurologic deficit are also uncommon and contribute to a lower occurrence of long-term morbidity and mortality in the AVM subgroup.

SUGGESTED READING FOR PART VI

Broderick J, Brott T, Kothari R, et al. The Greater Cincinnati/ Northern Kentucky Stroke Study: Preliminary first-ever and total incidence rates of stroke among blacks. *Stroke.* 1998; 29:415–421.

Broderick JP, Phillips SJ, O'Fallon WM, et al. Relationship of cardiac disease to stroke occurrence, recurrence, and mortality. *Stroke.* 1992;23:1250–1256.

Brown RD Jr, Petty GW, O'Fallon WM, et al. Incidence of transient ischemic attack in Rochester, Minnesota, 1985–1989. *Stroke.* 1998;29:2109–2113.

European Carotid Surgery Trialists' Collaborative Group: MRC European Carotid Surgery Trial. Interim results for symptomatic patients with severe (70–99%) or with mild (0–29%) carotid stenosis. *Lancet.* 1991;337:1235–1243.

Evans BA, Wiebers DO, Barrett HJM. The Importance of Symptoms in Predicting Risk for Subsequent Stroke Following an Initial Transient Ischemic Attack or Minor Stroke. In: Moore WS, ed. *Surgery for Cerebrovascular Disease.* 2nd ed. Philadelphia: WB Saunders, 1996:16–19.

Executive Committee for the Asymptomatic Carotid Atherosclerosis Study: Endarterectomy for asymptomatic carotid artery stenosis. *JAMA.* 1995;273:1421–1428.

Hackett ML, Anderson CS. Health outcomes 1 year after subarachnoid hemorrhage: An international population-based study. The Australian Cooperative Research on Subarachnoid Hemorrhage Study Group. *Neurology.* 2000;55:658–662.

Hop JW, Rinkel GJE, Algra A, et al. Case-fatality rates and functional outcome after subarachnoid hemorrhage—a systematic review. *Stroke.* 1997;28:660–664.

Ingall TJ, Whisnant JP, Wiebers DO, et al. Has there been a decline in subarachnoid hemorrhage mortality? *Stroke.* 1989;20:718–724.

Johnston SC, Gress DR, Browner WS, et al. Short-term prognosis after emergency-department diagnosis of transient ischemic attack. *JAMA.* 2000;284:2901–2906.

Meissner I, Wiebers DO, Whisnant JP, et al. The natural history of asymptomatic carotid artery occlusive lesions. *JAMA.* 1987;258:2704–2707.

North American Symptomatic Carotid Endarterectomy Trial Collaborators. Beneficial effect of carotid endarterectomy in symptomatic patients with high-grade carotid stenosis. *N Engl J Med.* 1991;325:445–453.

Petty GW, Brown RD Jr, Whisnant JP, et al. Ischemic stroke: Outcomes, patient mix, and practice variation for neurologists and generalists in a community. *Neurology.* 1998;50: 1669–1678.

Petty GW, Brown RD Jr, Whisnant JP, et al. Ischemic stroke subtypes: A population-based study of functional outcome, survival and recurrence. *Stroke.* 2000;31:1062–1068.

Petty GW, Brown RD Jr, Whisnant JP, et al. Ischemic stroke subtypes: A population-based study of incidence and risk factors. *Stroke.* 1999;30:2513–251.

Reed SD, Blough DK, Meyer K, et al. Inpatient costs, length of stay, and mortality for cerebrovascular events in community hospitals. *Neurology*. 2001;57:305–314.

Rothwell PM, Giles MF, Flossmann E, et al. A simple score (ABCD) to identify individuals at high early risk of stroke after transient ischaemic attack. *Lancet*. 2005;366:29–36.

Vernino S, Brown RD Jr, Sejvar JJ, et al. Cause-specific mortality after first cerebral infarction: A population-based study in Rochester, Minnesota. *Stroke*. 2003;34:1828–1832.

Whisnant JP, ed. *Stroke: Populations, Cohorts, and Clinical Trials*. Oxford: Butterworth-Heinemann, 1993.

Whisnant JP, Brown RD, Petty GW, et al. Comparison of population-based models of risk factors for TIA and ischemic stroke. *Neurology*. 1999;53:532–536.

Management and Rehabilitation After Stroke

Physical Therapy

Available data support the usefulness of a coordinated rehabilitation program for treating functional impairment that results from a stroke. The rehabilitation program should provide an environment of high motivation to help achieve the patient's maximal physical and psychological functional capacity and should be tailored to meet the needs of each patient and family. For planning and implementing this program most effectively, a coordinated, interdisciplinary team approach is required. Besides a physician who is knowledgeable in stroke rehabilitation, the composition of the team varies but often includes rehabilitation nurses, physical therapists, occupational therapists, speech therapists, psychologists, and social workers. The roles of key members of the multidisciplinary team (MDT) are usually as follows. The **consultant physician** coordinating the MDT should be a dedicated specialist with a specific interest in stroke. The doctor should monitor the patient medically for complications from the stroke and optimize management to prevent stroke recurrence and medical complications. Nursing staff should be shown how to handle stroke patients, without causing injury. They should be educated in rehabilitation principles, decubitus ulcer prevention, and management of continence. They should exercise emotional and psychological expertise in their interaction with stroke patients and their families. The nursing team provides other members of the MDT with information regarding the patient's progress in the care/treatment plans from their observation of the patient 24 hours a day. In addition, nurses must reinforce the plan of action implemented by other members of the MDT (such as the exercise and mobility plan initiated by the physical therapists). Nurse staffing levels should be sufficient to ensure the safety of stroke patients. **Physical therapists** should gain experience in managing stroke patients. In particular, the protection of the hemiplegic shoulder and arm should be emphasized, and this important activity should be followed by other members of the MDT. A major goal of the physical therapist is to optimize mobility. The **occupational therapist** should aim to enhance function, re-educate, and, if possible, re-apply the life role for the patient. The occupational therapist has an important role with regard to perceptive and cognitive assessments. A functional assessment, both in the hospital and in the patient's home, is essential in most cases. Therapy to optimize function should be ongoing. During the acute phase of the stroke, patients should be assessed for dysphagia either by the **speech/language therapist** or by the occupational therapist. This will require ongoing monitoring in the rehabilitation ward. For inpatients who are unable to swallow, an alternative feeding route should be commenced (if not already in place) soon after transfer to the rehabilitation ward. Patients with communication/language difficulty should receive ongoing speech therapy. A **social worker** should provide patient and caregiver support and initiate community support services at the time of discharge. They also facilitate the transition to skilled nursing facility care should that be necessary after the rehabilitation center stay. The **pharmacist** should review medications critically, collaborate with the other caregivers in providing a medication listing on discharge, assist staff in supervising a self-medication program, and provide assistance to patients and their families in promoting compliance. The **dietitian** should ensure that patients receive adequate nutrition and coordinate provision of feeding that is appropriate to patient needs. The dietitian should work closely with the speech/language therapist, particularly in cases in which alternative feeding is required. For inpatients with hyperlipidemia or diabetes, appropriate advice should be offered. It is also advisable to get a clinical **neuropsychologist** involved in the early evaluation and treatment of stroke survivors, especially young patients with cognitive deficit. Discharge planning should begin early in the course of admission and involve full collaboration with primary health care and local social services. Community-based rehabilitation services should develop partnerships with hospital-based stroke services.

Rehabilitation should be started with early, systematic, and realistic increases in the patient's activities and should be advanced in stages in a local hospital, in an outpatient clinic, at home, or in a specialized rehabilitation unit. The program must include rehabilitation that is specific to the deficit. For productive rehabilitation, the patient must willingly participate and have the cognitive ability to follow at least one-step commands and the memory to remember the lessons learned in therapy. For patients who have cerebrovascular disease and who have significant cardiac dysfunction (such as angina, arrhythmia, or myocardial infarction), the rehabilitation program should be combined with a cardiac rehabilitation program.

The **frequency of rehabilitation treatment** sessions varies with the setting and timing after a stroke and with the patient's response to therapy. Generally, therapy is provided twice daily in an inpatient setting; three times per week in an outpatient setting; and daily, when requested by a physician, in a nursing home setting. On the basis of the Mayo Clinic experience, approximately 50% of patients who survive ischemic stroke for 1 week are good candidates to benefit from physical therapy (the median number of sessions is 16); 40% benefit from occupational therapy (the median number of sessions is eight); and 13% benefit from speech therapy. Approximately 15% of patients eventually are transferred to a rehabilitation unit, in which the median duration of stay is about 32 days. Approximately half of the patients who survive for 6 months after stroke are partially or totally dependent in activities of daily living such as bathing, dressing, feeding, and mobility (including 10% of survivors who need long-term nursing care). About one third of patients who survive after stroke for 1 year are unable to remain independent, and this proportion remains relatively unchanged in survivors who are followed as long as 5 years.

Although the **duration of rehabilitation** therapy generally is determined by the patient's rate of functional recovery, the probability of improvement of movement in paralyzed limbs is maximal during the first month after stroke and decreases significantly after 6 months, whereas considerable improvement of speech, domestic and working skills, and steadiness can continue as long as 2 years. Recovery of arm movement is usually less complete than that of leg movement, and complete lack of any movement at onset of stroke or no measurable grip strength by 4 weeks is associated with a poor prognosis for return of useful arm function. However, functional recovery (lessening of disability or handicap), depending on both intrinsic neuronal recovery and adaptive recovery (the use of alternative strategies or adaptive equipment to perform an activity), often continues long after specific neurologic deficits have ceased to change. No established guidelines yet exist to help select patients for specific rehabilitation interventions.

Proper **positioning** in bed and repositioning (patients with hemiplegia should be turned every 1 to 2 hours, and side rails should be provided to prevent the patient from falling out of bed) help to prevent contractures and decubitus ulcers and should begin as soon as the patient has been admitted and the diagnosis made (Fig. 37-1). For alert patients, a trapeze should be put over the bed to enable them to change their own position.

Physical therapy in the form of passive exercises should begin as soon as the deficit is stable (a full, passive range of motion of paretic and nonparetic limbs should be performed for approximately 15 minutes at least three times a day, with special attention

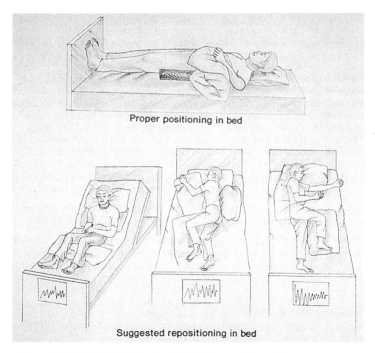

Proper positioning in bed

Suggested repositioning in bed

Figure 37-1.   Top: Positioning in bed for a patient who has had a stroke. Bottom: Suggested repositioning in bed.

to the shoulders, elbows, hips, and ankles), and active exercises and ambulation should be attempted as soon as the patient can tolerate them. These measures are important not only for maintaining and increasing limb function and mobility but also for preventing deep vein thromboses, especially in patients who are not receiving an anticoagulant (or antiplatelet) agent.

Patients who are alert and have a stable cardiovascular system should **sit up** in bed as soon as the neurologic deficit is stable (usually within the first or second day after onset of symptoms), except for conservatively treated patients with aneurysmal subarachnoid hemorrhage, in whom bed rest until definitive treatment or for at least 2 to 3 weeks is usually recommended. Patients who tolerate sitting up in bed may sit in a chair and then should be aided or instructed in a stepwise manner about how to **stand**; transfer to and from a wheelchair; **walk** (or push a wheelchair); and **perform other regular activities** of daily living, including eating, brushing teeth, washing, shaving, dressing, and undressing, as their neurologic status permits (sudden or intense activity should be avoided). During the early part of the exercise program, patients should be monitored closely, and special attention should be given to changes in blood pressure and heart function. For hemiplegic patients, the occupational therapist should cooperate closely with the physiotherapist, nursing staff, speech therapist, and the patient's spouse or family to provide retraining in basic self-care activities (such as feeding, dressing, and washing). The occupational therapist can individualize various types of upper extremity splints that can assist patients to increase their functional capabilities.

For prevention of **ulnar nerve compression palsy** and **shoulder–hand syndrome** (decreased mobility of the affected shoulder joint and edema over the hand and fingers with local tenderness over the shoulder and hand), the patient's weak arm should not be left to hang without support. (The treatment of shoulder–hand syndrome is discussed in Chapter 39). For patients with equinovarus deformity of the foot or flexion contracture of the paretic wrist and fingers, a foot-ankle plastic orthosis (a short or long leg brace) or a wrist-finger extension splint is commonly used (Fig. 37-2).

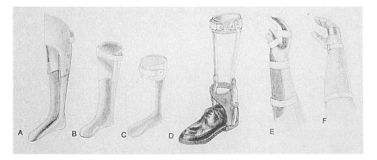

Figure 37-2.   A–D: Types of orthoses. E: Plastic positioning splint. F: Dorsal wrist cock-up positioning splint.

Selective gymnastic therapy in conjunction with point massage and autogenous training, heat therapy, cryotherapy, and acupuncture also may be instituted to **reduce spasticity.** Coordination exercises and frequent practice of standing and walking between parallel bars are required for patients with **poor coordination** (ataxia without paralysis) and **dysequilibrium.** If cognitive function is preserved in a patient with hemiparesis, then instructions in the use of various special devices (such as handrails along walls, quad canes, bedside table, specially designed card holders, typewriters, telephones, and other specific activity aids) can assist the patient in becoming more independent in the activities of daily living.

38

Speech Therapy

All patients with a communication problem that results from stroke should be referred for speech and language therapy assessment and treatment. A speech pathologist may also evaluate patients who have deficits in swallowing or thinking and are alert enough to participate. Intensive speech therapy is commonly indicated for motivated patients with dysphasia. The therapy to establish an effective means of communication is begun when the patient with dysphasia or dysarthria is awake, alert, and stable (the involvement of a speech therapist is generally very helpful). Communication techniques, alternatives, and therapies can be provided to the patient to enhance communication skills and to avoid the frustration that occurs when patients cannot communicate their needs adequately. The therapist may use verbal or nonverbal techniques, and communication may be facilitated by using a word board or by combining written and spoken language.

To be effective, auditory stimulation must be combined with visual stimulation, which should be sufficiently intense, clear, repetitive, and slow to assist the learning process according to the patient's functional status. Stimuli should be further tailored to be consistent with the patient's background, education, work history, and hobbies. The patient should hear speech frequently from conversation, radio, or television and be encouraged to respond (with adequate intervals of rest). Motivation by encouragement and other positive reinforcement is important. Drawing, copying, tracing letters and geometric designs, and various occupational therapies also are helpful. Where intelligible speech is not a reasonable goal, the speech and language therapist should augment speech attempts and enable communication through means other than spoken language. Improvement of speech can continue for 2 years and longer.

Other Chronic
Complications of Stroke

Common secondary impairments in patients who survive cerebral infarction or intracerebral hemorrhage are pain and edema in the hemiplegic arm, also known as **shoulder–hand syndrome** (5% to 10% of patients) or, less common, pain and edema in the leg. Edema in the paralyzed limb(s) may be relieved by elevation, pneumatic compression, or compression gloves. Treatment of painful joints in paralyzed limbs includes maintenance of appropriate passive range of motion within a pain-free arc(s) and proper positioning (cold or superficial heat should precede passive stretching). A paralyzed shoulder should be positioned in external rotation (forearm with supination and finger extension with abduction) and the hip in internal rotation and flexion with the knee and ankle in flexion.

Treatment with corticosteroids or nonsteroidal analgesics and a low-dose antidepressant (such as amitriptyline, 50 to 75 mg, in divided doses or at bedtime, especially for chronic pain associated with depression) or anticonvulsant agents (such as phenytoin, 100 mg daily; carbamazepine, 400 mg daily; or clonazepam, 0.5 mg daily) may also be considered. Local anesthetic agents (0.5% lidocaine hydrochloride given percutaneously, to 60 ml, or regional intravenous routes, 10 to 50 ml), stellate ganglion blocks (as many as seven to 10 treatments if the patient responds within three to four blocks), heat treatment of post-stroke arthropathy, transcutaneous nerve stimulation, and acupuncture also may be effective, especially for localized pain.

In patients who have **swallowing problems** that place them at risk for aspiration pneumonia and choking, short-term (to 4 to 6 weeks) use of nasogastric tube feedings until function returns or long-term use of a percutaneous feeding tube should be considered. Percutaneous placement of a feeding tube into the stomach or small bowel is particularly advisable for patients who have persistent, profound impairment of swallowing associated with bilateral hemispheric strokes or brainstem strokes.

Diplopia usually improves over time, and subtle deficits can be managed with prism glasses. For persistent diplopia that has been stable for >6 months, surgical correction may be considered.

Seizures can complicate cerebrovascular disorders beginning during the acute phase or many months after the event. Chronic convulsions are more often associated with lobar hemorrhagic stroke, cortical ischemic stroke, and subarachnoid hemorrhage. Treatment of seizure disorders in patients who survive stroke is similar to that for patients with epilepsy that results from other causes.

Spasticity and contractures may be controlled by standard physiotherapy techniques of repetitive muscle stretching through range-of-motion exercises, positioning, and handling (with splints). Either heat or ice massage may lead to a short-term reduction in spasticity. Although no medication has been uniformly useful in the treatment of spasticity, if physiotherapeutic measures are ineffective and the spasticity is marked, medical therapy that may be considered includes baclofen (starting with 5 mg twice daily and increasing, as tolerated, to 80 mg daily in two to four divided doses), diazepam (starting with 2 to 5 mg twice a day and increasing gradually, as tolerated), dantrolene sodium (starting with 25 mg and increasing, as tolerated, to 400 mg per day), and tizanidine in doses to 36 mg per day (not yet available in the United States). However, all of these drugs have potential side effects, including weakness or apparent weakness, which often develops as spasticity is lessened because the stiffness that is associated with spasticity may help support weak extremities, particularly the legs. Other possible side effects include drowsiness, gastric distress, and nausea with baclofen; sedation and cognitive clouding with diazepam; and nausea, drowsiness, and hepatotoxicity with dantrolene. Tizanidine may also produce systemic hypotension. If all of these measures fail, other potential therapeutic approaches include intrathecal administration of baclofen or morphine, peripheral nerve or spinal cord electrical stimulation (dorsal column stimulation), botulinum toxin injections, and various surgical procedures (such as cutting, lengthening, or transplanting tendons).

Patients with **urinary incontinence** should be evaluated for urinary tract infection. If no infection is present or if treatment does not resolve the incontinence, then postvoid residual urine volumes should be measured. Anticholinergic agents may be administered to patients with sterile urine and postvoid residual urine volumes <100 ml. If the urine is sterile and postvoid vol­umes are >100 ml, intermittent catheterization followed by a complete urologic evaluation is usually indicated. Urinary tract infections should be treated appropriately.

Cognitive deficits and depression are frequent complications of stroke and affect approximately 64% and 70% of all survivors, respectively. Cognitive deficits that are caused by stroke lead to 15% to 20% of dementias in the elderly, and severe depression occurs in approximately 33% of all patients after stroke (the risk for depression is particularly high in patients with damage in the dominant frontal hemisphere). Sexual dysfunction after stroke may result from depression, medication, paralysis, or fear. Reactive depression can often be helped substantially by encouraging verbalization of the patient's fears and anger. It is important for recovering individuals and their families to realize that most behavioral problems that develop as a direct result of stroke (such as inappropriate laughing, crying, or irritation with little provocation) usually do not last very long and often do not express the person's true feelings. Data suggest that the risk for depression after stroke is not affected by the stroke location. An emotional impact of stroke can be observed in approximately 25% of patients and may include anger, denial, anxiety, depression, and posttraumatic stress disorder. Some patients with mood disorders may require treatment by staff who are skilled in psychological approaches. There is evidence that family support services improve the quality of life for caregivers and reduce their potential for stress.

Psychotherapeutic agents and formal psychotherapy may be necessary for some patients (such as patients with considerable apathy, depression, indifference, or opposition to treatment). Agents used include nortriptyline hydrochloride (initially 25 mg once a day, as tolerated, and increased, as needed, gradually to 100 mg per day in divided doses), trazodone hydrochloride (initially 50 mg two to three times daily, as tolerated, and increased, as needed, by 50 mg per day every 3 to 4 days to 200 to 400 mg per day in divided doses), and selective serotonin reuptake inhibitors for depression and levodopa (0.5 to 1.0 g daily in divided doses with food) amantadine hydrochloride (100 mg per day) for behavioral problems such as inappropriate laughing or crying.

Family and Patient Education

Psychosocial therapy should be started with family members at the time of the patient's hospitalization and begin with the patient as soon as feasible. Family members should be given realistic, straightforward information and instructions to provide support for the patient and to develop a partnership for solutions to problems as early as possible. The family member who is closest to the patient should observe health personnel assisting the patient and practice under the supervision of a nurse or physical therapist. The physician should provide information and dispel myths regarding stroke to help provide the most positive yet realistic psychosocial environment for motivating, energizing, and inspiring the patient to move forward to return to a productive, useful life. Accurate and simply explained facts about the cause of the cerebrovascular event are essential for both the patient and the family, and both should understand that recovery from a stroke is often a slow process.

Family involvement becomes even more important when the patient is cared for at home after discharge from the hospital. Family members should provide encouragement, show confidence in improvement, and permit the recovering person to do as much as he or she can and to be as independent and vigorous as possible. It is important that the patient not become overly discouraged by failures. Patients need to be reassured that they are wanted and needed and that they are still important to the family and part of the social picture. They need to understand that many others have recovered from strokes and have been able to return to normal activities or continue to do very useful work. Giving the recovering person certain reasonable tasks (such as encouraging him or her to assume some household duties) is often helpful. It may also be very useful to assist the patient to develop new outside interests within his or her given capacities, particularly if the person is unable to return to gainful employment. Family counseling and education in the form of individual sessions or through regional family support groups are important to help the family overcome the stresses associated with new responsibilities and, sometimes, the depression that may occur in family members.

The physician should also be familiar with local driving guidelines and share this information with the patient and family. Generally, ongoing seizures and significant visual field deficit are considered to be absolute contraindications to driving; marked memory problems, poor concentration, and severe aphasia are relative contraindications to driving.

A treatment program that reduces the likelihood of further morbidity or mortality of patients after acute cerebrovascular events depends on (1) the pathophysiologic mechanism responsible for the event, (2) the degree of functional deficit (the degree of aggressiveness in the use of specific therapies varies inversely with the degree of residual functional deficit), and (3) the potential benefits and risks of the therapeutic method being considered.

If specific therapy for the underlying mechanism is available, appropriate measures should be provided, as outlined in Chapters 16 and 17. Correction of associated cerebrovascular risk factors with appropriate monitoring may also help to reduce the risk for a subsequent cerebrovascular event (see Chapters 24 to 31).

RESOURCES FOR PATIENTS

American Stroke Association
National Center
7272 Greenville Avenue
Dallas, TX 75231
Telephone: 888-478-7653
Web site: www.strokeassociation.org

National Stroke Association
9707 E. Easter Lane
Denver, CO 80112
Telephone: 800-787-6537
Web site: www.stroke.org

SUGGESTED READING FOR PART VII

Anderson C, Mhurchu CN, Rubenach S, et al. Home or hospital for stroke rehabilitation? Results of a randomized controlled trial. II: Cost minimization analysis at 6 months. *Stroke.* 2000;31:1032–1037.

Anderson C, Rubenach S, Mhurchu CN, et al. Home or hospital for stroke rehabilitation? Results of a randomized controlled trial. I: Health outcomes at 6 months. *Stroke.* 2000;31:1024–1031.

Carson AJ, MacHale S, Allen K, et al. Depression after stroke and lesion location: A systematic review. *Lancet.* 2000;356:122–126.

Dombovy ML, Basford JR, Whisnant JP, et al. Disability and use of rehabilitation services following stroke in Rochester, Minnesota, 1975–1979. *Stroke.* 1987;18:830–836.

Dromerick A, Reding M. Medical and neurological complications during inpatient stroke rehabilitation. *Stroke.* 1994;25:358–361.

Ernst E. A review of stroke rehabilitation and physiotherapy. *Stroke.* 1990;21:1081–1085.

Evans RL, Hendricks RD, Haselkorn JK, et al. The family's role in stroke rehabilitation: A review of the literature. *Am J Phys Med Rehabil.* 1992;71:135–139.

Feder M, Ring H, Rozenthul N, et al. Assessment chart for inpatient rehabilitation following stroke. *Int J Rehabil Res.* 1991;14:223–229.

Gibbons B. Stroke and rehabilitation. *Nurs Stand.* 1994;8:49–54.

Gladman J, Whynes D, Lincoln N. Cost comparison of domiciliary and hospital-based stroke rehabilitation. DOMINO Study Group. *Age Ageing.* 1994;23:241–245.

Hamilton BB, Granger CV. Disability outcomes following inpatient rehabilitation for stroke. *Phys Ther.* 1994;74:494–503.

Intiso D, Santilli V, Grasso MG, et al. Rehabilitation of walking with electromyographic biofeedback in foot-drop after stroke. *Stroke.* 1994;25:1189–1192.

Kalra L. Does age affect benefits of stroke unit rehabilitation? *Stroke.* 1994;25:346–351.

Kalra L. The influence of stroke unit rehabilitation on functional recovery from stroke. *Stroke.* 1994;25:821–825.

Mant J, Carter J, Wade DT, et al. Family support for stroke: A randomised controlled trial. *Lancet.* 2000;356:808–813.

Noll SF, Roth EJ. Stroke rehabilitation. 1. Epidemiologic aspects and acute management. *Arch Phys Med Rehabil.* 1994;75:S38–S41.

Oczkowski WJ, Ginsberg JS, Shin A, et al. Venous thromboembolism in patients undergoing rehabilitation for stroke. *Arch Phys Med Rehabil.* 1992;73:712–716.

Reding MJ, McDowell F. Stroke rehabilitation. *Neurol Clin.* 1987;5:601–630.

Reding MJ, McDowell FH. Focused stroke rehabilitation programs improve outcome. *Arch Neurol.* 1989;46:700–701.

Roth EJ. Heart disease in patients with stroke. Part II: Impact and implications for rehabilitation. *Arch Phys Med Rehabil.* 1994;75:94–101.

Sandin KJ, Cifu DX, Noll SF. Stroke rehabilitation. 4. Psychologic and social implications. *Arch Phys Med Rehabil.* 1994;75:S52–S55.

Shah S, Vanclay F, Cooper B. Efficiency, effectiveness, and duration of stroke rehabilitation. *Stroke.* 1990;21:241–246.

Teasdale TW, Christensen AL, Pinner EM. Psychosocial rehabilitation of cranial trauma and stroke patients. *Brain Inj.* 1993;7:535–542.

Teraoka J, Burgard R. Family support and stroke rehabilitation. *West J Med.* 1992;157:665–666.

Wade DT. Stroke: Rehabilitation and long-term care. *Lancet.* 1992;339:791–793.

Wild D. Stroke focus. Stroke: A nursing rehabilitation role. *Nurs Stand.* 1994;8:36–39.

Wolfe CD, Taub NA, Woodrow EJ, et al. Assessment of scales of disability and handicap for stroke patients. *Stroke.* 1991;22:1242–1244.

Appendixes

A

Clinical Anatomy of the Brain and Spinal Cord Vascular System

A-1. Brain and spinal cord vascular anatomy and syndromes

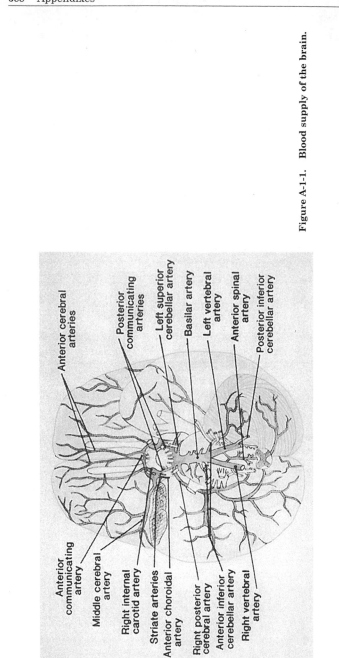

Figure A-1-1.   Blood supply of the brain.

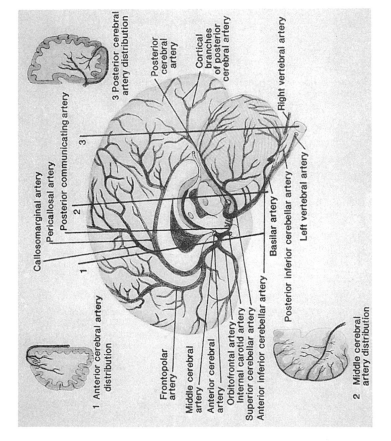

Figure A-1-2. Major cerebral arteries: distribution of blood supply.

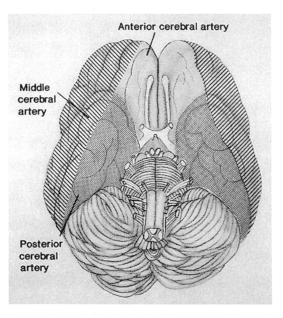

Figure A-1-3.   Major cerebral arteries: distribution of blood supply, view of base of the brain.

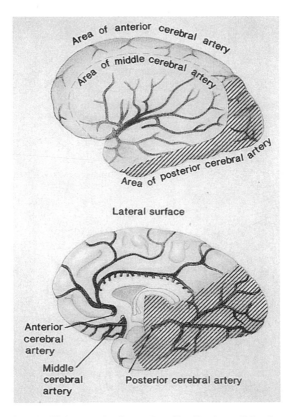

Lateral surface

Figure A-1-4.   Major cerebral arteries: distribution of blood supply, lateral views.

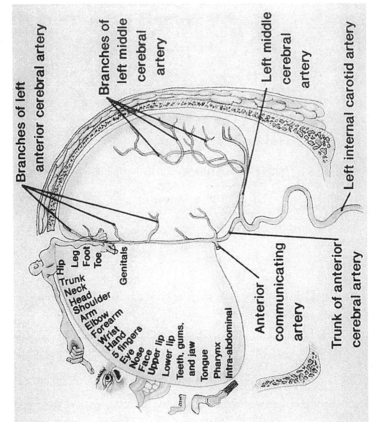

Figure A-1-5. Anterior and middle cerebral artery distribution to sensory fibers.

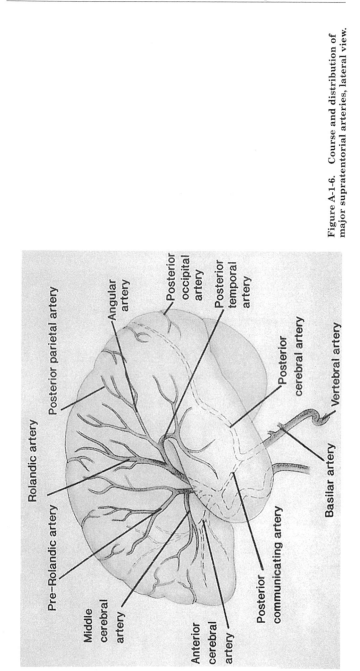

Figure A-1-6.   Course and distribution of major supratentorial arteries, lateral view.

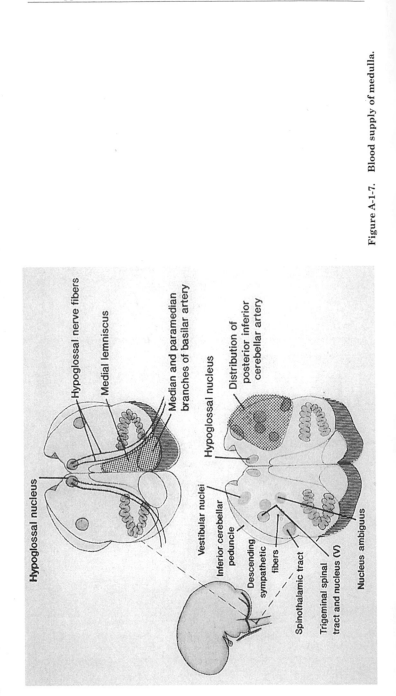

Figure A-1-7.   Blood supply of medulla.

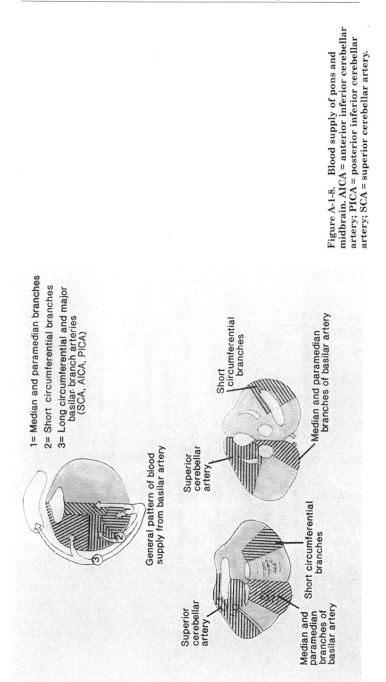

1 = Median and paramedian branches

2 = Short circumferential branches

3 = Long circumferential and major
    basilar branch arteries
    (SCA, AICA, PICA)

General pattern of blood
supply from basilar artery

Short
circumferential
branches

Median and paramedian
branches of basilar artery

Superior
cerebellar
artery

Superior
cerebellar
artery

Short circumferential
branches

Median and
paramedian
branches of
basilar artery

Figure A-1-8.   Blood supply of pons and midbrain. AICA = anterior inferior cerebellar artery; PICA = posterior inferior cerebellar artery; SCA = superior cerebellar artery.

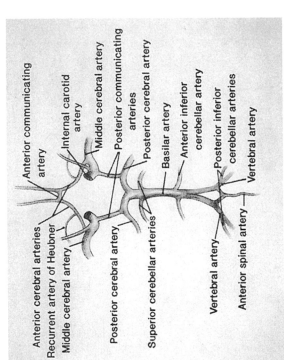

Figure A-1-9. Circle of Willis.

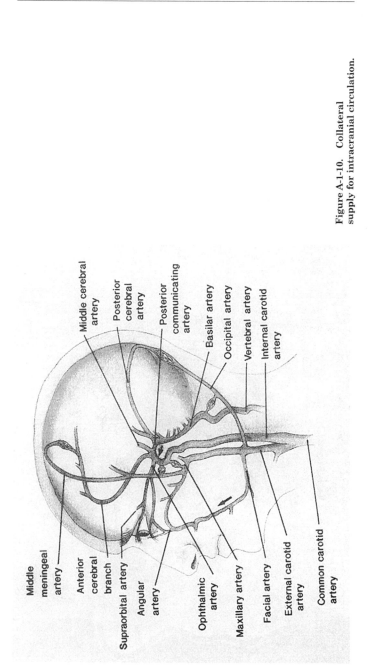

Figure A-1-10.   Collateral supply for intracranial circulation.

Middle meningeal artery

Anterior cerebral branch

Supraorbital artery

Angular artery

Ophthalmic artery

Maxillary artery

Facial artery

External carotid artery

Common carotid artery

Middle cerebral artery

Posterior cerebral artery

Posterior communicating artery

Basilar artery

Occipital artery

Vertebral artery

Internal carotid artery

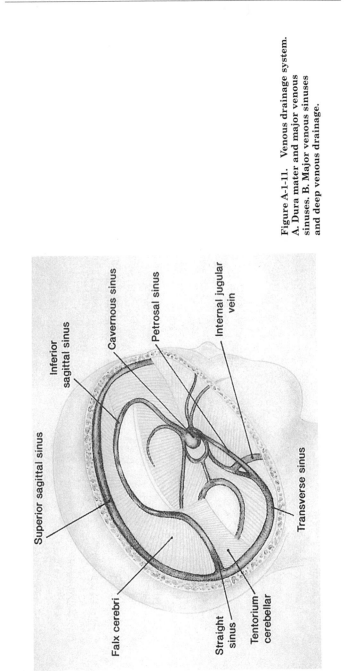

Figure A-1-11.   Venous drainage system. A. Dura mater and major venous sinuses. B. Major venous sinuses and deep venous drainage.

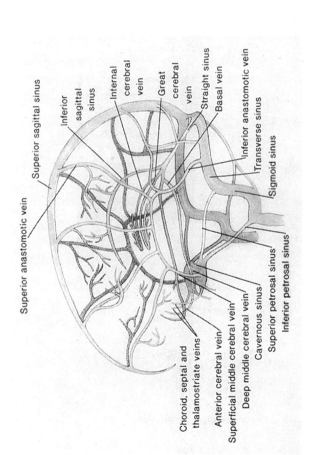

Superior anastomotic vein

Superior sagittal sinus

Inferior sagittal sinus

Internal cerebral vein

Great cerebral vein

Straight sinus

Basal vein

Inferior anastomotic vein

Transverse sinus

Sigmoid sinus

Choroid, septal and thalamostriate veins

Anterior cerebral vein

Superficial middle cerebral vein

Deep middle cerebral vein

Cavernous sinus

Superior petrosal sinus

Inferior petrosal sinus

B

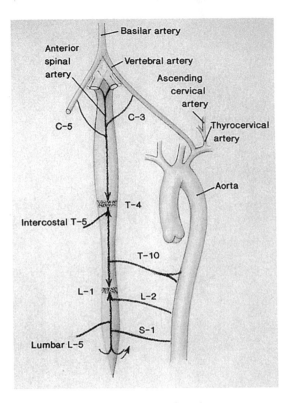

Figure A-1-12. Vascular supply to spinal cord.

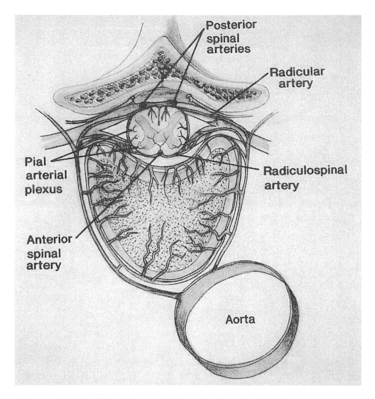

Figure A-1-13.   Vascular supply to spinal cord, axial view.

A-2.   Central nervous system ischemic vascular syndromes

Vessel	Major Structure(s) Supplied	Major Clinical Findings (Syndromes)
Brachiocephalic trunk	Right side of head, arm	Lower blood pressure in ipsilateral arm, other findings as for ICA syndrome
Common carotid artery	Each side of head	Findings as for ICA syndrome; poorly conducted heart sound along ICA, absence of superficial temporal artery pulse
Internal carotid artery	All structures of frontal, parietal, and temporal lobes; medial surfaces of the two hemispheres	Contralateral hemiparesis, hemianesthesia, hemianopia, aphasia; global aphasia (DH) or denial or hemineglect (NDH)
Ophthalmic artery	Orbit, forehead, dura of anterior fossa	Ipsilateral monocular blindness or amaurosis fugax
Anterior choroidal artery	Optic tract, cerebellum peduncle, two thirds of posterior limb of internal capsule, optic radiation	Findings as for middle cerebral artery syndrome (below) but language spared, pure motor or sensory stroke, ataxic hemiparesis, various intellectual deficits
Anterior cerebral artery	Medial aspects of cerebrum, superior border of frontal and parietal lobes	Weakness, clumsiness, and sensory loss affecting mainly distal contralateral leg
Small branches	Rostrum of corpus collosum, septum pellucidum, and lamina terminalis	Tactile anomia or ideomotor apraxia of limbs
Huebner's artery	Anterior limb of internal capsule, anterior portion of putamen, globus pallidum	Contralateral weakness of arm and face with or without rigidity or dystonia
Cortical branches	Major portion of mesial aspects of hemisphere, paracentral lobule	Contralateral weakness and sensory loss in leg; if bilateral, behavior disturbances

Artery	Location	Clinical features
Middle cerebral artery	Most of lateral surface of each hemisphere and deep structures of frontal and parietal lobes	Hemiplegia (face, arm, leg equally affected), hemianesthesia, hemianopia, aphasia (DH), hemineglect or dressing apraxia (NDH)
Upper division	Internal capsule (superior portion of anterior-posterior limb), corona radiata, external capsule, putamen, caudate nuclei (body)	Hemiplegia (face/arm more affected than leg), hemianesthesia or hemianopia, Broca's aphasia (DH) or spatial disorientation (NDH)
Lower division	Lateral surface of cerebral hemisphere at insula of lateral sulcus	Hemianopia or pure Wernicke's aphasia (DH) or other intellectual deficits (NDH)
Penetrating	Anterior limb of internal capsule, basal ganglia	Pure contralateral hemiplegia or hemiparesis
Cortical branches	Temporal, parietal, or frontal opercular surface of hemisphere	Monoparesis, discriminative and proprioceptive sensory loss, quadrantanopia, Broca's aphasia or Gerstmann's syndrome (DH), other intellectual deficits (NDH)
Vertebral artery	Midbrain, pons, medulla, and cerebellum	Various combinations of signs: ataxia, diplopia, vertigo, bulbar syndrome, facial weakness
Posterior-inferior cerebellar artery	Lateral medulla, cerebellum (posterior-inferior aspect); cranial nerves V, IX, X; vestibular nuclei; solitary nucleus/tract	Wallenberg's syndrome (alternating hemianesthesia, pharyngeal and laryngeal paralysis, dysphagia, hoarseness, decreased gag reflex, gait and ipsilateral limb ataxia) or Dejerine's syndrome
Anterior spinal artery	Caudal medulla (paramedian area), cranial nerve VII, solitary nucleus and tract, spinal cord (dorsolateral quadrants)	Radicular pain, loss of pain or temperature sensation, spastic weakness in legs with (cervical level) or without (below cervical level) focal atrophy and weakness of arms
Posterior spinal artery	Spinal cord (dorsal funiculus), dorsal gray horns	Loss of deep tendon reflexes and joint position sense, asterognosis at level involved

(Continued)

A-2. *Continued*

Vessel	Major Structure(s) Supplied	Major Clinical Findings (Syndromes)
Basilar artery	Pons, midbrain, cerebellum, occipital lobe, part of temporal lobe	Diplopia, coma, bilateral motor and sensory signs, cerebellar and cranial nerve signs
Short paramedian arteries	Medial basal pons (pontine nuclei, corticospinal fibers, medial lemniscus)	Paraparesis, quadriparesis, dysarthria, dysphagia, tongue hemiparesis and atrophy, gaze paralysis, cranial nerve VI palsy, contralateral hemiparesis; Millard-Gubler-Foville, Raymond-Cestan, Marie-Foix syndromes
Internal auditory artery	Auditory and facial cranial nerves	Vertigo, nausea, vomiting, nystagmus
Anterior-inferior cerebellar artery	Lateral aspect of pons and anterior-inferior cerebellum	Ipsilateral facial paralysis, taste loss on half of tongue, deafness or tinnitus, limb ataxia, contra-lateral sensory loss over body
Superior cerebellar artery	Lateral midbrain, superior surface of cerebellum	Ipsilateral cranial nerve VI and VII palsy, gait and limb ataxia, cerebellar signs, contralateral hemiparesis
Posterior cerebral artery	Entire occipital lobe, inferior and medial portion of temporal lobe	Hemianopia, quadrantanopia (macular vision spared), Gerstmann's syndrome, or cortical blindness
Small perforating arteries	Midbrain, posterior thalamus	Midbrain (Weber's, Benedict's) or thalamic (Dejerine-Roussy) syndromes
Cortical arteries	Occipital lobe (medial surface), uncus, fusiform, temporal lobe (gyrus), occipital pole	Hemianopia or quadrantanopia with sparing of macular vision, alexia or color anomia (DH), cerebral blindness (if bilateral lesions)
Pial spinal arteries	Nerve roots and spinal cord	Anterior or posterior spinal artery syndromes

DH = dominant hemisphere; ICA = internal carotid artery; NDH = nondominant hemisphere.

A-3. Symptoms of unruptured intracranial aneurysms

Artery Affected and Most Common Location	Major Structure(s) Involved (Compressed)	Clinical Findings[a]
Internal carotid artery Infraclinoid-intracavernous part	Cranial nerves III, IV, V, VI and pituitary fossa	Ipsilateral total ophthalmoplegia with small, poorly reactive pupil often associated with cranial nerve IV, V, VI palsy; facial pain or paresthesias or partial sensory loss; hypopituitarism; pulsatile noise in head
Supraclinoid part	Cranial nerves II, III; optic chiasm	Visual field defects associated with ipsilateral cranial nerve II palsy, decreased visual acuity, scotoma, optic atrophy or blindness; partial ophthalmoplegia due to cranial nerve III palsy
Middle cranial fossa, near petrous apex	Trigeminal ganglion; cranial nerves IV, VI	Raeder's paratrigeminal syndrome (unilateral oculosympathetic paresis—miosis and ptosis—associated with ipsilateral head, facial, or retro-orbital pain and cranial nerve IV and VI palsy)
Ophthalmic artery	Cranial nerve II, optic foramen, pituitary fossa	Ipsilateral painless loss of vision, optic nerve atrophy, x-ray enlargement of optic foramen, hypopituitarism
Anterior cerebral artery (at junction with anterior communicating artery)	Olfactory tract, optic chiasm, frontal lobes	Ipsilateral anosmia, bitemporal hemianopia (may begin with lower bitemporal quadrants); large aneurysm can produce intellectual deficits
Middle cerebral artery (at level of lateral fissure)	Lateral surface of cerebral hemisphere, surface between frontal and temporal lobes	Ipsilateral pain in or behind eye and in low temple associated with contralateral focal motor seizures, hemiparesis, dysphasia

(Continued)

A-3. Continued

Artery Affected and Most Common Location	Major Structure(s) Involved (Compressed)	Clinical Findings[a]
		(dominant hemisphere involvement), homonymous hemianopia or upper quadrantanopia
Posterior communicating artery (at junction with internal carotid artery)	Cranial nerves III, VI	Painful palsy of cranial nerve III (pain typically occurs above brow and radiates back to ear) with or without ipsilateral nerve VI palsy (cranial nerve III paresis usually incomplete)
Vertebral artery (on surface of medulla)	Cranial nerves IX, X, XI, XII	Ipsilateral Collet-Sicard, Villaret, Schmidt, Jackson, or Tapia syndromes and occasionally paralysis of cranial nerve VIII
Basilar artery (upper border of pons)	Cranial nerve V	Ipsilateral facial pain with or without tic douloureux
Anterior-inferior cerebellar artery	Cranial nerve VII and brainstem structures	Ipsilateral paralysis of all facial muscles, loss of taste, occasionally signs of hydrocephalus
Superior cerebellar artery (at vertebrobasilar junction)	Cranial nerve III and brainstem structures	Homolateral focal headache, occipital or posterior cervical location, associated with ipsilateral ptosis, divergent strabismus, horizontal-vertical diplopia, pupil dilation, ataxia
Posterior cerebral artery (proximal portion)	Midbrain structures	Focal ipsilateral headache (occipital or posterior cervical region), pseudobulbar signs, decreased level of consciousness

[a]Often mimic intracranial tumor at same location with slowly progressive focal neurologic signs. Virtually all aneurysms that cause symptoms other than rupture are 7 mm or more in size.

A-4.   Differential signs indicating hemispheric localization of intellectual deficits

Nondominant Hemisphere	Dominant Hemisphere	Bilateral Hemispheric Lesions
Prosopagnosia: inability to visually recognize well-known individuals	**Wernicke's aphasia:** difficulty understanding sentences when meaning depends on syntax, poor comprehension of spoken and written word but fluent speech with, sometimes, jargon and impaired repetition	**Impairment of analytic and remote memory**
Impairment of spatial orientation	**Broca's aphasia** (motor speech apraxia): good comprehension of spoken and written word but poor repetition, naming, and writing; nonfluent agrammatic speech	**Pseudobulbar palsy:** dysarthria, dysphagia, grasp, palmomental, sucking, snout, or rooting reflexes; increased jaw jerk; emotional lability; bulbar muscles spared
Anosognosia: ignores opposite hemiparetic side; denies weakness	**Conduction aphasia:** conversation relatively preserved, but cannot repeat word or sentences properly and makes phonemic, semantic, or paraphasic errors	**Akinetic mutism:** absence of any attempt at oral communication
Constructional apraxia: inability to copy geometric pattern	**Transcortical sensory aphasia:** repeats words or sentences well but unable to understand meaning of spoken or written words	**Palilalia:** repetition of last word or words of speech
Dressing apraxia: striking difficulty in dressing	**Transcortical motor aphasia:** nonfluent speech, preserved auditory comprehension, near normal ability to repeat phrases spoken by examiner	**Apraxia of gait:** loss of coordinated walking movements in absence of weakness, cerebellar disease, or sensory loss
Amusia: inability to identify auditory characteristics of music or identify songs by listening to them		**Paratonia** (gegenhalten): "plastic rigidity"—muscle tone increases in proportion to speed and strength of movement across a joint
Motor impersistence: inability to concentrate on a task, with consequent motor or verbal impersistence (e.g., on instruction, cannot hold breath or hold arm up for more than a few seconds)		

(Continued)

A-4. *Continued*

Nondominant Hemisphere	Dominant Hemisphere	Bilateral Hemispheric Lesions
Spatial acalculia: impairment of spatial organization of numbers—misalignment of digits, visual neglect (e.g., 124 as 24), digit inversion (e.g., 9 interpreted as 6), and reversal errors (e.g., 23 interpreted as 32)	**Global aphasia:** nonfluent, agrammatic speech, or mute, with impaired comprehension and repetition	**Pure anarthria or aphonia:** muteness with sparing of writing ability
Sensory aprosodia: poor perception of emotional overtones of spoken language	**Finger agnosia:** inability to identify specific fingers named by examiner	
	Color agnosia: inability to name colors or point to a color named by examiner	
	Acalculia: difficulty performing arithmetic calculations	
	Gerstmann's syndrome: agraphia, acalculia, right-left confusion, finger agnosia	
	Agraphia: inability to write properly	
	Echographia: compulsive copying of words and phrases	
	Apraxia of speech: automatic or reactive speech spoken without errors; volitional speech contains substitutions, repetitions, prolongations	

Glasgow Coma Scale

Test	Response	Score
Eye opening	Spontaneous	4
	Opens eyes to verbal stimulus	3
	Opens eyes to painful stimulus	2
	No response to any stimulus	1
Verbalization (verbal response)	Fully alert and oriented	5
	Confused	4
	Inappropriate	3
	Incomprehensible	2
	None	1
Motor response of nonparalyzed side	Normal (obedience to command)	6
	Localizes painful stimulus	5
	Withdrawal response to pain	4
	Flexion response to pain	3
	Extension response to pain	2
	None	1

Functional Status Scales (Stroke Severity Scales)

C-1. Barthel index[a]

Function	Score	Description
Feeding	10	Independent, able to apply any necessary device, eats in reasonable time
	5	Needs help (e.g., cutting) _____
Wheelchair or bed transfers	15	Independent, including placing locks of wheelchair and lifting footrests
	10	Minimal assistance or supervision
	5	Able to sit but needs maximal assistance to transfer _____
Personal toilet (grooming)	5	Washes face, combs hair, brushes teeth, shaves (manages plug if using electric razor) _____
Toilet transfers	10	Independent with toilet or bedpan; handles clothes; wipes, flushes, or cleans pan
	5	Needs help for balance, handling clothes or toilet paper _____
Bathing self	5	Able to use bathtub or shower or take complete sponge bath without assistance _____
Walking	15	Independent for 50 yd, may use assistive devices, except for rolling walker
	10	Walks with help for 50 yd
	5	Independent with wheelchair for 50 yd, only if unable to walk _____
Stairs, ascending and descending	10	Independent, may use assistive devices
	5	Needs help or supervision _____
Dressing and undressing	10	Independent, ties shoes, fastens fasteners, applies braces
	5	Needs help, but does at least half of task within reasonable time _____
Bowel control	10	No accidents, able to care for collecting device if used
	5	Occasional accidents or needs help with enema or suppository _____

C-1. *Continued*

Function	Score	Description
Bladder control	10	No accidents, able to care for collecting device if used
	5	Occasional accidents or needs help with device _____
		Total score _____

[a]The Barthel scale score 10 functions on a scale from fully dependent to independent. If performance of the patient is inferior to that described, the scores is 0; full credit is not given for an activity if the patient needs minimal help or supervision. Favorable outcome is usually defined as a score of 75–100.
Source: Adapted from Mahoney FI, Barthel DW. Functional evaluation: The Barthel index *Md State Med J*. 1965; 14:61–65.

DEFINITION AND DISCUSSION OF BARTHEL INDEX SCORING

Feeding

10 Independent. The patient can feed self a meal from a tray or table when someone puts food within reach. Patient must put on an assistive device (if needed), cut up food, use salt and pepper, spread butter, etc. Patient must accomplish this in a reasonable time.

5   Some help is necessary (e.g., cutting food), as listed above.

Moving from Wheelchair to Bed and Return

15 Independent in all phases of this activity. Patient can safely approach bed in wheelchair, lock brakes, lift footrests, move safely to bed, lie down, come to a sitting position on the side of the bed, change position of the wheelchair (if necessary to transfer back into it safely), and return to wheelchair.

10 Some minimal help is needed in some steps of this activity, or patient needs to be reminded or supervised for safety of one or more parts of this activity.

5   Patient can come to sitting position without help of second person but needs to be lifted out of bed or needs a great deal of help to transfer.

Doing Personal Toilet

5   Patient can wash hands and face, comb hair, clean teeth, and shave. Patient may use any kind of razor but must put in blade or plug in razor without help and take razor from drawer or cabinet. Female patients must put on own makeup, if used, but need not braid or style hair.

Getting on and off Toilet

10 Patient is able to get on and off toilet, fasten and unfasten clothes, prevent soiling of clothes, and use toilet paper without help. Patient may use wall bar or other stable object for support if needed. If necessary to use bedpan instead of toilet, then patient must be able to place bedpan on a chair, empty bedpan, and clean it.

5 Patient needs help because of imbalance or needs help handling clothes or in using toilet paper.

Bathing Self
5 Patient may use bathtub or shower or take complete sponge bath. Patient must be able to do all steps involved in whichever method is used without another person present.

Walking on a Level Surface
15 Patient can walk at least 50 yd without help or supervision. Patient may wear braces or prostheses and use crutches, canes, or walkerette but not rolling walker. Patient must be able to lock and unlock braces if used, assume standing position and sit down, place necessary mechanical aids into position for use, and dispose of them when sitting. (Putting on and taking off braces is scored under "dressing.")
10 Patient needs help or supervision in any of the above but can walk at least 50 yd with little help.

Propelling a Wheelchair
5 Patient cannot ambulate but can propel a wheelchair independently. Patient must be able to go around corners; turn around; maneuver the chair to a table, bed, toilet, etc. Patient must be able to push a chair at least 50 yd. (Do not score this item if patient receives score for walking.)

Ascending and Descending Stairs
10 Patient is able to go up and down a flight of stairs safely without help or supervision. Patient may (and should) use handrails, canes, or crutches when needed. Patient must be able to carry canes or crutches to ascend or descend stairs.
5 Patient needs help with or supervision of any of above items.

Dressing and Undressing
10 Patient is able to put on, remove, and fasten all clothing and shoelaces (unless necessary to use adaptions). Activity includes putting on, removing, and fastening corset or braces when these are prescribed. Special clothing such as suspenders, loafer shoes, or dresses that open in front may be used when necessary.
5 Patient needs help in putting on, removing, or fastening any clothing. Patient must do at least half of the work. Patient must accomplish this in a reasonable time. (Women need not be scored on use of brassiere or girdle unless these are prescribed garments.)

Continence of Bowels
10 Patient is able to control bowels and has no accidents. Patient can use suppository or take enema when necessary (as for patient who has spinal cord injury and has had bowel training).
5 Patient needs help in using suppository or taking enema or has occasional accidents.

Controlling Bladder

10   Patient is able to control bladder day and night. Patient who has spinal cord injury and wears external device and leg bag must put them on independently, clean and empty the bag, and stay dry day and night.

 5   Patient has occasional accidents or cannot wait for bedpan or get to the toilet in time or needs help with external devices.

A score of 0 is given in all of the above activities when the patient cannot meet the criteria as defined above.

C-2. Stroke Scale of National Institutes of Health-National Institute of Neurological Disorders and Stroke (NIH-NINDS)[a]

1. Date performed:
   _ _/_ _/_ _
   month day year

2. (a) Level of
   consciousness: Alert ( ) 0
   Drowsy ( ) 1
   Stuporous ( ) 2
   Coma ( ) 3
   (b) Level of consciousness questions:
   Answers both correctly ( ) 0
   Answers one correctly ( ) 1
   Incorrect ( ) 2
   (c) Level of consciousness commands:
   Obeys both correctly ( ) 0
   Obeys one correctly ( ) 1
   Incorrect ( ) 2

3. Best gaze: Normal ( ) 0
   Partial gaze palsy ( ) 1
   Forced deviation ( ) 2

4. Best visual: No visual loss ( ) 0
   Partial hemianopia ( ) 1
   Complete hemianopia ( ) 2
   Bilateral hemianopia ( ) 3

5. Facial palsy: Normal ( ) 0
   Minor ( ) 1
   Partial ( ) 2
   Complete ( ) 3

6. Best motor arm right: No drift ( ) 0
   Drift ( ) 1
   Cannot resist gravity ( ) 2
   No effort against gravity ( ) 3
   No movement ( ) 4

7. Best motor arm left: No drift ( ) 0
   Drift ( ) 1
   Cannot resist gravity ( ) 2
   No effort against gravity ( ) 3
   No movement ( ) 4

8. Best motor leg right: No drift ( ) 0
   Drift ( ) 1
   Cannot resist gravity ( ) 2
   No effort against gravity ( ) 3
   No movement ( ) 4

9. Best motor leg left: No drift ( ) 0
   Drift ( ) 1
   Cannot resist gravity ( ) 2
   No effort against gravity ( ) 3
   No movement ( ) 4

10. Limb ataxia: Absent ( ) 0
    Present in either upper or lower ( ) 1
    Present in both upper and lower ( ) 2

11. Sensory: Normal ( ) 0
    Partial loss ( ) 1
    Dense loss ( ) 2

12. Neglect: No neglect ( ) 0
    Partial neglect ( ) 1
    Complete neglect ( ) 2

13. Dysarthria: Normal articulation ( ) 0
    Mild to moderate dysarthria ( ) 1
    Near unintelligible or worse ( ) 2

14. Best language: No aphasia ( ) 0
    Mild to moderate aphasia ( ) 1
    Severe aphasia ( ) 2
    Mute ( ) 3

[a]A high score signifies a worse clinical state. Stroke severity is commonly divided into five groups: mild stroke (≤6), moderate stroke (7–10), moderately severe stroke (11–15), severe stroke (16–22), and very severe stroke (≥23). Source: Modified from Goldstein LB, Bertels C, Davis JN. Interrater reliability of the NIH stroke scale. *Arch Neurol.* 1989; 46:660–662.

NIH-NINDS STROKE GLOSSARY

Level of Consciousness

0   Fully alert, immediately responsive to verbal stimuli, able to cooperate completely
1   Drowsy, consciousness slightly impaired, arouses when stimulated verbally or after shaking, responds appropriately
2   Stuporous, aroused with difficulty (often painful stimuli must be applied), arousal usually incomplete, responds inadequately reverts to original state when not stimulated
3   Comatose, unresponsive to all stimuli or responds with reflex motor or autonomic effects

Level of Consciousness Questions

0   Patient knows age and month (only initial answer graded)
1   Patient answers one question correctly
2   Patient unable to speak or understand or answers incorrectly to both questions

Level of Consciousness Commands

0   Patient grips hand and closes or opens eyes to command
1   Patient does one correctly
2   Patient does neither correctly

Best Gaze

0   Normal
1   Partial gaze palsy, gaze abnormal in one or both eyes, but forced deviation or total gaze paresis is not present
2   Forced deviation or total gaze paresis not overcome by oculocephalic maneuver

Best Visual

0   Normal
1   Partial hemianopia, clear field cut
2   Complete hemianopia
3   Bilateral hemianopia

Facial Palsy

0   Normal
1   Minor (asymmetry with smiling and spontaneous speech, good volitional movement)
2   Partial (definite weakness but some movement remains)
3   Complete (no movement of entire half of face)

Right and Left Motor Arm

Patient is examined with arms outstretched at 90 degrees (if sitting) or at 45 degrees (if supine). Request full effort for 10 seconds. If patient's consciousness or comprehension is abnormal, then cue patient by actively lifting arm into position while giving request for effort.

0   No drift (limb holds 90 degrees for full 10 seconds)
1   Drift (limb holds 90 degrees but drifts before end of 10 seconds)

2   Cannot resist gravity (limb cannot hold 90 degrees for full 10 seconds, but some effort against gravity)
3   No effort against gravity (limb falls, no resistance against gravity)
4   No movement

Right and Left Motor Leg

While supine, patient is asked to maintain the leg at 30 degrees for 5 seconds. If patient's consciousness or comprehension is abnormal, then cue patient by actively lifting leg into position while giving request for effort.

0   No drift (leg holds 30 degrees for 5 seconds)
1   Drift (leg falls to intermediate position by end of 5 seconds)
2   Cannot resist gravity (leg falls to bed by 5 seconds, but some effort against gravity)
3   No effort against gravity (leg falls to bed immediately, no resistance against gravity)
4   No movement

Limb Ataxia

Finger-nose-finger and heal-to-shin tests are performed. Ataxia is scored only if clearly out of proportion to weakness. (Limb ataxia not testable in hemiplegia.)

0   Absent
1   Present is upper or lower limb
2   Present in both limbs

Sensory

Test with pin if patient's consciousness or comprehension is abnormal; score sensation normal unless deficit clearly recognized (e.g., clear-cut grimace asymmetry); without asymmetry, only hemisensory losses are counted as abnormal.

0   Normal, no loss of sensation
1   Mild/moderate (pinprick less sharp or dull on the affected side, or a loss of superficial pain with pinprick but patient aware of being tested)
2   Severe/total (patient unaware of being touched)

Neglect

0   None
1   Visual, tactile, or auditory hemi-inattention
2   Profound hemi-inattention to more than one modality

Dysarthria

0   Normal speech
1   Mild to moderate (slurs some words, understands with difficulty)
2   Unintelligible slurred speech (in the absence of or out of proportion to any dysphasia)

Best Language

0   Normal, no aphasia

1   Mild to moderate aphasia (word-finding errors, naming errors, paraphasias or impairment of communication by comprehension or expression disability)

2   Severe aphasia (fully developed Broca's or Wernicke's aphasia or variant)

3   Mute or global aphasia

C-3.   Modified Rankin disability scores[a]

Grade I	No significant disability; able to carry out all usual activities of daily living (without assistance). Note: this does not preclude the presence of weakness, sensory loss, language disturbance, etc., but suggests that these are mild and do not or have not caused patient to limit activities (e.g., if employed before, is still employed at same job).
Grade II	Slight disability; unable to carry out some previous activities but able to look after own affairs without much assistance (e.g., unable to return to previous job; unable to do some household chores but able to get along without daily supervision or help).
Grade III	Moderate disability; requires some help but able to walk without assistance (e.g., needs daily supervision, needs assistance with small aspects of dressing or hygiene, unable to read or communicate clearly). Note: ankle-foot orthosis or cane does not imply needing assistance.
Grade IV	Moderately severe disability; unable to walk without assistance and unable to attend to own bodily needs without assistance (e.g., needs 24-hour supervision and moderate to maximal assistance on several activities of daily living but still able to do some activities by self or with minimal assistance).
Grade V	Severe disability; bedridden, incontinent, and requires constant nursing care and attention.
Grade VI	Death

[a]No significant disability is usually defined as a score of 1–2, moderate to severe disability as a score of 3–5, and poor outcome as a score of 3–6.
Source: Modified from Rankin J. Cerebral vascular accidents in patients over the age of 60: II. Prognosis. *Scott Med J*. 1957; 2:200–215.

C-4.   Clinical grades of subarachnoid hemorrhage[a]

Hunt and Hess Scale

Grade	Criteria
I	Asymptomatic or minimal headache or stiff neck
II	Moderate to severe headache, stiff neck, no neurologic deficit other than cranial nerve palsy
III	Drowsiness, confusion, or mild focal signs
IV	Stupor, moderate to severe hemiparesis, possibly early decerebrate signs
V	Deep coma

World Federation of Neurological Surgeons (WFNS) Scale

WFNS Grade	GCS Score	Motor Deficit
I	15	Absent
II	13–14	Absent
III	13–14	Present
IV	7–12	Present or absent
V	3–6	Present or absent

GCS = Glasgow Coma Scale.
[a]Severe subarachnoid hemorrhage is usually defined as Hunt and Hess scale grade IV or V or as WFNS scale grade IV or V.
Source: From Hunt WE, Hess RM. Surgical risk as related to time of intervention in the repair of intracranial aneurysms. *J Neurosurg.* 1968; 28:14–19; and from Drake CG. Report of World Federation of Neurological Surgeons Committee on a universal subarachnoid hemorrhage grading scale (letter). *J Neurosurg.* 1988; 68:985–986.

Stroke and Cardiovascular Risk Profiles

D-1. Probability of stroke within 10 years for men who are aged 55–84 years and have no previous stroke[a]

Risk Factor	Points										
	0	1	2	3	4	5	6	7	8	9	10
Age (yr)	54–56	57–59	60–62	63–65	66–68	69–71	72–74	75–77	78–80	81–83	84–86
SBP (mm Hg)	95–105	106–116	117–126	127–137	138–148	149–159	160–170	171–181	182–191	192–202	203–213
Hyp Rx	No	Yes	Yes								
DM	No	Yes	Yes								
Cigs	No			Yes							
CVD	No			Yes							
AF	No				Yes						
LVH	No						Yes				

Points	10-Yr Probability (%)	Points	10-Yr Probability (%)	Points	10-Yr Probability (%)
1	2.6	11	11.2	21	41.7
2	3.0	12	12.9	22	46.6
3	3.5	13	14.8	23	51.8
4	4.0	14	17.0	24	57.3
5	4.7	15	19.5	25	62.8
6	5.4	16	22.4	26	68.4
7	6.3	17	25.5	27	73.8
8	7.3	18	29.0	28	79.0
9	8.4	19	32.9	29	83.7
10	9.7	20	37.1	30	87.9

AF = history of atrial fibrillation; Cigs = Smokes cigarettes; CVD = history of myocardial infarction, angina pectoris, coronary insufficiency, intermittent claudication, or congestive heart failure; DM = history of diabetes mellitus; Hyp Rx = under antihypertensive therapy; LVH = left ventricular hypertrophy on electrocardiogram; SBP = systolic blood pressure.

[a]Add points for risk factors listed (upper table), then add additional points for blood pressure level on antihypertensive therapy. Use lower table to obtain 10-year probability for stroke.

Source: From Wolf PA, D'Agostino RB, Belanger AJ, et al. Probability of stroke: A risk profile. From the Framingham Study. Stroke. 1991; 22:312–318.

D-2. Probability of stroke within 10 years for women who are aged 55–84 years and have no previous stroke[a]

Risk factor	Points										
	0	1	2	3	4	5	6	7	8	9	10
Age (yr)	54–56	57–59	60–62	63–65	66–68	69–71	72–74	75–77	78–80	81–83	84–86
SBP (mm Hg)	95–104	105–114	115–124	125–134	135–144	145–154	155–164	165–174	175–184	185–194	195–204
Hyp Rx	No (if yes, see below)										
DM	No		Yes								
Cigs	No			Yes							
CVD	No			Yes							
AF	No				Yes						
LVH	No						Yes				

If woman is currently under antihypertensive therapy, then add points according to SBP:

Risk Factor	Points										
	6	5	4	3	3	2	1	1	0	0	
SBP (mm Hg)	95–104	105–114	115–124	125–134	135–144	145–154	155–164	165–174	175–184	185–194	195–204

Points	10-Yr Probability (%)	Points	10-Yr Probability (%)	Points	10-Yr Probability (%)
1	2.6	11	11.2	21	41.7
2	3.0	12	12.9	22	46.6
3	3.5	13	14.8	23	51.8
4	4.0	14	17.0	24	57.3
5	4.7	15	19.5	25	62.8
6	5.4	16	22.4	26	68.4
7	6.3	17	25.5	27	73.8
8	7.3	18	29.0	28	79.0
9	8.4	19	32.9	29	83.7
10	9.7	20	37.1	30	87.9

AF = history of atrial fibrillation; Cigs = smokes cigarettes; CVD = history of myocardial infarction, angina pectoris, coronary insufficiency, intermittent claudication, or congestive heart failure; DM = history of diabetes mellitus; Hyp Rx = under antihypertensive therapy; LVH = left ventricular hypertrophy on electrocardiogram; SBP = systolic blood pressure.

[a]Add points for risk factors listed (upper table), then add additional points for blood pressure level on antihypertensive therapy. Use lower table to obtain 10-year probability for stroke.

Source: From Wolf PA, D'Agostino RB, Belanger AJ, et al. Probability of stroke: A risk profile. From the Framingham Study. *Stroke*. 1991; 22:312–318.

D-3. New Zealand cardiovascular risk prediction charts

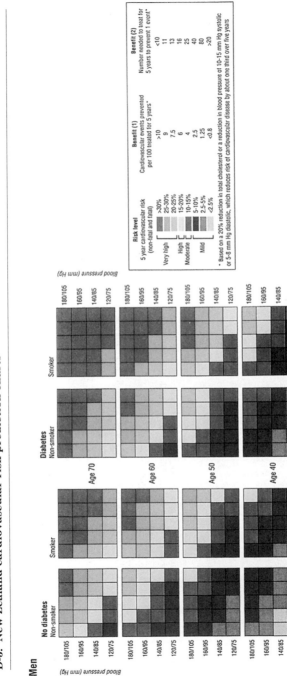

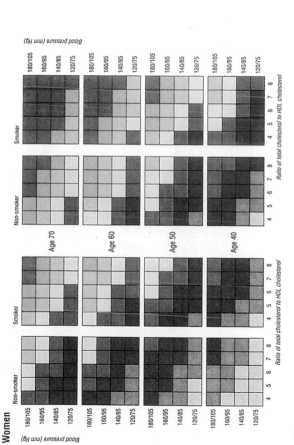

Source: Updated New Zealand cardiovascular disease risk-benefit prediction guide. *BMJ.* 2000; 320:709–710. Reprinted with permission.

Practice Guidelines for Management of Cerebrovascular Disease

E-1. Guideline for initial evaluation by telephone of a patient with cerebrovascular disease

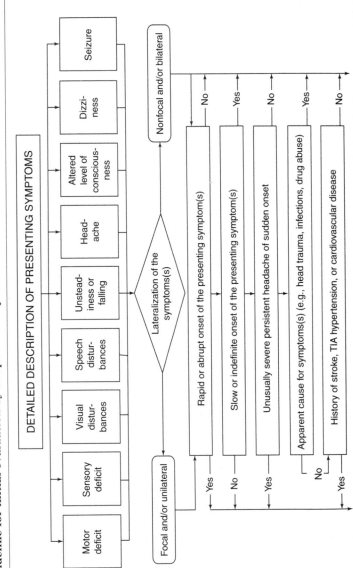

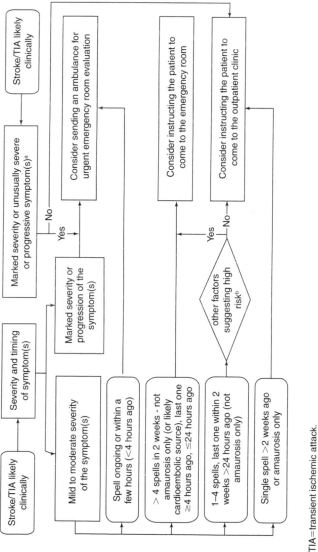

TIA = transient ischemic attack.

[a] Including evidence of other serious medical disorders that arise during the telephone interview.

[b] Probable cardioembolic source or causative arterial stenosis.

E-2. Guideline for transient ischemic attack/reversible ischemic neurologic deficit/minor ischemic stroke

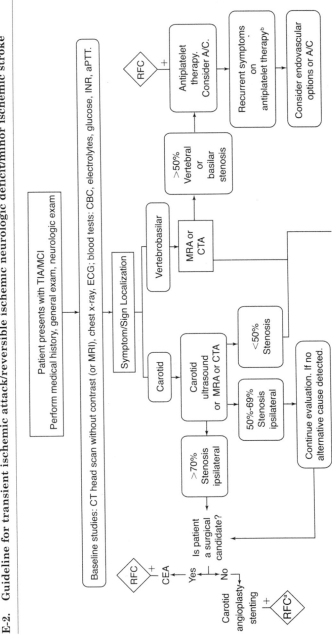

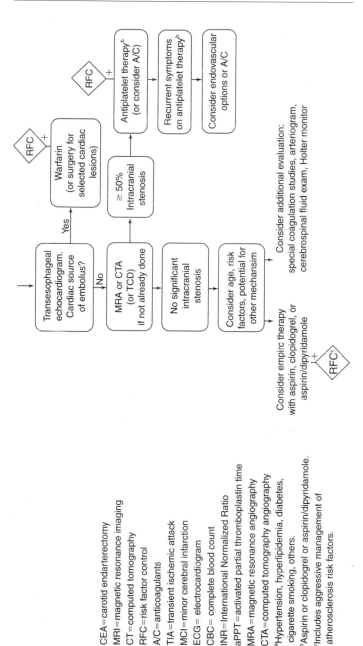

CEA = carotid endarterectomy
MRI = magnetic resonance imaging
CT = computed tomography
RFC = risk factor control
A/C = anticoagulants
TIA = transient ischemic attack
MCI = minor cerebral infarction
ECG = electrocardiogram
CBC = complete blood count
INR = International Normalized Ratio
aPPT = activated partial thromboplastin time
MRA = magnetic resonance angiography
CTA = computed tomography angiography
[a] Hypertension, hyperlipidemia, diabetes,
cigarette smoking, others.
[b] Aspirin or clopidogrel or aspirin/dipyridamole.
[c] Includes aggressive management of
atherosclerosis risk factors.

E-3. Guideline for major ischemic stroke

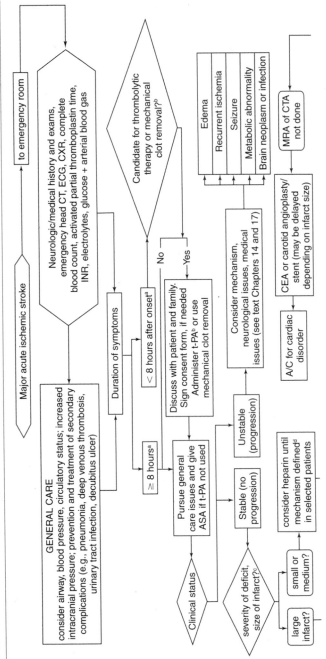

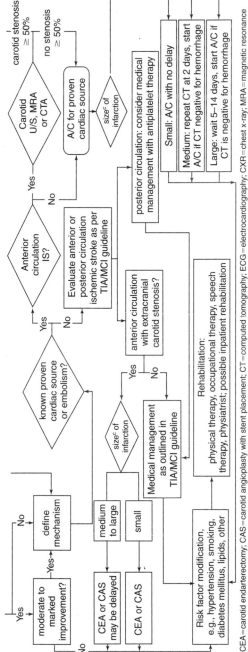

CEA=carotid endarterectomy; CAS=carotid angioplasty with stent placement; CT=computed tomography; ECG=electrocardiography; CXR=chest x-ray; MRA=magnetic resonance angiography; A/C=anticoagulants; OPG=oculopneumoplethysmography; TIA=transient ischemic attack; MCI=minor cerebral infarction; ASA=acetylsalicylic acid (aspirin); IS=ischemic stroke; U/S=ultrasound.

[a] Up to 12 hours if posterior circulation/basilar thrombosis.

[b] Patients most likely to benefit from intravenous t-PA include (1) ischemic stroke of < 3 hours' duration, (2) no hemorrhage or mass effect on head CT, (3) absence of uncontrolled hypertension, (4) absence of rapidly improving deficit. Consider intra-arterial t-PA up to 6 hours in middle cerebral artery and at least 12 hours in basilar artery. Mechanical clot retrieval up to 8 hours.

[c] Infarct size categorization: small, subcortical only and < 2 cm maximum diameter or less than one-half lobe; medium, up to one lobe; large, larger than one lobe.

[d] Especially if (1) cardiac source of embolism is likely, (2) large vessel with near occlusion with stuttering onset, (3) progressing ischemic stroke, (4) hypercoagulable state responsive to heparin, (5) no hemorrhage on head CT scan.

E-4.   Guideline for subarachnoid hemorrhage

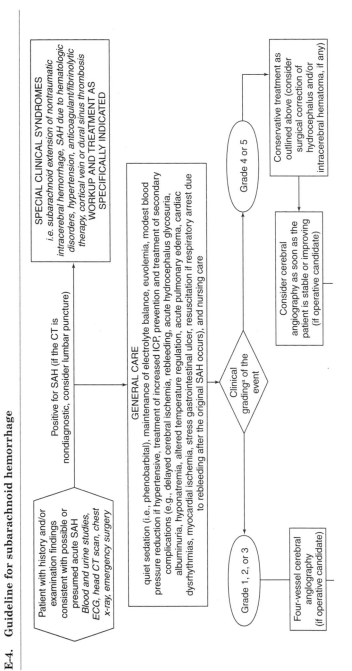

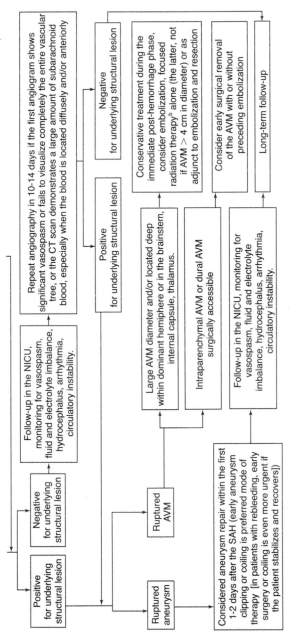

Repeat angiography in 10-14 days if the first angiogram shows significant vasospasm or fails to visualize completely the entire vascular tree, or the CT scan demonstrates a large amount of subarachnoid blood, especially when the blood is located diffusely and/or anteriorly

Negative for underlying structural lesion

Positive for underlying structural lesion

Conservative treatment during the immediate post-hemorrhage phase, consider embolization, focused radiation therapy[b] alone (the latter, not if AVM > 4 cm in diameter) or as adjunct to embolization and resection

Consider early surgical removal of the AVM with or without preceding embolization

Long-term follow-up

Follow-up in the NICU, monitoring for vasospasm, fluid and electrolyte imbalance, hydrocephalus, arrhythmia, circulatory instability.

Large AVM diameter and/or located deep within dominant hemiphere or in the brainstem, internal capsule, thalamus.

Intraparenchymal AVM or dural AVM surgically accessible

Follow-up in the NICU, monitoring for vasospasm, fluid and electrolyte imbalance, hydrocephalus, arrhythmia, circulatory instability.

Negative for underlying structural lesion

Positive for underlying structural lesion

Ruptured AVM

Ruptured aneurysm

Considered aneurysm repair within the first 1-2 days after the SAH (early aneurysm clipping or coiling is preferred mode of therapy [in patients with rebleeding, early surgery or coiling is even more urgent if the patient stabilizes and recovers])

SAH=subarachnoid hemorrhage; TCD=transcranial Doppler ultrasonography; NICU=neurologic intensive care unit; ECG=electrocardiography; CT=computed tomography; ICP=intracranial pressure; AVM=arteriovenous malformation.
[a]Hunt and Hess or WFNS clinical grades of SAH.
[b]Radiotherapy options of AVM treatment include gamma knife, linac, and proton beam.

E-5. Guideline for intracerebral/intraventricular hemorrhage

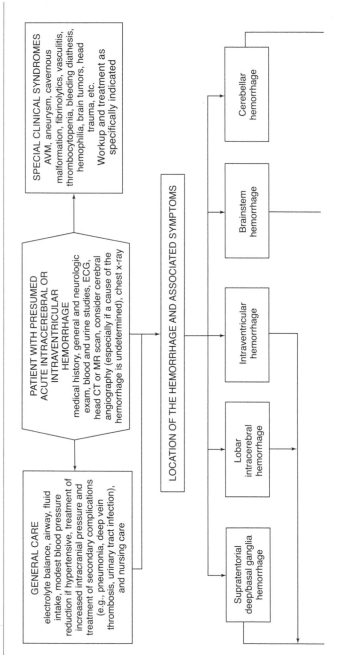

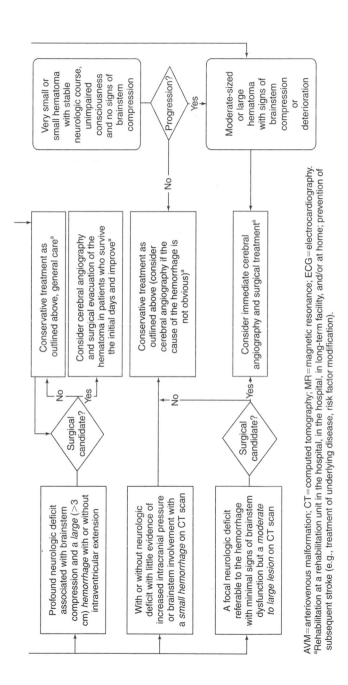

AVM=arteriovenous malformation; CT=computed tomography; MR=magnetic resonance; ECG=electrocardiography.
[a]Rehabilitation at a rehabilitation unit in the hospital, in the hospital, in the long-term facility, and/or at home; prevention of subsequent stroke (e.g., treatment of underlying disease, risk factor modification).

E-6.   Guideline for asymoptomatic carotid artery stenosis

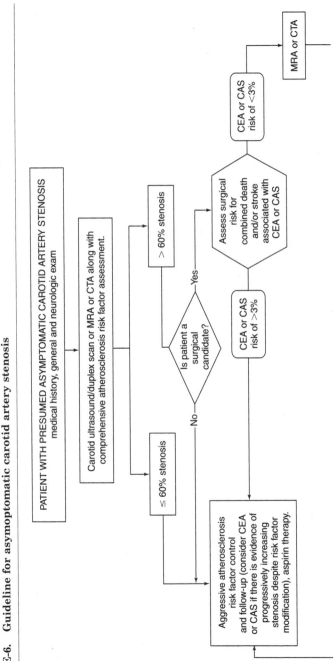

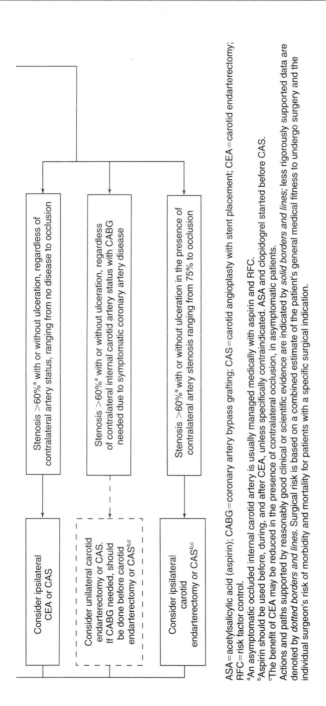

ASA=acetylsalicylic acid (aspirin); CABG=coronary artery bypass grafting; CAS=carotid angioplasty with stent placement; CEA=carotid endarterectomy; RFC=risk factor control.

[a]An asymptomatic occluded internal carotid artery is usually managed medically with aspirin and RFC.

[b]Aspirin should be used before, during, and after CEA, unless specifically contraindicated. ASA and clopidogrel started before CAS.

[c]The benefit of CEA may be reduced in the presence of contralateral occlusion, in asymptomatic patients.

Actions and paths supported by reasonably good clinical or scientific evidence are indicated by *solid borders and lines*; less rigorously supported data are denoted by *dotted borders and lines*. Surgical risk is based on a combined estimate of the patient's general medical fitness to undergo surgery and the individual surgeon's risk of morbidity and mortality for patients with a specific surgical indication.

Outline of Diets Low in Fat and Cholesterol and Table of Ideal Body Weight

F-1. Low-fat, low-cholesterol diet

Food	Anytime	Sometimes	Avoid
Fruits and vegetables	Any fresh, juiced, frozen, canned, or dried	Avocado, olives	Coconut; vegetables in cheese, cream or butter; French-fried vegetables
Grains (breads, cereals, rice, pasta, and baked goods)	Bread, bagels, breadsticks, English muffins, pita bread, plain rolls, corn tortillas, hot and cold tortillas, hot and cold cereals, rice, bulgur, pasta, popcorn (plain or light microwave), pretzels, no-oil tortilla chips, fat-free and low-fat crackers and cookies	Biscuits, muffins (from mix), cornbread, low-fat granola, pancakes, waffles, French toast, packaged rice mixes, popcorn (regular, microwave, or buttered), low-fat or reduced-fat snack foods	Doughnuts, croissants, sweet rolls, commercial muffins, granola, egg noodles, stuffing, regular chips, crackers, pies, cakes, cookies
Diary products	Skim and 1%-fat milk, buttermilk, nonfat dry milk, fat-free yogurt and cheese, fat-free or low-fat cottage cheeses	2%-fat milk, 4%-fat cottages cheese, reduced-fat and part-skim milk cheeses, low-fat yogurt, frozen yogurt, ice milk, sherbet	Whole milk, whole milk yogurt and cheeses, ice cream (regular and gourmet)
Meat, eggs, and meat substitutes	Any finfish or shellfish (except shrimp), water-packed tuna, surimi, poultry, ground turkey	Shrimp, oil-packed fish, fish sticks, poultry (with skin), ground beef (extra lean and lean), eggs (4/wk)	Fried fish or poultry, USDA prime beef, pork, or lamb (rib, brisket, shoulder, porterhouse, T-bone),

(Continued)

F-1. *Continued*

Food	Anytime	Sometimes	Avoid
	(without skin), USDA choice or select beef (round sirloin, tenderloin, flank, ground round), lamb (leg), pork (center-cut ham, loin chops, tenderloin), Canadian bacon, low-fat luncheon meats, dried beans and peas, lentils, egg substitutes, egg whites, tofu, tempeh, soy and textured protein meat substitutes, fat-free meat substitutes		organ meats, regular ground beef, sausage, bacon, most regular luncheon meats, peanut butter, nuts
Fats	Polyunsaturated oils (corn, sunflower, soybean, sesame, cottonseed), monounsaturated oils (canola, olive, peanut), margarine, reduced-fat margarine, reduced-fat salad dressing, fat-free sour cream	Regular salad dressing, mayonnaise, reduced-fat sour cream, reduced-fat cream cheese, sour half-and-half	Coconut oil, palm and palm kernel oils, shortening, lard, butter, cream, half-and-half, sour cream, cream cheese, gravy, most nondairy creamers

F-2. Very-low-fat, very-low-cholesterol diet

Anytime

Fruits and Vegetables

Fresh, frozen canned, dried, or juiced: apples, apricots, bananas, blackberries, blueberries, cantaloupe, cherries, cranberries, currants, dates, figs, gooseberries, grapefruit, grapes, honeydew, kiwis, lemons, limes, mangoes, mulberries, nectarines, oranges, peaches, pears, pineapples, plums, pomegranates, prunes, raisins, raspberries, star fruits, strawberries, tangerines, watermelon, fruit ices, sorbets

Fresh, frozen, canned, dried, or juiced: artichokes, asparagus, beans (green, wax, lima) beets, broccoli, brussels sprouts, cabbages, carrots, cauliflower, celery, collards, corn, cucumbers, dandelion greens, eggplant, escarole, fennel, garlic, kale, kelp, leeks, lentils, lettuce, mushrooms (button, cup, flat, chanterelle, morel, oyster, shiitake, etc.), mustard greens, okra, onions, parsnips, peas, peppers (bell, chile), potatoes (baked, mashed), radishes, rutabagas, snow peas, spinach, sprouts (alfalfa, mustard, bean, radish), squash, sweet potato (baked, mashed), Swiss chard, tomato, turnips, turnip greens

Grains

Whole-grain breads, bagels, breadsticks, English muffins, pita bread, plain rolls, hot and cold whole-grain cereals (corn, oats, rye, wheat, barley, bulgur, millet, quinoa, buck-wheat), rice (brown, white, wild), grits, macaroni, pasta, non-egg noodles, corn tortillas, air-popped popcorn, pretzels, fat-free crackers, fat-free cookies, fat-free muffins

Dairy

Fat-free nondairy desserts, nonfat, soy, milk, nonfat rice milk, soy shakes, fat-free cheese substitutes

Fats

Fat-free chocolate, fat-free salad dressing, fat-free nondairy creamer

Miscellaneous

Fat-free vegetarian chili and other soups (split pea, lentil, vegetable)

Beans, Eggs, Meat Substitutes

Beans (kidney, garbanzo, pinto, black, brown, white, great northern, mung, navy, red, Mexican, lima), lentils, peas (split, black-eyed), soybean products (tofu, tempeh, miso), Seitan (wheat gluten), egg whites, fat-free meat substitutes,[a] including veggie burgers, veggie hot dogs, veggie Canadian bacon, veggie chicken, veggie turkey with or without vegetarian gravy, and veggie breakfast strips, links and patties

(Continued)

F-2. *Continued*

Sometimes

Fruits and Vegetables

Avocado, coconut, olives, vegetables in low-fat cheese sauce,[b] vegetables in low-fat cream sauce[a]

Grains

Very-low-fat snack foods, low-fat snack foods (low-fat popcorn, low-fat chips, crackers, cake),[b] egg noodles

Dairy

Skim milk, nonfat yogurt, fat-free sour cream, fat-free cream cheese, fat-free cottage cheese, low-fat yogurt,[b] low-fat sour cream,[b] low-fat cream cheese,[b] low-fat cottage cheese,[b] low-fat cheese[b]

Fats

Low-fat salad dressing, olive oil and other vegetable oils with little saturated fat and no cholesterol

Miscellaneous

Vegetarian pot pie with meat substitute, low-fat vegetarian enchiladas, low-fat vegetarian burritos, roasted vegetable pizza with vegetarian or low-fat cheese topping

Beans, Eggs, Meats Substitutes

Nuts (peanuts, walnuts, pecans almonds, Brazil nuts, etc.), seeds (sesame, pumpkin, sunflower, etc.), egg substitute,

textured vegetable protein,[b] veggie burgers,[b] meatless breakfast strips,[b] links and patties,[b] meatless ground beef substitutes,[b] meatless chicken breast,[b] patties,[b] kebabs,[b] meatless Buffalo wings, meatless Salisbury steak,[b] meatless cocktail wieners,[b] meatless fish fillet,[b] meatless salmon steaks,[b] lentil loaf[b]

Avoid

Fruits and Vegetables

Fried vegetables, vegetables in regular cheese, cream sauce, or butter, vegetables in margarine

Grains

Regular cake, regular chips, chow mein noodles, regular cookies, regular crackers, croissants, doughnuts, granola, regular muffins, pies, regular popcorn, regular snack foods, stuffing, sweet rolls

Dairy

Whole or 2% milk, whole or reduced-fat yogurt, reduced-fat or regular cheese, ice cream, cream, reduced-fat or regular sour cream, reduced-fat or regular cream cheese, reduced-fat or regular cottage cheese

Fats

Most margarines, regular salad dressings, oils with large amounts of saturated fat (coconut, palm, palm kernel, etc.), butter, lard, shortening, regular nondairy creamers, regular or milk chocolate

Meats, Eggs

Meat (including poultry, fish, and seafood), egg yolks

[a]As long as it contains no saturated fat or cholesterol.
[b]As long as they are < 7 g of total fat, and < 2 g of saturated fat, and < 5 mg cholesterol per serving.

F-3. Metropolitan Height and Weight Tables

Men[a]

Height Ft	Height In.	Small frame	Medium frame	Large frame
5	2	128–134	131–141	138–150
5	3	130–136	133–143	140–153
5	4	132–138	135–145	142–156
5	5	134–140	137–148	144–160
5	6	136–142	139–151	146–164
5	7	138–145	142–154	149–168
5	8	140–148	145–157	152–172
5	9	142–151	148–160	155–176
5	10	144–154	151–163	168–180
5	11	146–157	154–166	161–184
6	0	149–160	157–170	164–188
6	1	152–164	160–174	168–192
6	2	155–168	164–178	172–197
6	3	158–172	167–182	176–202
6	4	162–176	171–187	181–207

Women[b]

Height Ft	Height In.	Small frame	Medium frame	Large frame
4	10	102–111	109–121	118–131
4	11	103–113	111–123	120–134
5	0	104–115	113–126	122–137
5	1	106–118	115–129	125–140
5	2	108–121	118–132	128–143
5	3	111–124	121–135	131–147
5	4	114–127	124–138	134–151
5	5	117–130	127–141	137–155
5	6	120–133	130–144	140–159
5	7	123–136	133–147	143–163
5	8	126–139	136–150	146–167
5	9	129–142	139–153	149–170
5	10	132–145	142–156	152–173
5	11	135–148	145–159	155–176
6	0	138–151	148–162	158–179

[a]Weights at ages 25–59 years, based on lowest mortality. Weight in pounds, according to body frame (in indoor clothing weighting 5 lb, shoes with 1-in heels).
[b]Weights at ages 25–59 years, based on lowest mortality. Weight in pounds, according to body frame (in indoor clothing weighting 3 lb, shoes with 1-in heels).
Source: From Metropolitan Life Foundation: Height and Weight, Table 1. *Stat Bull Metrop Life Found.* 1983; 64:2–9.

Subject Index

Figures are indicated by page numbers followed by *f*; tables are indicated by page numbers followed by *t*